BSAVA Manual of Companion Animal Nutrition & Feeding

First Edition

Edited by

Noel C. Kelly
MVB, M Appl Sc (Food Science), MRCVS
Blacklion Pet Hospital
Greystones, Co Wicklow, Ireland

and

Josephine M. Wills
BVetMed, PhD, MRCVS
WALTHAM Centre for Pet Nutrition
Melton Mowbray, Leicestershire, England

Iowa State University Press / Ames

Published by:
British Small Animal Veterinary Association
Kingsley House, Church Lane
Shurdington, Cheltenham
Gloucestershire
United Kingdom
GL51 5TQ.

Published in the United States by:
Iowa State University Press
Ames, Iowa 50014-8300.

Typeset and Printed by:
Fusion Design, Fordingbridge, Hampshire, UK.

ISBN 0-8138-1983-0

Contents

Contributors

Ronald Shand Anderson, BVMS, PhD, MRCVS
Department of Veterinary Clinical Science and Animal Husbandry, Faculty of Veterinary Science, Veterinary Field Station, Leahurst, Neston, South Wirral, L64 7TE, UK

David Church, BVSc, PhD, MACVSc
Department of Veterinary Clinical Sciences, University of Sydney, Sydney, Australia 2006

Mike Davies, BVet Med, Cert VR, Cert SAO, FRCVS
GTI Veterinary Systems Ltd, Spitfire House, Old Farum Park, Salisbury, Wiltshire SP4 6EB, UK

Susan Donoghue, VMD, Dip ACVN
Nutrition Support Services, Inc., Route 1 Box 189, Pembroke, VA 24136, USA

Andrew T.B. Edney, BA(Hons), BVetMed, MRCVS
Crocket Cottage, 22 Crocket Lane, Empingham, Rutland LE15 8PW, UK

Dominique Grandjean, DVM, PhD
Unite de Médécine de L'Elevage et du Sport, Département d'Elevage et Pathologie des Equidés et Carnivores, Ecole Nationale Vétérinaire d'Alfort, 94700 Maisons-Alfort, France

Edward James Hall, MA, Vet MB, PhD, MRCVS
University of Bristol, Department of Clinical Veterinary Science, Division of Companion Animals, Langford House, Langford, Bristol BS18 7DU, UK

John G. Harte, MVB, MRCVS
WALTHAM Centre for Pet Nutrition, Waltham-on-the-Wolds, Leicestershire LE14 4RT, UK

Richard Harvey, BVSc, MRCVS
Godiva Referrals, 207 Daventry Road, Cheylesmore, Coventry CV3 5HH, UK

Åke A. Hedhammar, DVM, MSc, PhD
Department of Medicine and Surgery, Swedish University of Agricultural Sciences, Box 7037, S- 750 07 Uppsala, Sweden

Noel C. Kelly, MVB, M Appl Sc (Food Science), MRCVS
Blacklion Pet Hospital, Greystones, Co Wicklow, Ireland

James K. Kirkwood, BVSc, PhD, MRCVS
Veterinary Science Group, Institute of Zoology, Regent's Park, London NW1 4RY, UK

Martin P.C. Lawton, BVetMed, CertVOphthal, CertLAS, C Biol, MIBiol, FRCVS
12 Fitzilian Avenue, Harold Wood, Romford, Essex RM3 0QS, UK

Alastair Macartney, BSc, PhD
WALTHAM Aquacentre, Waltham-on-the-Wolds, Leicestershire LE14 4RT, UK

Peter J. Markwell, BSc, BVetMed, MRCVS
WALTHAM Centre for Pet Nutrition, Waltham-on-the-Wolds, Leicestershire LE14 4RT, UK

Hein P. Meyer, DVM, DipECVIM
Department of Clinical Sciences of Companion Animals, Faculty of Veterinary Medicine,
Utrecht University, PO Box 80.154, NL-3508 TD Utrecht, The Netherlands

James G. Morris, MAgrSc, BSc, PhD
Department of Molecular Biosciences, School of Veterinary Medicine,
University of California, Davis, CA 95616, USA

Jan Rothuizen, DVM, PhD, DipECVIM
Department of Clinical Sciences of Companion Animals, Faculty of Veterinary Medicine,
Utrecht University, PO Box 80.154, NL-3508 TD Utrecht, The Netherlands

David Senior, BVSc, Dip ACVIM
Professor and Head, Veterinary Clinical Sciences, School of Veterinary Medicine,
Louisiana State University, Baton Rouge, LA 70803-8410, USA

Bryn J. Tennant, BVSc, CertVR, PhD, MRCVS
Capital Diagnostics, Bush Estate, Penicuik, Midlothian E1126 0QE, UK

Graham Tobin, BSc, PhD
Harlan Teklad, Shaws Farm, Blackthorn, Bicester, Oxon OX6 0TP, UK

Andrew G. Torrance, MA, Vet MB, PhD, Dip ACVIM, Dip ECVIM-CA, MRCVS
Bloxham Laboratories Ltd., George St, Teignmouth, Devon TQ14 8AH, UK

David A Williams, VetMB, PhD, MRCVS, DipACVIM
Purdue University, Department of Veterinary Clinical Sciences, 1248 Lynn Hall,
West Lafayette, IN 4707 1248, USA

Josephine M. Wills, BVetMed, PhD, MRCVS
WALTHAM Centre for Pet Nutrition, Melton Mowbray, Leicestershire LE14 4RT, UK

Foreword

The proper feeding of companion animals is a science which many practitioners admit is not well understood by them.

This addition to the BSAVA Manual series will give all those who have an interest in nutrition and feeding of pets the opportunity to increase their knowledge of this important topic. It will ensure that they can give both the correct advice on feeding in health and the appropriate nutritional management in sickness to the many species included in the manual.

The concise way in which the feeding requirements of dogs, cats, small pets and exotic species, including reptiles and ornamental fish, are presented, and with clinical nutrition considered on a systematic basis, means that the user will very rapidly be able to find the answers to problems which arise daily. This can only lead to better practical management of the nutritional care of our patients.

Once again the BSAVA has been able to call on twenty four authors of outstanding international repute to contribute to this volume. The editors, Noel Kelly and Josephine Wills, both of whom are also authors, are to be congratulated on producing a manual which complements so well the recognised wealth of information in the Manual series. The BSAVA *Manual of Companion Animal Nutrition and Feeding* will bridge the gap between the science and practice of the subject.

John Robert Dalton BVMS MRCVS
President BSAVA 1995-96

Editors' Foreword

This manual is a handbook for veterinary practitioners and students, biological scientists and nutritionists, with an interest in nutrition and feeding of companion animals. It addresses the ever increasing dimension of dietary management, in both health and disease, in the daily conduct of companion animal practice.

The editorial objective has been to bridge the knowledge gap between theoretical nutrition and the practical feeding of healthy or sick animals. This has been achieved in a concise way, systematically covering food types, dietary needs and appropriate feeding of dogs, cats, other small mammals, reptiles, birds and fish in health and sickness.

Basic principles of nutrition and feeding, together with evaluation of food types available are outlined practically but comprehensively in Part 1. Part 2 addresses the feeding of healthy dogs and cats appropriate to life stage and life style, from reproduction and lactation through puppyhood and kittenhood to adult maintenance, performance, and old age.

In Part 3, clinical nutrition of the dog and cat is presented, taking a systematic approach to nutritionally associated illness. The underweight and obese animal, and those having systemic disease, orthopaedic and skin problems, are approached by assessment of pathological status, dietary strategy, and finally evaluation of success. Methodology of feeding the sick animal, intensive nutritional care and support, receive detailed attention.

A very useful and informative section is found in Part 4 on the nutritional requirements and disorders of small pets and exotics including reptiles. Appropriate food types are discussed, as are feeding methods and techniques. The difficult area of nutrition of captive free-living wild animals receives attention in this section as does the nutrition and feeding of ornamental fish.

A very practical feature of this book is found in the appendices, in which salient details from many of the chapters are summarised in tabloid form for quick reference.

Noel Kelly

Josephine Wills

Acknowledgements

The Editors would like to express their sincere thanks to all the contributors to this manual. Not only is their hard work in writing each chapter appreciated, but also their patience during the delay between their contributions and production of the finished Manual.

In addition, we are grateful to Fiona Taylor and Jane French, for their excellent help with manuscript preparation, and Fusion Design for advice on layout and graphics.

Our thanks to all those involved with the evolution of this project, for their help and encouragement, particularly Harvey Locke and Simon Petersen-Jones.

And finally, thanks to our other halves, for their tolerance when the editors took this manual on holiday with them.

Noel Kelly

Josephine Wills

Mineral	Function	Imbalance causes:
Calcium (Ca) and Phosphorus (P)	Calcium and phosphorus are the major minerals involved in maintaining the structural rigidity of bones and teeth. Calcium is also essential for normal blood clotting and for nerve and muscle function. Phosphorus is involved in many enzyme systems and is also a component of the 'high energy' organic phosphate compounds. These are mainly responsible for the storage and transfer of energy in the body.	The absolute concentrations of these minerals in the diet are of paramount importance, but the ratio of calcium to phosphorus is also of great significance. The minimum calcium:phosphorus ratio for growth is generally considered to be about 1:1. For adult animals it is somewhat less critical. Imbalance in this ratio, where calcium is much less than phosphorus, leads to a marked deficiency of calcium in relation to bone formation. *Calcium deficiency* – Nutritional secondary hyperparathyroidism, causing skeletal deformities and lameness in the growing animal. Hypocalcaemia in lactating bitches (particularly of the toy breeds) causes eclampsia, with nervous disturbances. *High levels* of calcium and phosphorus or a very high ratio are also harmful: conditions such as hip dysplasia, osteochondrosis syndrome, enostosis and wobbler syndrome have been related to excessive calcium intake in the growing dog.
Magnesium (Mg)	Required for healthy bones and teeth; normal functioning of heart and skeletal muscle and nervous tissue; sodium and potassium metabolism; many essential enzyme reactions, particularly those concerned with energy metabolism.	*Deficiency* – Muscular weakness and in severe cases, convulsions. Dietary deficiency unlikely. *Very high intakes* – Associated with an increased incidence of Feline Lower Urinary Tract Disease.
Potassium (K)	Required for acid-base balance and osmoregulation of the body fluids, nerve and muscle function and energy metabolism.	*Deficiency* – Muscular weakness, poor growth and lesions of the heart and kidney. Naturally occurring deficiencies are rare, but can occur in cats if fed diets containing urinary acidifiers with a marginal potassium content.
Sodium (Na) and Chloride (Cl^-)	Being the major electrolytes of body water, they are required for acid-base balance and osmoregulation of the body fluids. Chloride is also an essential component of bile and hydrochloric acid (which is present in gastric juice).	*Deficiency* – Fatigue, exhaustion, inability to maintain water balance, decreased water intake, retarded growth, dry skin and hair loss. Excess will cause greater than normal fluid intake and it has been suggested that some dogs with hypertension may benefit from a diet lower in sodium.

Table 1.1: *Macro-minerals.*

acids. Signs of protein deficiency include poor growth or weight loss, rough and dull hair coat, anorexia, increased susceptibility to disease, muscle wasting and emaciation, oedema and finally death. Deficiency of a single essential amino acid results in anorexia and subsequent negative nitrogen balance.

Cats exhibit a number of nutritional peculiarities, many of which are reflected in their protein and amino acid requirements (see Chapter 3). Not only do they have a higher maintenance protein requirement than many other mammals, but they are also particularly sensitive to an arginine-deficient diet and they have a specific dietary need for the amino-sulphonic acid, taurine.

Dietary protein in excess of the body's requirements is not laid down as muscle but is, instead, converted to fat and stored as adipose tissue. Protein is a precious raw material and one which should be used as efficiently as possible.

Mineral	Function	Imbalance causes:
Iron (Fe)	An essential component of: the oxygen-carrying pigments, haemoglobin (in blood) and myoglobin (in muscle); many enzymes (haem enzymes) which are involved in cell respiration.	*Deficiency* – Anaemia with weakness and fatigue. *Toxicity* – Anorexia and weight loss in dogs.
Copper (Cu)	Copper is involved in the formation and activity of red blood cells; as a co-factor in many enzyme systems; and in normal pigmentation of skin and hair.	*Deficiency* – Anaemia due to impaired absorption and transport of iron and decreased haemoglobin synthesis. Bone disorders can also occur. *Toxicity* – May also cause anaemia due to competition between copper and iron for absorption sites in the intestine. Copper toxicosis in Bedlington Terriers is an inherited defect which causes hepatitis and cirrhosis. Other breeds may also be affected, including West Highland White Terriers and Dobermann Pinschers (Thornburg *et al.*, 1985 a,b). For these breeds, foods with high copper contents and copper-containing mineral supplements should be avoided.
Zinc (Zn)	An essential component of many enzyme systems, including those related to protein and carbohydrate metabolism, and is essential for maintaining healthy coat and skin. Zinc is required by all animals, but the zinc requirement is particularly affected by the other components of the diet. For example, a high dietary calcium content or a vegetable protein-based diet can dramatically increase the zinc requirement and this latter effect may be related to that reported for iron absorption.	*Deficiency* – Poor growth, anorexia, testicular atrophy, emaciation and skin lesions. Poor skin or coat condition can occur in companion animals due to a marginal deficiency, where the animal is not obviously unwell. *Toxicity* – Zinc is relatively non-toxic.
Iodine (I)	An essential component of thyroid hormones, which regulate basal metabolism in the body, and this is its only recognised function.	*Deficiency* – Goitre (enlargement of the thyroid gland) is the principal sign of iodine deficiency although other factors may also produce goitre. Hypothyroidism has been reported in dogs and iodine deficiency has also been observed in zoo felids, domestic cats, birds and horses. Clinical signs include skin and hair abnormalities, dullness, apathy and drowsiness. There can also be abnormal calcium metabolism and reproductive failure with fetal resorption. *Toxicity* – Acute effects similar to those of a deficiency. The high doses in some way impair thyroid hormone synthesis and can produce so-called iodine myxoedema or toxic goitre. Anorexia, fever and weight loss has been reported in cats (National Research Council, 1986).

Mineral	Function	Imbalance causes:
Selenium (Se)	An obligatory component of glutathione peroxidase, the enzyme which protects cell membranes against damage by oxidising substances. The action of selenium is closely interrelated with that of vitamin E, such that the presence of one nutrient can 'spare' a deficiency of the other. Selenium may also have other roles, including protection against lead, cadmium and mercury poisoning and has been implicated as an anti-cancer agent.	*Deficiency* - Many effects but one described in dogs is degeneration of skeletal and cardiac muscles. Effects of deficiency in other species include reproductive disorders and oedema. *Toxicity* - Highly toxic in large doses; the difference between the recommended allowance and the toxic dose may be quite small.
Manganese (Mn)	Involved in many enzyme-catalysed reactions and is required for carbohydrate and lipid metabolism and cartilage formation.	*Deficiency* - Defective growth, reproduction and disturbances in lipid metabolism.
Cobalt (Co)	An integral part of the vitamin B_{12} molecule.	*Deficiency* - Unlikely to occur if adequate vitamin B_{12} present in diet.

Table 1.2: *The main trace minerals.*

Fat

Dietary fats consist mainly of mixtures of triglycerides, where each triglyceride is a combination of three fatty acids joined by a unit of glycerol. The character of each fat is determined largely by the different fatty acids in each. Fatty acids may be described as **saturated**, where there are no double bonds between carbon atoms, or **unsaturated**, where one or more double bonds are present. Those containing more than one double bond are referred to as **polyunsaturated**. Most fats contain all of these types but in widely varying proportions.

Dietary fat has several roles. It serves as the most concentrated source of energy in the diet and gives an acceptable texture to food. However, its most important functions are as a provider of essential fatty acids (EFA) and as a carrier for the fat-soluble vitamins A, D, E and K. There are currently three recognised EFA, all of which are polyunsaturated; linoleic, α-linolenic and arachidonic acids. Linoleic and α-linolenic acids are the parent compounds from which the more complex, longer chain compounds (derived FA) can be made. The cat is unusual in that it is unable to convert sufficient of the parent EFA into longer chain derivatives and therefore requires a dietary source of arachidonic acid, which in practical terms means a requirement for FA of **animal** origin.

Fatty acids are involved in many aspects of health, including kidney function and reproduction. They are essential components of cell membranes and they are necessary for the synthesis of prostaglandins. Signs associated with EFA deficiency in dogs and cats include dull, scurfy coat, hair loss, fatty liver, anaemia and impaired fertility.

It should be noted that diets high in polyunsaturated fatty acids (PUFA) may become rancid through oxidation, which can lead to the destruction of other nutrients. Vitamin E is an antioxidant vitamin which protects these PUFA from degradation.

Carbohydrate

Carbohydrates provide the body with energy and may be converted to body fat. This group includes the simple sugars (such as glucose) and the complex sugars (such as starch) which consist of chains of the simpler sugars.

All animals have a metabolic requirement for glucose, but provided the diet contains sufficient glucose precursors (amino acids and glycerol), most animals can synthesise enough to meet their metabolic needs without a dietary source of carbohydrate. During pregnancy and lactation, there are increased demands for glucose, but recent work has shown that in the dog, dietary carbohydrate is not required, even at this stage, if there is a sufficient supply of gluconeogenic amino acids.

Sugars and **cooked** starches are economical and easily digested sources of energy whereas uncooked starches are less readily digested. Some species (some dogs, for example) may find sugars palatable but others, such as the cat, do not respond to the taste of sugars. The value of disaccharides such as sucrose or lactose is limited in most animals by the activity of the intestinal disaccharidases, such as sucrase and lactase. In particular, the activity of lactase declines with age and an excessive consumption of lactose-containing products can lead to diarrhoea.

Dietary Fibre

Dietary fibre, or roughage, is the term applied to the group of indigestible polysaccharides such as cellulose, pectin and lignin. They are usually associated with plant material and typically constitute the cell walls of plants. These materials generally escape digestion and pass through the digestive tract relatively unchanged. The role of dietary fibre in the animal depends to a large extent on the physiology of the animal's digestive tract, but in most species, a limited amount of dietary fibre may provide bulk to the faeces, regularising bowel movements and thus helping to prevent constipation or diarrhoea.

Micro-Nutrients

Minerals

Minerals are inorganic nutrients, which are sometimes referred to collectively as 'ash'. They may be divided into macro-minerals (which are required in relatively large amounts) and trace elements or micro-minerals (which are required in relatively small or trace amounts). Electrolytes are minerals in their salt form as found in the body tissues and fluids.

The functions of the macro-minerals and the main trace minerals are shown in Tables 1.1 and 1.2. In addition, a number of trace elements have been demonstrated as necessary for normal health in mammals, although specific requirements have not been established for companion animals (Table 1.3). It appears that the amounts required in the diet are very low and the likelihood of a deficiency of any of these nutrients in a normal diet is consequently almost non-existent. Conversely, as with the majority of the trace elements, these substances are all toxic if fed in large quantities, although the amounts which can be tolerated vary from one element to another. Arsenic, vanadium, fluorine and molybdenum are the most toxic, whereas relatively large amounts of nickel and chromium can be ingested without adverse effects.

Vitamins

Vitamins are organic compounds which help to regulate the body processes. Most vitamins cannot be synthesised in the body and must, therefore, be present in the diet. They may be classified as **fat-soluble** (vitamins A, D, E and K) or **water-soluble** (B-complex vitamins and vitamin C). A frequent intake of water-soluble vitamins is necessary since they are poorly stored in the body, with excesses being lost via the urine. The fat-soluble vitamins are stored to a much greater extent and consequently, a daily intake is less critical. However, because they are stored, the risk of toxicity arising through excessive intake is far greater with the fat-soluble vitamins.

The functions of the fat-soluble vitamins are summarised in Table 1.4. The B-complex vitamins are used to form co-enzymes (co-factors) which are involved with normal metabolic function, especially energy metabolism and synthetic pathways. They are now usually referred to by their chemical names rather than by a letter/number combination (Table 1.5). Ascorbic acid (vitamin C) is required for many intracellular reactions and protein synthesis, but most mammals (except man, other primates and the guinea pig) can synthesise it from glucose. There is no dietary requirement for vitamin C in normal, healthy companion animals, but a dietary source may be beneficial under certain circumstances (such as stress or high activity levels) or in certain individuals.

Water

An animal's requirement for water is at least as important as that for any other nutrient; life may continue for weeks in the absence of food but only for a few days, or even hours, when water is not available. Water performs many vital functions within the body and the body water content is regulated within quite narrow limits. A daily intake is necessary to replace obligatory water losses from the body which occur mainly via the urine, faeces, skin and lungs and in productive secretions such as milk.

Water is taken into the body in several forms: as fluid drunk, as a component of food, or as metabolic water (that released during the breakdown of protein, fat and carbohydrate). The daily water intake of any individual will depend on a number of factors including the moisture content of the food, environmental temperature, level of activity and physiological state. A plentiful supply of fresh drinking water should, therefore, always be available.

Element	Involvement
Chromium	Carbohydrate metabolism, closely linked with insulin function
Fluoride	Teeth and bone development, possibly some involvement in reproduction
Nickel	Membrane function, possibly involved in metabolism of the nucleic acid RNA
Molybdenum	Constituent of several enzymes, one of which is involved in uric acid metabolism
Silicon	Skeletal development, growth and maintenance of connective tissue
Vanadium	Growth, reproduction and fat metabolism
Arsenic	Growth, also some effect on blood formation, possibly haemoglobin production

Table 1.3: *Additional trace elements.*

Vitamin	Function	Imbalance causes:
Vitamin A (retinol)	Component of the visual pigments (which transmit light) in the eye and is important for proper vision. Involved in cell differentiation and maintenance of normal cell structure, so is important for sustaining healthy skin, coat, all mucous membranes and for normal bone and teeth development.	*Deficiency* - Abnormalities of the squamous epithelium (usually manifest as seborrhoeic coat conditions); xerophthalmia (excessive dryness of the eye); night blindness; increased susceptibility to microbial infections; crusting lesions of the external nares and accompanying nasal discharge; infertility. Deficiencies are uncommon, but cats require a source of pre-formed vitamin A, which is found only in animal tissue. *Toxicity* - Liver damage; painful bone disease resulting in the formation of bony exostoses and ankylosis of joints, particularly in the cervical vertebrae and the long bones of the forelimb. Cats are particularly susceptible and the problem usually arises following prolonged oversupplementation of the diet with vitamin A (in cod liver oil, for example) or by feeding large quantities of liver.
Vitamin D	Metabolites stimulate calcium absorption in the intestine and, in conjunction with parathyroid hormone, stimulate resorption of calcium from bone. Requirements are closely linked to the dietary concentrations of calcium and phosphorus. Vitamin D_3 may be synthesised from lipid compounds in the skin following exposure to sunlight.	*Deficiency* - Extremely rare, but frequently confounded by a simultaneous calcium and phosphorus imbalance. Causes rickets in the young animal and osteomalacia in the adult, characterised by a failure of mineralisation of newly formed osteoid. In the young animal, endochondral ossification of the growth plates is disturbed, giving rise to the typically enlarged metaphyses, particularly of the radius, ulna and ribs. *Toxicity* - Hypercalcaemia which, if prolonged, results in extensive calcification of the soft tissues, lungs, kidneys, and stomach. Deformations of the teeth and jaws can also occur and death can result if the intake is particularly high.
Vitamin E	Acting with selenium, protects cell membranes against oxidative damage. The requirement for vitamin E is increased when dietary levels of polyunsaturated fatty acids (PUFA), which are easily oxidised, are high.	*Deficiency* - Pansteatitis (yellow fat disease) in cats - a painful inflammatory condition of body fat (especially subcutaneous fat). Can be induced by feeding diets of oily fish, which are rich in PUFA, or rancid fat. Skeletal muscle dystrophy, reproductive failure and impairment of the immune response in dogs. *Toxicity* - Unlikely to occur and relatively high doses may be tolerated.
Vitamin K	Regulates the formation of several blood-clotting factors (factors VII, IX, X and XII).	*Deficiency* - Simple deficiency unlikely to occur, since in normal, healthy animals the requirement for vitamin K is met by bacterial synthesis in the intestine. Hypoprothrombinaemia and haemorrhage may occur in some animals when bacterial synthesis is suppressed, or if vitamin K antagonists (such as warfarin or other coumarin compounds) are present in the diet. *Toxicity* - Low toxicity but very large intakes can produce anaemia and other blood abnormalities in young animals.

***Table 1.4:** Fat-soluble vitamins.*

Vitamin	Function	Imbalance causes:
Thiamin (Aneurin, Vitamin B_1)	Involved in carbohydrate metabolism. Requirement is dependent on the carbohydrate content of the diet.	*Deficiency* - Anorexia, neurological disorders (especially of the postural mechanisms) followed ultimately by weakness, heart failure and death. Can occur, especially in cats, as a result of feeding large amounts of certain types of raw fish which contain the enzyme thiaminase. In addition, the vitamin is progressively destroyed by high temperatures and under certain conditions of processing. *Toxicity* - Low toxicity.
Riboflavin (B_2)	A constituent of two co-enzymes which are essential in a number of oxidative enzyme systems. Essential for cellular growth.	*Deficiency* - Eye lesions, skin disorders and testicular hypoplasia. *Toxicity* - Not reported.
Pantothenic acid	A constituent of co-enzyme A which is essential for carbohydrate, fat and amino acid metabolism.	*Deficiency* - Depressed growth, fatty liver, gastrointestinal disturbances (including ulcers), convulsions, coma and death. Naturally occurring deficiencies unlikely. *Toxicity* - Not reported.
Niacin (Nicotinamide and Nicotinic acid)	A component of two important co-enzymes, the nicotinamide adenine dinucleotides, which are required for oxidation-reduction reactions necessary for the utilisation of all the major nutrients.	*Deficiency* - Pellagra in humans and blacktongue in dogs and cats; characterised by inflammation and ulceration of the oral cavity with thick, blood-stained saliva and foul breath. *Toxicity* - Not considered toxic.
Pyridoxine (Vitamin B_6)	Involved in a wide range of enzyme systems associated with nitrogen and amino acid metabolism.	*Deficiency* - Anorexia, weight loss and anaemia. Irreversible kidney damage in cats. *Toxicity* - Not considered toxic.
Biotin	Required for a variety of reactions involving the metabolism of fats and amino acids. Important in maintaining the integrity of keratinised structures, such as the skin and hair.	*Deficiency* - Dry, scaly skin with dull, brittle hair, hyperkeratosis, pruritus and skin ulcers. Unlikely to occur since the daily requirement is normally met by intestinal bacterial synthesis. However, a deficiency may develop following the prolonged use of oral antibiotics or by feeding of large amounts of raw egg white containing avidin, a protein which binds biotin.
Folic acid (Pteroylglutamic acid, Folacin)	Important for a number of reactions including the synthesis of thymidine, a component of DNA. Maturation of red blood cells in bone marrow.	*Deficiency* - Anaemia and leucopenia, but unlikely to occur since most of the daily requirement can be met by intestinal bacterial synthesis.
Vitamin B_{12} (cyanocobalamin)	Function is closely linked to that of folic acid. Also involved in fat and carbohydrate metabolism and in the synthesis of myelin.	*Deficiency* - Pernicious anaemia and neurological signs.
Choline	A constituent of phospholipids which are essential components of cell membranes. Also the precursor of acetylcholine, a neurotransmitter chemical.	*Deficiency* - Unlikely to occur, but experimentally causes fatty infiltration of the liver.

***Table 1.5:** B-complex vitamins.*

A BALANCED DIET

A balanced diet can be defined as a diet which allows no net gain or loss of nutrients from the body to maintain a state of metabolic equilibrium. This diet will supply all the key nutrients needed to meet the daily needs of the recipient animal together with the quantity of energy required to sustain the animal's life stage. The provision of a balanced diet must inevitably include considerations of a number of factors which are all interlinked, including nutrient content, energy content, digestibility and palatability of the food.

The fundamental requirement for all species is for energy: if this need is coupled to the requirement for an individual nutrient then providing the correct quantity of energy also maintains the correct nutrient balance. When all key nutrients are balanced to the energy content of the diet, then animals requiring a higher plane of nutrition (as in gestation or lactation) will inevitably receive a higher intake of all key nutrients when they increase the amount of food consumed to meet their energy demands.

Nutrient Balance

Nutrient requirements are bounded by a minimum and, in some cases, a maximum value. In other words, the amount of nutrient needed in the diet must lie on a 'plateau' between deficiency on one hand and toxicity on the other (Figure 1.1). The main criteria for what constitutes a complete diet can therefore be summarised thus:

- The content of each nutrient must be on the plateau
- Each nutrient must be present in the correct ratio to the energy content of the diet
- Each nutrient must be at the correct ratio to other nutrients (where appropriate)
- Each nutrient must be in a form that is useable by the animal for which the diet is made.

Nutrient Interactions

Deficiencies of a specific nutrient may occur as a result of interactions with other components of the diet, which reduce their bioavailability. For example, excessive amounts of phytate (as can be found in cereal-based diets) will interfere with the intestinal absorption of zinc and high levels of calcium will reduce the absorption of both copper and zinc. The absorption of iron is known to be influenced by a number of factors. Ferrous iron is better absorbed than ferric iron and iron contained in foods of animal origin tends to be better absorbed than that from vegetable sources.

The availability of biotin is reduced in the presence of the protein, avidin, in raw egg white; thiamin is broken down by the enzyme thiaminase which is present in certain types of raw fish. Vitamin E is a natural antioxidant and levels may be depleted where the diet contains rancid (oxidised) fat; furthermore, higher dietary levels of vitamin E are needed when the diet is high in polyunsaturated fats, which are easily oxidised. The requirement for vitamin E is also dependent on the dietary level of selenium, since the presence of one can offset a deficiency of the other to some degree.

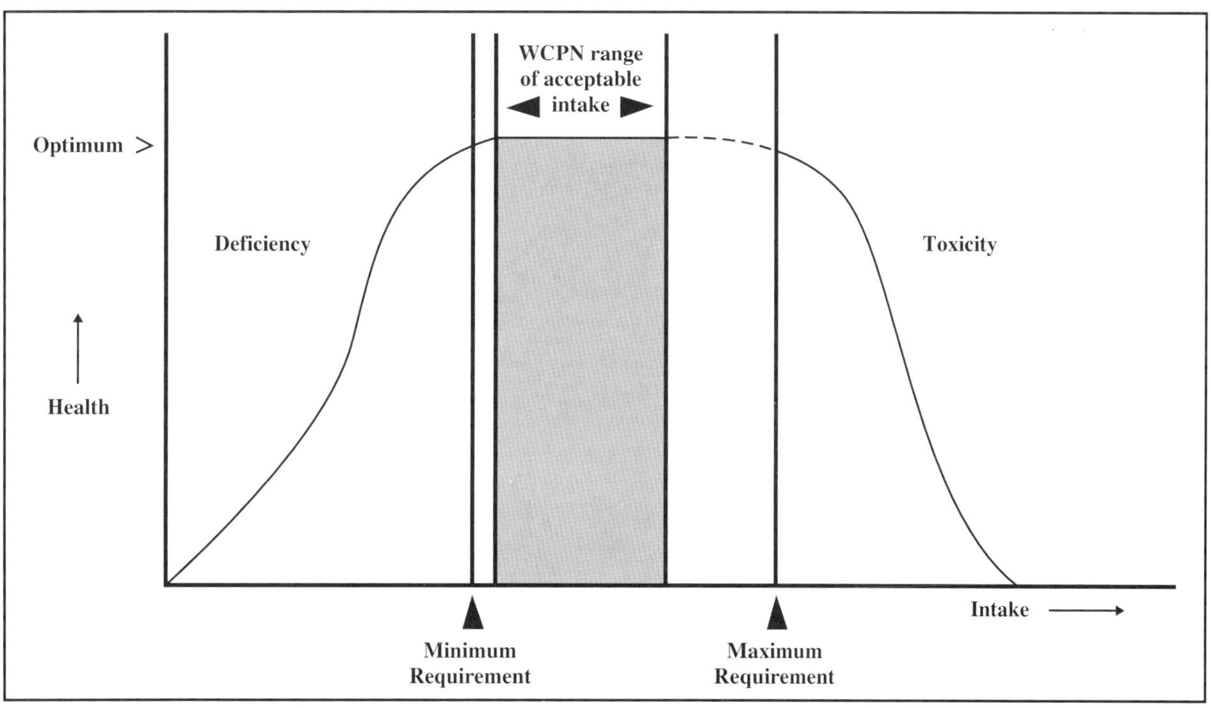

Figure 1.1: *Nutrient intake and nutritional adequacy.*

WCPN = Waltham Centre for Pet Nutrition

A further example of how overall dietary composition will affect the requirement for a particular nutrient, is that of potassium. The requirement for potassium is increased with high levels of dietary protein.

Digestibility

For nutrients to be of any use to the animal, they must be biologically active, that is the animal's digestive system must be able to extract the nutrient from the food and incorporate it into its metabolic pool. Simply analysing foodstuffs for total nutrient content does not give information on digestibility, and this must be measured by the collection of faeces and urine over a fixed period of time. Factors which affect the digestibility of a substance include chemical composition of the food, its state of subdivision and its method of preparation or processing.

Palatability

The palatability of food is a complex subject including a knowledge of the factors affecting appetite and behaviour, as well as an understanding of taste, smell and texture of food and their inter-relationships. The importance palatability cannot be overemphasised since a food which is left uneaten, whatever its nutrient content, is of no nutritive value to the animal.

First impressions of a food are always important and food must always be presented in a manner appropriate to the size of the animal. Cats and small dogs prefer food in small pieces which are not too sticky, whereas larger dogs are able to eat foods with a much broader spectrum of shape and size.

Smell and taste are necessary sensory components of any meal and animals with poor appetites can often be tempted to eat by providing strong-smelling foods, particularly if the food is warmed to about 35°C. Cats can distinguish between sweet and bitter tastes but show neither a positive nor negative response to the addition of glucose in their food. In general, meat is very palatable to dogs and cats and its acceptance can often be further enhanced by the addition of fat, especially animal fat.

Most animals enjoy variety in their diet, although they may be initially suspicious of a food which differs markedly from their previous diet. Above all it is important to recognise that, like humans, all animals are individuals with their own dietary likes and dislikes.

Species	Food Type and ME Equation
Cat	Canned $(P \times 3.9 + F \times 7.7 + C \times 3.0) - 5$ Dry $(P \times 5.65 + F \times 9.4 + C \times 4.15)\ 0.99 - 126$ Semi-moist $P \times 3.7 + F \times 8.8 + C \times 3.3$
Dog	All $P \times 3.5 + F \times 8.5 + C \times 3.5$

Table 1.6: *Calculation of metabolisable energy in cat and dog foods (kcal/100g food[1]).*

P *Protein g/100 g of food*
F *Fat (acid ether extract) g/100g of food*
C *Carbohydrate (calculated by difference) g/100 g of food*
[1] *For result in kJ/100g food, multiply by 4.184*

FOOD ENERGY

The body obtains energy by oxidising food but the energy is released gradually by a series of complex chemical reactions, each regulated by an enzyme. Many of these enzymes require the presence of vitamins or minerals in order to function properly.

No animal is able to utilise **all** the energy from its food. Energy intake is therefore considered at three different levels: gross energy (GE), digestible energy (DE) and metabolisable energy (ME). **Gross energy** of ingested food is the amount of heat released when the food is totally oxidised in an environment of pure oxygen. This is the maximum amount of energy that can be released and is assessed by bomb calorimetry. Although a substance may have a high GE content, it is of no use unless the animal is able to digest and absorb it. **Digestible energy** is the energy available from a food when it has been absorbed into the body after digestion in the digestive tract and is calculated as GE minus faecal losses.

Some of the absorbed food energy may be only partially available to the tissues, with the remainder (mainly in the form of end products of protein metabolism) being lost in the urine. The energy which is ultimately utilised by the tissues is known as ME and is calculated as DE minus urinary losses.

The DE and ME contents of foods depend both upon their composition and upon the species which consumes them. The digestive systems of animals differ markedly between species and even two fairly similar animals, such as the dog and the cat, show differences in digestibility values when fed the same food (Kendall *et al.*, 1982). In addition to these species differences there will be variations between individual animals in their own metabolic efficiency.

The only way to obtain a meaningful measurement of the ME content of food is thus to feed it to as large a group as possible and measure energy (by calorimetry) of food, faeces and urine. This is a costly and time consuming exercise, which is not possible without specialised facilities. Therefore, over the years, simple formulae have been developed which give reasonable approximations of the ME in a food from its carbohydrate, fat and protein contents, allowing for the losses in absorption and efficiency. Table 1.6 lists the equations used to calculate the ME content of commercially prepared cat and dog foods.

Utilisation of Food Energy

Energy is used to perform muscular work, processes such as breathing and physical activity to maintain body temperature. Energy expenditure can be divided into two parts: basal metabolic rate (BMR), which keeps the body 'ticking over', and thermogenesis. BMR includes processes such as respiration, circulation and kidney function and it may be affected by many factors including body weight and composition, age and hormonal status. Thermogenesis is simply an increase in metabolic rate over the basal level and includes the cost of digesting, absorbing and utilising nutrients (sometimes called the 'thermic effect of food' or 'dietary induced thermogenesis'), of muscular work or exercise, of stress, or of maintenance of body temperature in a cold environment. Certain drugs or hormones may also be the cause of thermogenesis. In contrast to BMR, the degree of thermogenesis can vary widely and may cause large variations in daily output. Thermogenesis is capable of rapid adaptive response to changes in the internal or external environment.

The energy density of the diet must be high enough to enable the dog or cat to obtain sufficient calories to maintain energy balance. This is the principal factor determining the quantity of food eaten each day and thus the amount of each nutrient ingested by the animal. Nutrient requirements are usually expressed in terms of the ME concentration so that the values are applicable to any type of food or diet regardless of its water content, nutrient content or overall energy value.

Energy Requirements

Energy expenditure or requirements can ultimately be measured in terms of heat loss or heat production and this fact leads to the key concept in the calculation of energy requirement for different animals. Clearly, it is most convenient to express energy needs in terms of body weight, which is a familiar and easily measurable quantity. However, heat loss varies not with body weight, but with body surface area (BSA), a quantity which is difficult to assess accurately.

Nevertheless, as BSA varies with the square of linear dimensions, and body weight with the cube (i.e. volume), heat loss **should** vary with body weight (W) adjusted mathematically in line with these two factors; $W^{2/3}$ or $W^{0.67}$. The body weight thus modified is often referred to as the **metabolic** body weight or body size. It should be possible to use this value to compare energy requirements of animals with widely differing body weights. This is particularly relevant for dogs, which are unique in that there is such a wide variation in body weight within a single species. The equation currently recommended for calculation of the **average** requirements of dogs is as follows:

$$E = 110\ W^{0.75}\ \text{kcal/day (or } 460\ W^{0.75}\ \text{kJ/day)}$$

where W is body weight in kg. This type of equation is referred to as an **allometric** equation; it relates size to a function which, in this case, is energy requirement. The values obtained assume a moderate amount of activity for a dog in a temperate climate.

Energy requirements do, however, also vary with the body **type** and in feeding studies in dogs, it has been shown that breed conformation affects the *in vivo* requirements of the individual. For example, Newfoundlands need less than the predicted amounts whereas Great Danes need more. These two breeds have approximately the same body weight, but have very different body composition, hair type (coat) and shape.

For cats and other species in which there is a relatively narrow range of body weight, it might be expected that energy requirements could be related directly to body weight with little error. Nevertheless, even in cats a logarithmic relationship to body weight has been reported with larger cats displaying a lower energy requirement per unit of body weight than smaller ones (Earle and Smith, 1991).

Energy Balance

An animal is said to be in energy balance when its expenditure of energy is equal to its intake, with the result that the level of energy stored in the body does not change. The following equation is derived from the Law of Conservation of Energy:

Energy stored = energy intake - energy expenditure

In the adult dog or cat, energy is stored predominantly as fat with some increase in lean tissue (fat-free mass). In the growing or pregnant animal the emphasis shifts to the accumulation of lean tissue. Fat is stored as adipose tissue and these deposits are easily observed in the obese animal. It is also possible to decrease energy stores, by reducing the intake until it is less than energy output. This reverses the equation:

Expenditure - intake = loss of energy from stores

Under these conditions of negative energy balance, the body has to catabolise its own tissues to meet its energy needs; as the stores are gradually depleted, the animal becomes thinner and body weight decreases.

Energy balance is achieved by the matching of input and output **over long periods**. A very small imbalance maintained over a long period of time will cause obesity (if the net difference is positive) or wasting (if the net difference is negative). For example, a 35kg dog will require about 1580kcal per day (6620kJ) according to the predictive equation (see above). If this estimate is wrong by only 100kcal/day (418kJ) (about 30g of dog biscuit), then it could result in an increase of 2–3kg bodyweight if maintained over a year.

The principal mechanism of control of energy balance is thought to be via regulation of intake, although some variation of output is also thought to be important. Regulation of intake is thought to fit a negative feedback mechanism to a greater or lesser degree (see below). Intake is capable of precise control in contrast to expenditure which appears to act as a crude buffer, opposing any change to the energy content of the body.

FACTORS AFFECTING FOOD INTAKE

It is the energy requirement of the animal and the energy density of the food which primarily determine the quantity of food eaten each day (see above).

Although very palatable foods may disturb the control of intake, many animals fed bland foods regulate energy intake very precisely. Even when the same food is given in dilute form (using water or some non-digestible material to alter the energy density) compensation usually occurs rapidly and completely to a new, appropriate level of food intake.

As previously indicated, food intake is thought to be regulated primarily via a negative feedback mechanism. There are several feedback elements which may signal change, such as plasma nutrient or metabolite levels. Any discrepancies against set reference points indicate change in energy stores and stimulate neural and hormonal activity which may initiate or inhibit feeding.

The neural response involves 'feeding centres' in the brain which are probably not discrete 'hunger' and 'satiety' centres as once thought, but bundles of neurons covering several areas. Stimulation of these by electrodes can cause satiated animals to eat or prevent hungry animals from eating.

The hormonal response is more complex. Insulin stimulates feeding but it is not known whether this is a direct effect on the central nervous system or from peripheral hypoglycaemia. Glucagon has the opposite effect to insulin, inhibiting feeding, as do oestrogens and luteinising hormone. All these hormones have roles other than the stimulation or inhibition of feeding, and are not the sole agents governing intake.

In addition to neural and hormonal mechanisms there are other, more direct stimuli to feeding. Contractions of an empty stomach are thought to cause the sensation of hunger and provoke feeding, whereas gastric distension inhibits eating.

This model provides a useful framework to the theories of regulation of energy intake. However, the full explanation is still elusive and allowance must be made for some control of energy expenditure to regulate energy balance. In most cases regulation is successful. Disturbances occur when highly palatable titbits are offered and the appetite for a particular food drowns out physiological satiety signals: this seems to affect dogs rather more than cats which suffer much less often from obesity.

PREPARED PET FOODS

Raw Materials

The pet food industry uses a range of raw materials of animal, cereal and vegetable origin, which are almost entirely the by-products of the human food industry or are surplus to human requirement. Reputable pet food manufacturers do not use diseased tissue, or other materials which are unfit for human consumption, in the preparation of their products. They do not use materials which originate from animal species which are not normally acceptable in the human food chain. Where raw materials of animal origin are imported from abroad, this is only permitted from countries with a satisfactory animal health status.

Quality

Prepared pet foods from reputable pet food manufacturers come with a guarantee of nutritional adequacy, quality and safety. This is ensured not only by legislation, but also by the strict self-governing policies that are imposed by the national and international trade associations and the individual companies themselves.

Typical Analysis

Recipes used vary widely between individual pet food manufacturers. EC regulations dictate that the concentrations of the following nutrients must be declared as percentages in the product: protein, oil, fibre and ash. The 1991 Feeding Stuffs regulations also require a statement of the percentage moisture in the product, if this is over 14%. These values can be used to compare nutrient values between different products but it is important always to compare like with like. The important aspect is the level of nutrient that is ingested by the animal. This depends on energy and the energy content is proportional to the dry matter content.

Declaration of energy content on the label may offer some advantages but is a very complex issue. The energy content depends on the protein, fat and carbohydrate contents of the product (i.e. the energy-containing nutrients). The main challenge is to find an acceptable way to calculate the available or metabolisable energy (ME) of the food from these constituents. The ME content depends both upon the composition of the food and the animal which is eating it. For example, the digestive system of the dog seems to be more efficient than that of the cat. Thus, the **same food** fed to dogs or cats will yield different ME values in the two species. Until an agreed method has been finalised which gives a ME value for pet foods which is neither misleading nor over-complicated, the EC has ruled that energy declarations on pet foods are illegal. This reinforces the importance of reliable feeding recommendations.

DIETARY SUPPLEMENTATION

Contrary to many advertisements and popular beliefs, young animals and lactating females do not require large quantities of minerals and vitamins. Provided they are fed a balanced diet appropriate to their life stage, their needs will be met as their food intake increases to meet their energy requirements. There is no advantage to be gained by overdosing.

Supplementation should be undertaken with care as this may unbalance an otherwise balanced diet, and many nutrient interactions can result in a reduced availability of specific nutrients. This can lead to the possibility of toxicities, as may readily occur with vitamins A and D, for example. Dietary supplementation can be expensive and is unlikely to be of benefit in non-deficient animals.

However, the value of vitamin/mineral supplements used in moderate amounts should not be dismissed. They can act as an insurance for those individual animals who may experience difficulties in either absorption or utilisation of specific nutrients. Although they are unnecessary when a commercially prepared pet food is fed, supplements are likely to be required in order to nutritionally balance home-prepared diets. In addition, they have a psychological benefit for people who need to give what they see as extra care. Nevertheless, in cases of diet-related nutrient deficiencies, it is considered preferable to correct the deficient diet itself rather than to rely on blanket supplementation.

REFERENCES:

Earle KE and Smith PM (1991). Digestible energy requirements of adult cats at maintenance. *Journal of Nutrition* **121,** S45-S46.

Kendall PT, Holme DW and Smith PM (1982). Comparative evaluation of net digestive and absorptive efficiency in dogs and cats fed a variety of contrasting diet types. *Journal of Small Animal Practice* **23,** 577-587.

Legrand-Defretin V (1993). Energy requirements of dogs and cats - what goes wrong? *International Journal of Obesity* **18** (suppl.1), S22-S28.

National Research Council (1986). *Nutrient Requirements of Cats.* National Academy Press, Washington D.C.

Thornburg LP, Einger WL, McAllister D and Hoekema DJ (1985a). Copper toxicosis in dogs, Part 1: copper-associated liver disease in Bedlington Terriers. *Canine Practice* **12** (4), 41-45.

Thornburg LP, Dennis GL, Olwin DB, McLaughlin CD and Gulbas NK (1985b). Copper toxicosis in dogs, Part 2: the pathogenesis of copper-associated liver disease in dogs. *Canine Practice* **12** (5), 33-38.

CHAPTER TWO

Food Types and Evaluation

Noel C. Kelly

INTRODUCTION

In the developed economies of Europe the vast majority of pet owners feed industrially prepared commercially available food to their dogs and cats. It is vital then that an informed choice of food type is made to provide a complete and balanced diet appropriate to life stage nutrient requirements.

To provide effective dietary evaluation as a service to clients, the practising veterinarian must have a working knowledge of these requirements, familiarity with the food types available, and their capacity to satisfy the animal's nutritional demand.

Key elements in adopting a proactive role are recognition of the owners' concern about correct feeding for their pets, food type and presentation, interpretation of label information and nutritional claims. Raw material ingredients have a major impact on pet food quality, so that a fundamental understanding of their significance is important, for both industrially and home prepared food.

In this discussion we will look at the following topics:

1) Commercially available food types.
2) Product and dietary evaluation.
3) Label information interpretation.
4) Home-prepared food.

Understanding the practical aspects of feeding the different food types and their probable contribution to the diet will facilitate confident and comfortable discussion in the consulting room.

COMMERCIALLY AVAILABLE FOOD TYPES

Physical Form

Classification within the grocery trade is based on the moisture content, which determines the form of the product presented, processing technology, preservation, packaging and shelf life.

Table 2.1 gives the commonly presented forms of commercially available pet food, moisture and dry matter content. Table 2.2 gives comparable values for some fresh meats and offal.

Function

Descriptive terms based on function or strategic positioning in the overall dietary plan of the dog and cat define pet food products into specific functional groups.

- **Complete and balanced** – Canned, semi-moist or dry, nutritionally complete for dog or cat. These may be claimed to be complete nutrition for specific life stages or for all life stages. The life stage orientation or intended purpose of the food and the intended species should be clearly stated.

Classification	Moisture %	Dry matter %	Packaging and Presentation
Moist	72-85	15–28	Can, 'plastic pot', foil tray Formed or loaf type product
Semi-moist	15-30	70-85	Sachets, cellophane wrap (sausage type) chunks, burgers, 'meat-ball' 'chewy sticks'
Dry	5-12	88-95	Bags and boxes Expanded particles, biscuit snacks, mixed meal

Table 2.1: *Broad classification based on moisture content.*

Meat type	Moisture %	Dry matter %
Beef	74	26
Lamb	70	30
Chicken	74	26
Mince	60	40
Liver	68	32
Dressed tripe	88	12

Table 2.2: *Comparative values for meat and offal.*

- **Complementary** - Canned, semi-moist, or dry foods which do not meet the known nutritional requirements for the species when fed alone. They may be intended as a major part of the diet, such as complementary canned or mixer, in which case the additional food type needed to complete the ration should be stated, together with life stage or purpose orientation and intended species.

Snacks and treats are also often described as complementary foods:

Snacks: Usually incomplete, palatable foods for intermittent or occasional variety in the diet, commonly prepared for cats, and useful for tempting sick or inappetent animals. However, snacks intended to be fed as part of a dietary regimen are often formulated as complete.

Treats: Very often dry or semi-moist products given as rewards, or for a strategic purpose such as dental health.

- **Veterinary dietary products** - Supplied through veterinary surgeons. Moist or dry complete food types for the treatment or management of dietary problems and pathological conditions, or to supply special needs. (Usually industrially prepared, these food types may however be prepared with home-made recipes.)

Food Type Characteristics

Tables 2.3 and 2.4 give typical nutrient compositions of food types and Table 2.5 their processing, preservation and common ingredients.

Moist Foods

Traditionally canned, now available also in plastic pots, foil trays and 'plastic cans' these products have a moisture content range of 72–85% as fed or 'as is'. The high water content, whilst not implying suboptimal quality, means that these products have less nutrients per 100g than other food types so that more must be eaten to satisfy energy and nutrient needs, with a significant impact on feeding costs. It is however because of their moisture content and ingredients' form that these products are the most palatable of the commercially available pet foods. Protein content ranges from 7% to 9% in dog food and 8% to 11% in cat food on an 'as fed' basis. Fat content ranges from 3% to 9% for dog food and 3% to 5% for cat food depending on the ingredient source. Carbohydrate range is 2–13% in dog food and 1–7% in cat food. Energy content varies from 65kcal (273kJ) ME to 130kcal (546kJ) ME per 100g of cat or dog food. Protein, fat and energy content tend to be at the upper end of the range in puppy and kitten food.

Digestibility of moist food types for both dogs and cats is high, being 80–85% for most nutrients in quality products.

Meaningful comparison between food types as to their energy and nutrient content should be made on a dry matter (DM) basis.

The contents vary from all meat with high protein and fat to almost all vegetable/cereal type similar to dry or soft-moist products on a dry matter basis. Complete and complementary products are available for dogs and cats in this category.

Appearance and Shape

- **Loaf** - ground cereal and chopped meat, fish, poultry, giving solid meatloaf-like appearance typical of 'ration' type products (see below).

- **Formed** - ground cereal and chopped or comminuted meat, pre-formed. They may be meat-based, fish-based, meat and cereal or fish and cereal food types, in a balanced formulation or a complementary mainly meat (gourmet) type. Their appearance in the can or on serving may be as balls, shapes or chunks together with gelling agents and mineral/vitamin supplements in gravy or jelly.

- **All meat** - meat and meat by-products, mineral/vitamin supplement with or without gravy or jelly.

Quality balanced canned (moist) products are usually higher in animal source proteins and in animal fat, but lower in carbohydrate than dry or semi-moist products. Energy density is highest, on a dry matter (DM) basis, of all commercially available food types. Palatability seems to be directly related to the meat or fish content, those with high cereal being less palatable. The meat-based products contain mainly cooked meat, poultry or fish and their by-products, in chunks or unformed, and with gravy or jelly.

Although these food types may be fed on their own if balanced, usually, with the exception of the complete 'ration' type, they are fed as a complementary food to

Dog Foods

Dry complete

Nutrient	% As fed	Range	% DM
Carbohydrate	44	(35-60)	48
Protein	24	(18-30)	28
Fat	12	(6-20)	11
Moisture	8	(8-12)	-
Ash	8	(7-8)	9
Fibre	4	(4-6)	5.6
Energy ME kcal/100g*	350		360

Semi-moist

Nutrient	% As fed	Range	% DM
Carbohydrate	43	(35-50)	59
Moisture	23	(15-50)	-
Protein	19	(17-25)	26
Fat	6	(6-12)	9
Ash	6	(5-8)	7.5
Fibre	3	(3-3.5)	4.5
Energy ME kcal/100g*	280		380

Moist (Canned) meat-based

Nutrient	% As fed	Range	% DM
Moisture	80	(72-85)	-
Protein	8	(7-9)	40
Fat	5	(3-9)	35
Carbohydrate	4	(2-13)	15
Ash	2	(0.9-3)	7.5
Fibre	0.5	(0.5-1)	2.5
Energy ME kcal/100g*	80		400

Moist (Canned) ration (animal by-products and cereal)

Nutrient	% As fed	Range	% DM
Moisture	76	(74-80)	-
Carbohydrate	12	(5-13)	50
Protein	6	(6-8)	25
Fat	2	(2-4)	8
Ash	2	(2-6)	8
Fibre	2	(2-4)	8
Energy ME kcal/100g*	80		400

Table 2.3: *Typical nutrient composition of dog foods 'as fed' and in DM (listed in decreasing order of magnitude – rounded off values).*

* *(1kcal = 4.184kJ)*

Cat Foods

Dry complete

Nutrient	% As fed	Range	% DM
Carbohydrate	46	(35–50)	50
Protein	30	(25–33)	32
Moisture	7	(7–10)	-
Fat	6	(6–12)	7.5
Ash	7	(6–7.5)	7.5
Fibre	3	(2–4)	3.2
Energy ME kcal/100g*	360		400

Semi-moist

Nutrient	% As fed	Range	% DM
Carbohydrate	48	(45–50)	60
Moisture	21	(15–30)	-
Protein	17	(17–25)	21.5
Fat	6	(6–12)	7.5
Ash	6	(5–7)	7.5
Fibre	2.0	(1–3)	2.5
Energy ME kcal/100g*	270		340

Moist (Canned) meat-based

Nutrient	% As fed	Range	% DM
Moisture	84	(75–84)	-
Protein	8	(8–11)	50
Fat	4.5	(3.5–6)	28
Carbohydrate	1.8	(1–7)	11
Ash	1.2	(1–2.5)	7
Fibre	1	(0.5–1.0)	6
Energy ME kcal/100g*	70		350

Moist (Canned) ration (animal by-products and cereal)

Nutrient	% As fed	Range	% DM
Moisture	80	(75–83)	-
Protein	8	(7–9)	40
Fat	6	(4–6)	30
Carbohydrate	2.9	(2–3)	14.5
Ash	2	(1.8–2.4)	10
Fibre	1	(1.0–1.8)	5
Energy ME kcal/100g*	80		400

Table 2.4: *Typical nutrient composition of cat foods 'as fed' and in DM (listed in decreasing order of magnitude).*

* *(1kcal = 4.184kJ)*

Food Type	Process/Preservation	Ingredients
Dry complete: Expanded particles Biscuit-shaped or kibbled Meal type	 Extrusion cooked (steam/pressure) Shaped and dried Baked Cooked ingredients, coarse mixed	 Cereal grains, soya meal, meat and bone meal, meat meal, fish meal, fresh meat, fats and oils, 'digest', minerals, vitamins, antioxidants
Mixers: Expanded particles	 Extrusion cooked and dried	 Cereal grains, fat, minerals, vitamins
Semi-moist: Shaped particles, meat-balls, burgers	 Extrusion cooked and shaped, low pH, low A_w	 Cereal grains, meat and meat by-products, fresh meat, fats, sugars, salts, humectants e.g. glycerol, organic acids, preservatives, minerals/ vitamins
Moist: **Canned ration type** Cereal and meat 'loaf'	 Heat cooked and sterilised	 Cereal grain, meat by-products soya flour (TVP), fish, fishmeal, vegetable gum (guar) and other gelling agents e.g. carageenan
Canned meat-based with shaped elements such as soya chunks, textured vegetable protein and gelled alginate chunks known as 'analogue'	 Heat cooked and sterilised	 Meat, meat by-products, poultry, poultry by-products, fish, soya flour, gelling and thickening agents such as carrageenan, guar, alginates

Table 2.5: *Processing and preservation of industrially prepared pet foods – dog and cat.*

dogs with a good quality mixer biscuit, the latter supplying cereal-based carbohydrate as a cheaper energy source. Some minerals and vitamins are supplied by the moist product but these are complemented by the appropriate mixer.

Ration type canned products contain mainly cereal grain, soya, meat and poultry or fish and their by-products. Quality palatable rations with high energy density can be produced which are complete and balanced, based on a good choice of raw material ingredients. The latter may help to prevent the development of fixed food preferences exhibited by pets fed on food types with a single or few predominant ingredients. Ration type foods are formulated to supply a complete and balanced diet.

Semi-moist (soft-moist)

Semi-moist food types are available as 'complete and balanced', and as snacks or treats for dogs and cats. They are presented as 'minced pieces', burgers, balls or chunks, ranging in moisture content from 15% to 40%. The latter determines consistency which varies from a moist meat-like texture (25–30% moisture) to a firm drier type (15% moisture). Major nutrient levels are protein 17–25%, fat 6–12% and carbohydrate 35-50%. Energy content is approximately 270kcal (1134kJ) ME/100g food but this will vary with the moisture content. Raw materials such as meat, meat by-products, soya flour, vegetable protein, cereals, fats and sugars also influence appearance and texture. These products invariably more closely resemble dry food types than moist in their nutrient content. They do however tend to have a higher proportion of animal protein and a higher energy density on a dry matter basis than do dry foods. The carbohydrate complement is mainly as disaccharides (sucrose), with a lower level of the starch type found in dry products.

Digestibility of the constituent nutrients is high (80–85%).

Humectants such as sugars, salts, glycerol are incorporated to reduce water availability (A_w) or water activity (A_Δ) below that conducive to bacterial and fungal growth in or on the food. This retards microbiological spoilage. Further processing aids used to augment this are the addition of mould and yeast inhibitors such as potassium sorbate and organic acids to inhibit bacterial proliferation further by lowering the pH of the food system. Semi-moist products are relatively stable at room temperature and humidity and so may be exposed on an *ad libitum* basis without spoilage. Be aware however that the high palatability of some of these food types may encourage their consumption to excess, thereby over-riding the energy intake governing system, leading to obesity in dogs and cats.

'As fed', on a volume basis, semi-moist products have the highest caloric density, having a lower moisture content than canned and fewer air spaces than extruded dry products.

Semi-moist is not the most viable of the commercially prepared pet food sectors but it does have a niche market, particularly in the snacks and treats area.

Dry

Dry foods for dogs and cats are usually in the form of extrusion cooked expanded particles - see Figures 2.1 and 2.2. (Meal types of flaked cooked cereals and dried meat are however still commercially available for dogs - see Figure 2.3, as are kibbled biscuit, baked and broken.)

Dry foods may be 'complete and balanced' for all life stages or indeed segmented, with specific life stage orientation. They contain cereal, cereal by-products, animal or vegetable protein, meat and bone meal, fish meal, soya meal, fats, minerals and vitamins in different combinations. Nutrient levels 'as fed' range from 20% to 27% protein, 7% to 12% fat and 35% to 50% carbohydrate in dry dog food and 30% protein or more in cat food, with emphasis on protein and fat of animal origin for this species. Fresh meat ingredients may be incorporated in these products. Products for dogs and cats have surface applied palatability agents such as 'digest', a liquid or powdered hydrolysed form of animal tissues such as liver or intestines from chicken or rabbit. Fat is also sprayed on the surface following extrusion which further enhances palatability.

Energy content is typically about 350kcal (1470kJ) ME/100g food for a maintenance product.

'Mixer biscuit' for dog and cat is more commonly extruded particle or flake products than baked biscuit as the name might imply. The latter type of baked, shaped biscuits are available as 'crunchy' snacks, treats or rewards - see Figure 2.5. Their cooked flavours and fat content promote palatability. Some of these are oriented towards promoting dental health by physical abrasive action.

Quality 'mixers' are cereal based with little protein concentrate but are supplemented with minerals, trace elements and vitamins commensurate with energy content and are formulated to complement meat-based canned (moist) products. Poor quality (often cheaper) 'mixers' are mainly cooked cereals with just enough fat added for the cooking process and may well need supplementation with minerals and vitamins even when fed with quality moist products.

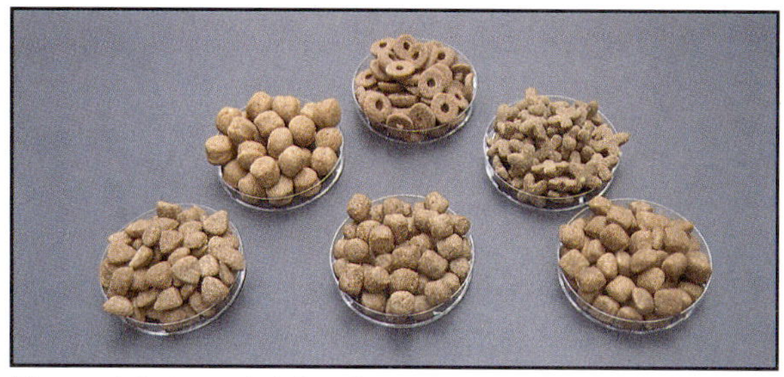

Figure 2.1: *Extruded dog diets.*

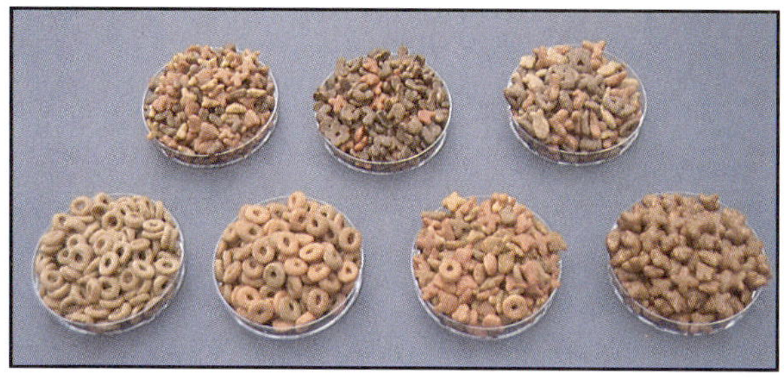

Figure 2.2: *Extruded cat diets.*

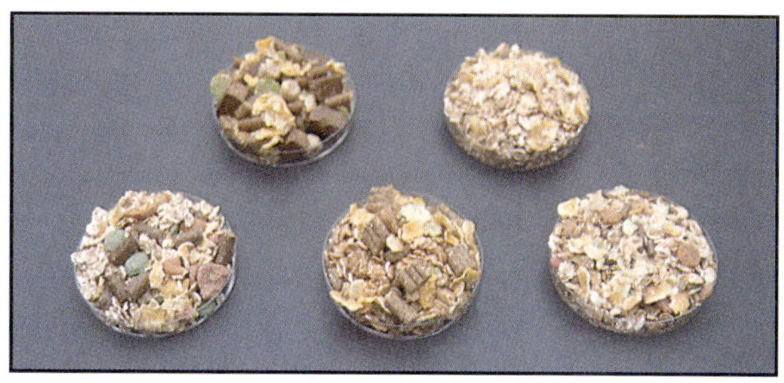

Figure 2.3: *Coarse mix dog diets.*

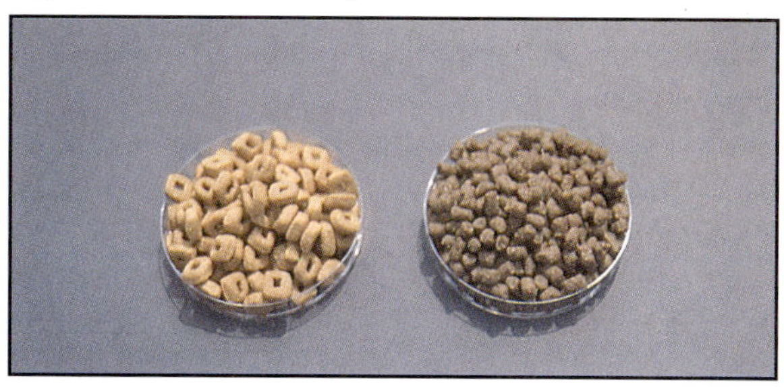

Figure 2.4: *Extruded puppy diets.*

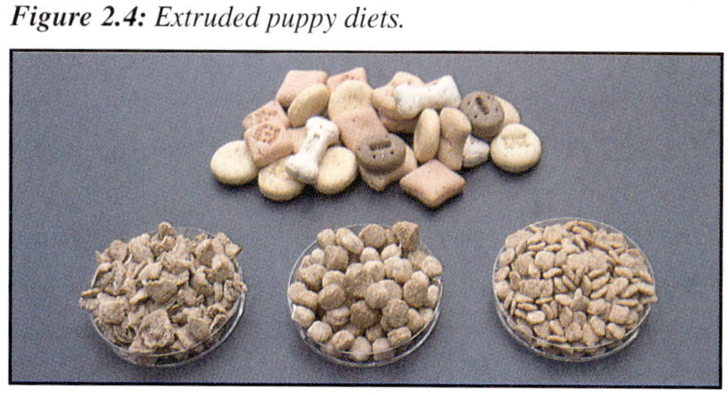

Figure 2.5: *Dog mixers & biscuits.*

Dry foods for dogs and cats are usually a less expensive feeding option than their moist or semi-moist counterparts. However more recent trends to further market segmentation have seen the entry of 'super premium' food types, many of which are life stage or lifestyle orientated, and this has considerably narrowed the cost advantage for this type of dry product.

Nutrients and energy per unit weight 'as fed' are greater in dry than in moist food types so that less weight of product is required to supply equivalent nutrient amounts.

Digestibility

Quality dry foods, unless significantly high in fibre have good digestibility which may be comparable or lower than moist products.

Dry foods are better digested by dogs than they are by cats possibly reflecting differences in gastrointestinal structure and function. They are usually less palatable than moist or semi-moist but this varies with ingredients, processing practices and palatability enhancement by surface application of fat and 'digest' following extrusion. There are technological constraints on the incorporation of fresh abattoir materials and fat level inclusion in the extrusion cooking, process and packaging considerations limit the amount of compensatory surface applied fat following the extrusion process. Maintenance type dry foods may be of limited acceptability and digestibility for small and toy breeds and also for pets in special demand situations such as lactation, work/stress or illness. This type of product can be suitably enriched with proteins, fat, minerals and vitamins, preferably from another balanced source such as a canned product, to meet these situations. 'Super premium' dry food types may however be more nutrient and energy dense with protein and fat levels of up to 30% and 22%, respectively, for dog food, whilst cat food may have 35% protein and 22% fat. These food types have high digestibility and may result in reduced stool volume. They may have an energy content of up to 400kcal (1680kJ) ME/100g food.

Best popular or premium brand dry foods may be lower in digestible fibre than cheaper ones and are comparable to quality canned (moist) foods in digestibility of nutrients. These parameters may well be reflected in stool pattern and consistency, with well formed firm stools being produced twice daily for a quality, highly digestible product, whilst a poor quality product may result in several bulky stools daily.

Because of the cereal content, starch is an important energy source in dry foods which make them a cheaper and suitable food for maintenance in the dog.

Availability of essential fatty acids (EFA), especially linoleic for the dog and arachidonic for the cat, may be less than optimal from some complete dry foods following prolonged storage in adverse conditions of warm, damp environments or exposure to daylight. This is particularly pertinent if tallow (beef fat) is used as the fat source, having only about 2% as linoleic acid. Total fat may be less than 10% so that rancidity on storage may render the low level of EFA less available. Even in the domestic situation this phenomenon could be significant with the advent of bulk buying, especially for the small dog or cat, if food is stored in an open pack in a warm humid kitchen for a prolonged period, of 6 months or more. Quality dry dog food will use a rich source of linoleic acid such as soya oil (50% linoleic) which gives an assurance of keeping quality with a predicted shelf life ('best before') of 18 months.

Dry food types are simple to feed and easily stored.

PRACTICAL GUIDELINES FOR FEEDING DIFFERENT FOOD TYPES

Industrially Prepared

Canned (moist) complementary – Feed with an equal volume of good quality mixer.

Balanced meat-based and **ration** type canned (moist) products may be fed on their own as a balanced diet.

Semi-moist complete food types may be fed to dogs and cats as their sole nutrition or they may be fed to complement a canned product.

Complete dry food can be fed 'as is' in the dry state or moistened with water @ 1 part water to 4 parts food on a volume basis. Cats prefer dry products without added water but this should be freely available.

Dry mixer – Feed in equal volume with complementary canned dog food.

Home-Prepared

Cooked fresh meat should be fed on an equal **weight** basis with a quality 'mixer' which is usually balanced for minerals relative to its energy content.

Cooked fresh meat should be mineral supplemented, especially when the carbohydrate portion of the diet is not a 'mixer', but rice, potato, bread or pasta. Ground egg shell, bone meal, sterilised bone flour, dicalcium phosphate may all be suitable, while proprietary mineral/vitamin tablets are usually inadequate in this situation to supply sufficient calcium (Donoghue, 1992) (see section on home-made diets). Vitamin supplementation is also advisable in this situation with particular attention to thiamin and vitamins A and E.

Feeding Regimen

Frequency and amount of feeding for dogs varies with life stage, physiological state, body size and practical considerations. Cats are occasional feeders and tend to return to their food several times a day, possibly up to 12 times in a 24 hour period if fed *ad libitum* (Sohail, 1983). This however must be modified to suit the household routine and cats adapt their intake to suit their needs on time limited exposure to food (Kanarek, 1975). Two to three times a day feeding seems adequate for most cats for maintenance.

Semi-moist and dry food types are relatively stable on short-term exposure at room conditions and may be exposed 'free choice' to dogs and cats. Moist foods or moistened dry food should not be left on offer for protracted periods as they tend to dry out, become less palatable and undergo spoilage.

Determining the amount of a particular food type to be fed appropriate to the animal's size, life stage and lifestyle is not a pure science. Individual variation is considerable, particularly in dogs and this is reflected in the high incidence of obesity evident in the canine population, even among those fed in accordance with guidelines on pet food labels. ME is the most appropriate measure of the metabolically useful energy in the diet but it is rarely measured directly and information is scant on the available energy from the ingredients and food type. Therefore rigid regimens are not practicable and owners should be educated as to how they can monitor bodily condition manually as well as by periodic weight recording on platform scales at the clinic. Feeding guidelines are usually based on National Research Council estimates of ME available to dogs and cats from protein, carbohydrate and fat in feed ingredients commonly used in pet foods. Products which have been assessed for performance in feeding colonies of varied breed type and size have the best assurance of valid guidelines.

Substituting One Balanced Food Type with Another for Equivalent Maintenance

1) Determine the amount of the food type currently being fed.
2) Calculate or read off label (if given) the energy content of the amount being fed.
3) Calculate or read off data sheet or label (if given) the equivalent energy in a given amount of the 'new' food type and substitute this in the feeding regimen phased incrementally over a 4 day period.
4) Check body condition and weight at 1 month. If results are poor review food choice or feeding regimen.

'Rules of Thumb'

1) Commercially available food types have an approximate ME value of **400kcal (1680kJ)/100g** on a **Dry Matter** basis. Table 2.6 gives approximate energy values for commonly fed commercial and table food types.

(Dog food)

2) A teacup holds about 100g (3.5oz) of complete dry food or of mixer ≅ 350kcal (1470kJ) ME.
3) A 400g can will hold about 140g of 'mixer' ≅ 500kcal (2100kJ) ME
4) A 170g (6oz) pack of semi-moist food type ≅ 425kcal (1785kJ) ME
5) A 400g can of canned (moist) dog food ≅ 330kcal (1386kJ) ME*

Food type	Weight/measure	Energy (kcal ME)[1]
Canned meat-based dog food	400g can	320
Canned ration type dog food	400g can	330
Canned meat-based puppy food	400g can	400
Canned cat food	400g can	280
Canned kitten food	400g can	340
Complete dry	100g cup[2]	350
Mixer biscuit	100g cup[2]	350
Lean meat	100g	130
Mince beef medium fat	100g	200
Liver	100g	160
Tripe	100g	150
Egg (whole)	100g (two large eggs)	163
Milk	122g (half cup)[2]	80
Rice (cooked)	175g (1 cup)[2]	185
Bread (white)	100g (4 slices)	250

Table 2.6: *'Rule of thumb' energy values for food types 'as fed'.*

1 1kcal = 4.184kJ; 2 An 8 fl. oz cup.

(Cat food)

6) A teacup full of complete dry cat food ≅ 330kcal (1386kJ) ME

7) A 40g (1.5oz) pack of semi-moist food ≅ 110kcal (462kJ) ME

8) A 400g can of canned (moist) cat food ≅ 300kcal (1260kJ) ME*
A 180g can of canned (moist) cat food ≅ 140kcal (588kJ) ME
A 90g can of canned (moist) cat food ≅ 70kcal (294kJ) ME

*Puppy and kitten foods tend to have a higher energy content having about 400kcal (1680kJ) ME and 350kcal (1470kJ) ME, respectively, per 400g can.

'Hands on' Determination of ME Value of Pet Food

We can determine the ME value of pet food for practical purposes by **one** of the following ways:

1) Read it off the label or data sheet if given (not a regulatory requirement - to be voluntary in USA. Energy declarations on pet foods labels are illegal in EC until an acceptable methodology of calculation is agreed).

2) Calculate it from the typical analysis.[†]

3) Use 'rule of thumb' values for the different food types (as listed earlier or see Table 2.6).

4) Check with the manufacturer.

5) For home-made food types refer to Table 2.7.

[†]The ME supplied by a food type can be 'guestimated' using rough formulae derived from analytical data:

For the dog:

ME(kcal/100g[‡]) = Protein(g)x3.5 + fat(g)x8.5 + Carbohydrate(g)x3.5

(Carbohydrate is not usually stated in the typical analysis but can be approximately estimated in g/100g by difference:

100 - moisture = DM. DM - (protein + fat + ash) = carbohydrate).

For the cat different factors are suggested by the NRC (1986) for the different food types to calculate the ME kcal/100g[‡]:

Moist:	(Protein** x 3.9 + Fat** x 7.7 + CHO** x 3.0) - 5
Semi-moist:	Protein x 3.7 + Fat x 8.8 + CHO x 3.3
Dry:	(Protein x 5.65 + Fat x 9.4 + CHO x 4.15) 0.99 - 126

** g/100g of food.

To determine the approximate ME supplied by a cat food.

For example a **canned** cat food having a typical analysis of:

Protein 9.2% Oil 3.0% Ash 2.5% Moisture 80% (i.e. 20% DM) will have:

20g DM/100g 'as fed' or 80g DM in a 400g can.

Carbohydrate (CHO) content will be
20 - (9.2+3.0+2.5) = 5.3g/100g 'as fed'.

ME kcal/100g[‡] = (Protein x 3.9 + Fat x 7.7 + CHO x 3.0) - 5

kcal from	Protein:	9.2 x 3.9 = 36kcal
	Fat:	3.0 x 7.7 = 23 kcal
	CHO:	5.3 x 3.0 = 15.9kcal
		75kcal - 5

ME from nutrients/100g = 70kcal (approximately)

ME from a 400g can 'as fed' ≅ 300kcal[‡]

(This food supplies 0.70kcal/g and the protein contributes about 50% of total calories.)

PRODUCT AND DIETARY EVALUATION

Commercially available complete pet foods are formulated to provide the necessary nutrients in the correct proportions. Feeding a balanced diet maintains nutritional and metabolic equilibrium.

This is effected by feeding food of optimal acceptability, nutrient content, digestibility, and nutrient to energy ratio appropriate to the animal's needs. This means that the food is eaten in appropriate quantity and digested efficiently enough to supply the energy and nutrient requirements of the animal.

When the energy requirement has been satisfied, it is of vital importance that the quantity of food consumed also supplies the animal's requisite protein, fat, minerals and vitamins.

Commercially available complete food types from manufacturers with the appropriate technological excellence, nutritional knowledge, and quality assurance based on feeding trials conducted according to recognised protocols, are most

‡ *1kcal = 4.184kJ*

likely to be adequate in this respect. This should preclude or contraindicate supplementation with minerals or vitamins.

Industrially prepared pet foods are formulated from various raw materials. Multi-ingredient interaction in food processing involving prolonged heating, such as the canning process, and in extrusion cooking, exposure to high temperature and pressure, affect nutrient bioavailability, which is a salient factor determining dietary balance. Bioavailability of taurine for example is compromised in processing of canned cat food and must be catered for adequately in the formulation. Thiamin and other process sensitive nutrients must also be considered. It follows therefore that the experience curve, technical and nutritional knowledge of the manufacturer are of paramount importance to insure against excessive processing losses and inadequate availability of vital nutrients. Properly conducted product feeding trials are the only real validation of adequacy in this respect. It is also important however to avoid toxic nutrient excesses such as vitamins A and D or mineral imbalance.

Food	kcal[1]	Protein	Fat	Moisture	Calcium	Phosphorus	Measure[2]
Meat							
Mince	200	18	21	60	0.01	0.16	
Beef	120	20	4.6	74	0.007	0.18	
Pork	104	20	7.1	71	0.008	0.20	
Lamb	160	20	8.8	70	0.007	0.19	
Heart	197	15	15	70	0.02	0.18	
Chicken	120	20	4.3	74	0.005	0.2	
Chicken skin	223	16	17	66	0.01	0.17	
Giblets	103	17	3.0	78	0.01	0.22	
Offal							
Lungs	100	17	4	73	0.01	0.19	
Spleen	120	17	6.5	75	0.03	0.22	
Kidney	86	15	2.6	79	0.02	0.25	
Liver	163	21	7.8	68	0.001	0.36	
Green tripe	154	12	11	76	0.01	0.10	
Dressed tripe	63	9	3.0	88	0.08	0.04	
Milk products							
Whole	65	3.5	3.5	87	0.12	0.09	1 cup = 244g
Skimmed	59	3.6	0.1	90	0.12	0.10	
Dry non-fat	363	35.6	0.8	3.0	1.31	1.02	1 cup = 68g
Cheddar cheese	398	25	32	37	0.75	0.48	1 inch cube = 17g
Cottage cheese	106	13.6	4.2	78	0.01	0.15	1 cup = 225g
Egg							
Whole	163	12.9	11	74	0.02	0.2	1 egg = 50g
White	51	10.9		87.6	0.01	0.15	1 = 33g
Yolk	348	16.0	30	51.1	0.14	0.57	1 = 17g
Cooked rice	106	2.1	0.1	73.4	0.02	0.06	1 cup = 175g
Bread							
White	270	8.7	3.2	35	0.08	0.01	1 slice = 25g
Wholemeal	243	10.5	3.0	36	0.10	0.23	1 slice = 28g
Fat							
Beef fat (trimming)	736	5.2	15.2	trace	0.05		
Lard	902	0	100	0	0	0	T = 15g
Margarine	720	0.6	81	15	0.02	0.02	T = 15g
Cooking oil	884	0	100	0	0	0	T = 15g

Table 2.7: *Typical nutrient content of table foods often fed to dogs and cats (g/100g 'as fed'). (Adapted from Small Animal Clinical Nutrition III Eds. LD Lewis, ML Morris and MS Hand. Mark Morris Associates, Topeka, Kansas.)*

1 1kcal = 4.184kJ; 2 1 cup = 8 fl.oz. T = 1 level tablespoon.

Linoleic acid content (%) of fat and oils *Beef fat 1, Lard 10, margarine 25, soyabean oil 52, corn oil 53, safflower oil 72.*

Guidelines for Selection and Recommendation of Pet Foods

Practical Considerations

- Decide on feeding strategy for the puppy or kitten from an early age based on potential adult size, owner's preference for food type, economic dictates and avoidance of fixed food preference in pets.
- Because of the relative palatability advantage of moist food types, changing to a dry food for maintenance may prove difficult later.
- Feed by 'eye and hand' as label instructions are guidelines only.
- Feeding of very palatable food types 'free choice' to dogs, such as gourmet type selected meat ingredient moist products, or of meat-based semi-moist products to cats, may over-ride the intrinsic energy intake control mechanism and lead to obesity.
- Fixed food preferences may occur in dogs and cats fed gourmet type single or limited ingredient formulations and home-prepared selected meat rations giving rise to feeding management problems later.
- Toy breeds and 'finicky' feeders need more palatable, nutrient dense food types because of their low volume intake. Some complete dry maintenance food types may well be unsuitable for these animals because of their physical form, bulk and, particularly, limited palatability.
- Large breeds will prove more costly to feed. The high carbohydrate content of complete dry foods usually means a cheaper feeding option.
- Select the food type for the specific need and life stage as it is wasteful to feed a growth or performance type product to the adult dog or cat in maintenance.

Further Selection Parameters

- Note the basis for nutritional claims on the label. Those proven by feeding trials conducted according to established protocols e.g. AAFCO (Association of American Feed Control Officials) are usually more valid than those based on chemical analysis or calculated values albeit claiming NRC (National Research Council) compliance.
- Don't overlook 'in house' knowledge of food types and brands supporting our patients in good health and appearance over time.
- Keep in mind selected products for each life stage of dogs and cats in which you have confidence. Periodic reviews of analysis and ingredients by reference to label or to manufacturer are indicated as these may well change.
- Manufacturer reputation, experience curve, commitment to nutritional research and *in vivo* product evaluation are cogent considerations in the selection of prepared pet foods for recommendation to our clients.
- When we have confidence in product performance on the basis of critically applied parameters or personal 'hands on' experience we should not hesitate to recommend them by brand name. It is far more laudable to endorse a quality product than to allow our clients to gravitate to suboptimal or to patently poor nutrition for their pet.

Selection of Veterinary Diets for Disease Entity Management

- Manufacturing practice must be based on the highest quality standards.
- Food types should be of guaranteed fixed formulation.
- Manufacturers should have 'in house' colony feeding facilities.
- Sound clinical studies supporting the efficacy of therapeutic diets in the treatment and management of disease in dogs and cats are desirable but not often available for specific conditions (Morris and Rogers, 1991). Accumulation of naturally occurring affected groups of animals and their response in paired studies pose logistical problems. Reported controlled studies often refer to models, not naturally occurring cases of disease (Morris and Rogers, 1991).
- Lack of palatability or acceptability may render the use of these products impracticable, particularly in advanced pathological conditions such as chronic renal impairment (see home-made alternatives later in text).

Veterinary diets, however, are generally formulated on the basis of very sound nutritional, biochemical and pathophysiological data. They can very often make a measurable contribution to the management of disease conditions.

However there is universal recognition in manufacturing, and veterinary circles that more clinical efficacy data are needed from controlled, paired studies to substantiate implied benefits in the adjunctive management of disease in dogs and cats. Whilst benefits of reducing diets and struvite dissolution regimens in the dog and cat may be self evident with intrinsic controls, we lack evidence for example that high dietary protein results in progression of renal disease in dogs (Brown, 1994), or that reduction of protein intake is conducive to preservation of renal structure or function. Thus the imposition of a restricted dietary protein intake on dogs with mild renal impairment is a questionable regimen without reference to clinical and biochemical indications (see Chapter 11).

Assessment of Adequacy

Claims for adequacy for commercially available food types may be based on a number of alternative requirements.

- **Chemical profile** by calculation from ingredients' level and type which is then compared with known values (e.g. AAFCO) and nutrient profile tables. This method does not monitor or cater for ingredient quality or variation, processing losses or bioavailability of nutrients and so is not an exacting requirement.
- **Analysis** and comparison with a recognised recommended nutrient profile (e.g. NRC) for the appropriate life stages. Whilst some assessment is made of nutrients and of nutrient losses, their bioavailability is not evaluated.
- **Feeding trials** (e.g. AAFCO) which are the most exacting validation of claims. These vary in stringency from maintenance to the more exacting 'all life stages' catering for gestation, lactation and growth. Digestibility studies to determine *in vivo*, overall and individual nutrient digestibility of prepared pet foods enhance considerably claims of adequacy, particularly if the latter are based on calculated chemical profile or on analysis only, without actual feeding trial validation.

There are no official protocol standards for proving adequacy of veterinary/dietary food types and the onus devolves on the manufacturer.

Commercial Segmentation

Quite apart from physical form and function the market positioning of pet foods is segmented as follows, with cost and potential quality increasing with order of listing:

- Generic
- Private label
- Popular national brand
- Premium brand.

Generic: Plainly packaged, these are of low cost which may well reflect cheaper raw materials of lower quality. Nutritional adequacy claims are made on the basis of chemical analysis or calculated values only and are not validated by feeding trials. As they tend to be low in fat and quality animal-sourced protein these products may lack palatability resulting in poor acceptability. This can have significant impact in growth situations in which puppies or kittens may in fact take in less food than they need for normal growth. The need for supplementation may then eliminate the cost advantage.

Private label: 'House brand' products are manufactured for retail multiples to a given formulation at competitive manufacturing costs. Product quality will vary with the marketing strategy of the retail company, which may be focused on quality, differentiated, or merely low cost, high volume. The claims for adequacy may be made on the basis of analysis with or without digestibility studies. Feeding trials may sometimes be required but the onus usually devolves on to the manufacturer.

Popular national brand: These branded products are usually nutritionally adequate for the purpose for which they are formulated having been critically evaluated by feeding trials according to approved protocols. A detailed nutrient profile has usually been chemically assayed for trace elements. Ingredients and palatability may vary between different branded products from the same manufacturer.

Premium brands: Premium brands have a focus on quality and are often sold through supermarkets or selected outlets such as pet shops and veterinary clinics. More recently sub-segmentation has seen the development of life stage and lifestyle 'super premium' orientated products. These are usually manufactured from quality raw materials, are of high digestibility and palatability, and are assessed for nutritional adequacy by feeding trials. Designation of 'Premium' and 'Superpremium' seems to be rather arbitrary, devolving more on manufacturers' product description than on any strictly regulated criteria.

Specific Indicators of Suitability of Food Types

Having looked at selection guidelines in the broader context, let us now look at specific indicators.

Quality: Quality may be defined as the degree of excellence of the product for its intended purpose. In pet food this devolves on the nutrient type, level, digestibility and most significantly bioavailability. It is the latter parameter which raises the most pertinent questions concerning critical nutrients in prepared multi-ingredient pet food.

Dogs and cats need nutrients to remain healthy, not specific food types. These nutrients, in commercially available pet food are derived from raw materials which supply the ingredients listed on the label. It is the propensity of these raw materials to supply nutrients with a chemical profile most suited to the digestive systems of the dog and cat, and which can most closely approximate the metabolic requirements of these species, that ultimately determines pet food quality. It can be seen that poor grade or unsuitable raw materials will not produce a quality product, irrespective of pet food type. It also follows that the typical analysis found on the label says little or nothing about quality. The ingredients list is a better indicator as it at least gives us the raw material source of nutrients. However we can get wide variation in nutrient composition of by-product ingredients.

In a canned (moist) dog food an animal protein source should be among the first two ingredients listed, whilst in a complete dry dog food it should be among the first three.

In cat food an animal protein source should invariably head the ingredients list because of the special nutrient requirements of this species.

High ash (mineral content), low fat content and poor quality protein sources such as cereal grains may indicate inferior quality pet food.

Table 2.8 gives raw materials used in pet foods and their contribution to the diet.

Quality may be compromised by suboptimal manufacturing practices or storage conditions. Poorly sealed or poorly lined bags and unlaquered cans may affect the quality of the food.

Descriptive term	Example	Contribution to diet
Meat (muscle)	Skeletal, tongue, diaphragm, heart, oesophagus	Animal fat, protein, and energy
Meat by-products	Lung, spleen, kidney, brain, blood, bone, intestine	Animal fat, protein and energy
Meat meal, meat and bone meal, fish meal, blood meal	Dry rendered product from animal tissues	Animal fat, protein and energy
Cereals	Corn, wheat, oats, barley, corn gluten meal	Carbohydrate (starch), cereal protein, energy and fibre
Soya meal, soya flour	Vegetable source protein including TVP (textured vegetable protein)	Vegetable protein Textured/chunks
Animal fat, vegetable oil	Tallow, chicken fat, corn oil, soya oil	Fats, fatty acids, essential fatty acids and energy
Egg	Egg powder	Protein of high biological value
Milk	Skim milk powder, whey	Milk protein
Grain hulls, root crops	Bran, beet pulp	Dietary fibre
Humectants	Sugars, salts, glycerol	Reduction of water availability Energy
'Digest'	Chicken or rabbit from hydrolysed liver or intestines	Flavour and palatability Some protein and fat
Preservatives	Sodium benzoate Sodium and potassium sorbate	Retard spoilage from moulds and bacteria
Flavours	Natural and artificial and 'nature identical' flavours, process reacted flavours, key character compounds	Improvement of organoleptic appeal (taste, smell, mouthfeel)
Colouring agents	Natural and artificial colouring such as caramel and titanium dioxide	Improvement of appeal to the owner
Aromas	Natural and artificial aromas and tones	Improvement of appeal to both owner and animal
Vitamins, minerals	Vitamin and mineral premixes	Nutrients and dietary balance
Antioxidants	Natural such as vitamin E (natural or synthetic tocopherals), gallate esters, butylatedhydroxyanisole or hydroxytoluene	Prevents rancidification of fats

Table 2.8: *Raw materials in pet food.*

National Research Council-recommended nutrient requirements for dogs and cats are stated in terms of 'available nutrients' (NRC, 1985, 1986). Chemical analysis, though complying with recommended nutrient levels, is no guarantee of bioavailability. Pet foods with similar label claims for nutritional adequacy based on chemical analysis can vary widely in performance (Huber *et al.*, 1986,1991) due to differences in nutrient availability from processed mixed ingredient food types. Fresh unprocessed nutrients or purified and semi-purified nutrient constituents are more predictably available. NRC data are derived from the latter and so difficulties arise in extrapolation to industrially processed pet food.

Trace element availability may be a problem in certain products and indeed zinc deficiency has been referred to in the USA as 'generic dog food disease' (Morris and Rogers, 1991). Excess phytate from cereals may reduce mineral availability (NRC, 1985). Heat and alkaline pH in the canning process may compromise nutrients such as thiamin giving rise to clinical signs in cats and kittens (Morris and Rogers, 1991). A recent outbreak of thiamin deficiency in cats in a UK cattery has been attributed to a diet of complementary cat food which was shown on analysis to contain inadequate amounts of thiamin (see Chapter 10). Methionine deficiency has been reported in queens and kittens on a high fat canned diet with poor quality protein source from chicken feet and heads (Morris and Rogers, 1991). This problem was compounded by the reduced intake due to high energy (fat) content. Copper and zinc deficiency have been observed in cats and kittens on a diet with vegetable based protein source (Morris and Rogers, 1991). Almost all of the incriminated products in this study complied with recommended parameters for chemical analysis.

In assessing adequacy of different dry dog foods all claiming to be 'complete and balanced for all life stages' on the basis of 'meeting or exceeding nutrient requirements as established by the NRC', Huber *et al.* (1991) found that one of three foods evaluated had suboptimal growth performance for puppies in their first 5 weeks of the test period relative to those groups fed on two other foods, despite similar intake levels and satisfactory chemical analysis. The indications were that digestibility and bioavailability of nutrients were the problem. Furthermore skin lesions consistent with zinc deficiency were observed in puppies fed this product even though the zinc level was adequate on chemical analysis. Again bioavailability was the limiting factor. This may be compromised by a high calcium and also by a high phytate level predisposing to decreased zinc absorption particularly in cereal based diets. The NRC recommends levels for **bioavailable** nutrients, so most diets tend to exceed the calcium requirements by the addition of calcium concentrates and indeed this was the case in this particular study, resulting in decreased bioavailability of zinc.

A previous study by Huber, Wilson and McGarity (1986) assessing three privately branded and one national brand dry dog foods with the same claims and analysis on the labels, found different feeding values particularly for one of the private brand products which had poor digestibility.

Analytical values are not invariably useful in assessing adequacy and should not be the sole basis for evaluation.

Pet food which has not been critically assessed by feeding trials, can however be sold legally under current regulation.

Why nutrient deficiencies may occur in industrially prepared pet food:

a) **Inadequate knowledge of canine or feline nutrition.** Exact nutrient requirements may not be known with certainty and availability from food systems may be difficult to predict unless ascertained from feeding trials. This is true of taurine availability in cat food. Whilst NRC recommendations suggest 400 mg/kg feed for growth and 500mg/kg feed for reproduction, this may not be adequate in commercially available foods (Pion *et al.*, 1987) as clinical signs of deficiency may be seen in cats on certain commercially available foods that were taurine deficient. The effect of process engineering parameters on the bioavailability of this nutrient is not fully assessed and documented.
   Recent studies have indicated that biosynthesis of L-carnitine may be limited or inadequate in certain animals and so supplementation with crystalline L-carnitine may be necessary in the industrial preparation of pet foods as the requirement may not be met by the normal levels in the feedstuff ingredients (Hilton, 1989).

b) **Nutrient losses in processing, thermal and transport abuse and storage.** Processing of all three main types of industrially prepared pet food is potentially destructive to vitamins. Composition of ingredients, moisture, pH, heat and storage all influence the level of potency of vitamins which may be compromised even though the formulation appears to be adequate (Adams, 1981). Vitamin A may be reduced by 20% to 30% in extruded cat food and less so in canned and semi-moist food types. By contrast thiamin losses would appear to be significantly higher in canned foods than in extruded feed types. This vitamin is added to canned foods to compensate for losses in the prolonged heating process.

Heat, light, moisture and adverse storage conditions adversely affect quality in food types which are not hermetically sealed and fatty acid availability will diminish through oxidative processes and rancidification of fats.

c) **Errors in formulation.** Formulations used by manufacturers which rely solely on compliance with analytical parameters, and ignore nutrient availability may produce specific nutrient deficiencies. We may get a zinc deficiency for example by nutrient interaction compromising bioavailability (Czarneki, 1986) or a low potassium level which can produce polymyopathy in cats (Dow *et al.*, 1987).

We can see from the overview of pet food evaluation that compliance with recognised criteria for nutrient requirements based on calculated chemical profile or on actual chemical analysis does not constitute an assurance of adequacy. The latter can only be validly based on digestibility and recognised feeding trial studies. However it must be said that occurrence of clinical nutritional deficiencies in pets fed on foods determined as being complete by analysis would appear to be rare.

LABEL INFORMATION INTERPRETATION

The label is a reference from which useful information can be derived which may help us to make a value judgement on the product it describes.

In simple terms the label conveys:

- That it is pet food, its type and flavour.
- Its intended use - for dog or cat.
- Whether complete or complementary (product description).
- Promotional and advertising graphics and words.
- Nutritional information and legally required nutritional analysis.
- Feeding guidelines.
- Ingredients list.
- The manufacturer, or whom it is made for, net weight, best before date.

As veterinarians we are primarily interested in the ingredients and their source, the typical analysis, the probable energy content and the basis for the claim of nutritional adequacy.

We cannot accurately assess quality from label information in terms of true digestibility of nutrients or overall digestibility of the food, the bioavailability of nutrients nor the actual available energy. Nor can we tell the biological value of the protein source (eg. chicken muscle or feet and heads). Furthermore the basis of the nutritional adequacy claim is not always clear from the label.

We **can** tell:

- The ingredients, their source and their probable contribution to food value.
- The approximate ME content calculated from the typical analysis or as stated on the label if given (see page 37).
- The protein and fat level and their broadly designated source.
- The moisture and ash level.
- The nutritional adequacy claim and its basis if clearly stated.
- The date of manufacture and 'best before' date.
- Additives (if added) in the groups preservatives, antioxidants and colours.
- Batch number.
- The net weight.

Regulatory Influence

In the **UK** pet food labelling is regulated by the implementation of **EC** directives through the Feeding Stuffs Regulations (HMSO, 1991) under the control of the Ministry of Agriculture and by the Office of Fair Trading under the Trades Descriptions Act. This legislation regulates particularly the important information appearing in the statutory statement pertaining to ingredients listing and description, declaration of additives, the typical analysis and product description. 'Best before' date, net weight and batch number must also appear on the pack but not necessarily in the statutory statement.

In the USA the state and federal officials formed the Association of American Feed Control Officials (AAFCO), an advisory body which together with the Pet Food Institute (PFI), the National Feed Ingredients Association and the American Feed Industry Association all have input to the Uniform State Feed Bill. The Bill regulates labels, additives, ingredients, statements of adequacy and describes AAFCO test protocols for proving a claim and is enforced by state feed control officials. The Food and Drugs Administration (FDA) regulates manufacturing practice and the United States Department of Agriculture (USDA) ensure properly marked labels (Remillard, 1991).

The Principal Display Panel

The label mainly consists of the Principal Display Panel (PDP) and the Statutory Statement. The information of interest to us on the PDP conveys the species for which the food is intended in words (Dog Food or

Cat Food) or a picture, and the predominating ingredients and flavours are specified by the 'namer' as follows: 'beef' (70–100% beef), 'beef dinner' (10–70% beef), 'beef flavour' (beef to impact significantly on taste and flavour). If two or more main ingredients are stated e.g. 'salmon and tuna', together they constitute 10% to 70% of the ingredients and each individually greater than 3% (Burger and Thompson, 1994).

The Statutory Statement

The ingredients are listed here by name e.g. 'chicken', or category as defined by regulation, for example 'meat and animal derivatives' (meaning fresh or frozen fleshy parts, all parts of the carcase and processing derivatives. Similar categories pertain to eggs, milk or derivatives of these). These categories give wide scope to the manufacturer. Listing may be in descending order by weight, or ingredients in each category by weight or as percentage of the total product.

The **Typical Analysis** (Guaranteed Analysis in USA) is located here on the statutory statement also, giving protein, oil (fat), fibre, ash, and moisture (if the latter is more than 14%). The Guaranteed Analysis used in USA products gives minima and maxima for protein, fat, and fibre, and so levels of these nutrients will vary.

In assessing label information particularly with regard to the quality assurance and the basis for the product description, if in doubt veterinarians should contact the manufacturer. Should the information not be forthcoming then the validity may be in doubt. Ideally the ingredient raw materials should be of approved quality as defined by a recognised body such as AAFCO in its official publication.

All inclusive terms such as 'meat by-products', 'cereal grain products', 'meat and animal derivatives', though legal, are not specifically descriptive enough to enable us to compare pet foods. The difference between 'meat meal' and 'meat and bone meal' is not obvious as both contain some proportion of bone.

In a moist product ingredients are listed 'as is' so that ingredients with a high water content such as meat by-products (70% moisture) will be listed first even though incorporation level on a dry matter basis may be lower than cereals (10% moisture) listed later, as on a weight/volume basis the latter ingredients weight less. Expressed on a DM basis, cereals could be more prominent. Thus, more meaningful representation of product composition would be achieved by converting ingredients to a dry matter basis (Remillard, 1991).

In a dry product all the ingredients have approximately the same DM content so that the ingredients list is a better indicator of prominence.

Some ingredients may be broken down into multiple categories. In a list such as 'meat and bone meal, ground corn, rice, flaked corn and corn flour', corn may well be the major ingredient and not meat and bone meal as listed.

In EC countries additives in the preservative, antioxidant and colours categories which have been added must be stated. However those which may be present in preprocessed ingredients in small amounts, on the 'carry over' principle may not need to be declared, so that preservatives or antioxidants, albeit in small amounts, may be present but not stated.

In the EC states, fat-soluble vitamins A, D, E, and copper are also listed when added and the 'best before' date usually corresponds with the predicted shelf life for these vitamins.

Despite regulation, all the necessary information necessary to evaluate a product critically is not yet appearing on labels in Europe or the USA. With the objective of encouraging more comprehensive information on pet food labels in Canada, a voluntary certification scheme is monitored by the Canadian Veterinary Medical Association for manufacturers who comply with recommended manufacturing, labelling and substantiated claims' standards (Allard, 1988). Detailed ingredients lists are required, not just groupings.

Also, ME values determined by actual digestibility studies, protein digestibility, and proof of adequacy by feeding trials are desirable for confidence and quality assurance pertaining to products having a central role in nutrition for our dogs and cats. More critical clinical trial studies are also desirable to substantiate implied benefit in the treatment and management of disease entities by strategic use of veterinary diets.

HOME-PREPARED FOOD

This includes a variety of home-cooked foods (fresh meat, offal, dairy products, eggs, cereals, vegetables, pulses, fish) used in combination to provide a varied diet for total nutrition, or on a varietal basis to supplement or augment normal feeding regimens.

Many owners feed home-prepared food to their dogs and cats for different reasons:

- They adopt a traditional approach being among a minority of owners not using industrially prepared food.
- Induced preference in pets by exposure to home-cooked food from kitten or puppyhood.
- Anthropomorphism ascribing human food predilection to pets.
- Finicky feeders will 'hold out' for tasty home-cooked treats.
- Home-produced 'elimination diets' may work better in food related disease, such as skin problems (see Chapter 14).
- Poor owner perception of industrially prepared food as 'unwholesome' or as unappetising.

- Veterinary diets may lack palatability or acceptability particularly in advanced illness, necessitating home-prepared feeding.
- Advantage is taken of readily available food in the home or from a catering source.

Home-Sourced Foods

Ingredients used in home-made diets for pets should be fit for human consumption. The quality depends on the source and digestibility of nutrients. High protein quality and biological value pertain to eggs, dairy sources, meat and fish.

Meat and fish are also rich sources of fats/oils, iron and B vitamins but low in calcium and vitamins A and D. Fats from meats are highly digestible in dogs and cats and provide a high energy source. Fats differ in their degree of saturation: beef > lamb > pork > poultry > fish. Generally the more unsaturated, the better the source of essential fatty acids. Meats are not a balanced food unless fed in whole carcase form or ground whole in the case of fish.

Whole milk is virtually a complete food but is low in iron and vitamin D. It gives us quality protein, energy from fat and lactose and is a good source of calcium, phosphorus, a number of trace elements and vitamins A and B complex. Skimmed milk is low in these vitamins having had the fat separated. Cream and cheese with a high fat content are good sources of vitamin A, while cottage cheese is low in fat and a good source of quality protein.

Eggs supply excellent quality protein of high biological value, from both white and yolk. The yolk also is high in fat and fat-soluble vitamins. Eggs are best fed cooked for hygienic reasons and to destroy avidin.

Cereals and vegetables generally lack palatability for dogs and cats. They are however, a good source of energy for these animals and are widely used in commercially available and home-prepared pet food. The proteins from cereals and vegetables are usually of lower biological value with some exceptions such as soya bean. Starch from these sources must be cooked to improve digestibility for dogs and cats. Legumes such as beans, soya and green peas contain complex carbohydrates and sugars of poor digestibility which predispose to flatus production in the large intestine and soya should be heat-treated to inactivate anti-trypsin and haemagglutinins. However, appropriately prepared peas, beans and pulses in moderate amounts are useful to provide protein, energy and B vitamins. 'Greens' and carrots are useful for 'bulk' particularly in a weight reducing role.

Vegetable oils are rich in essential fatty acids notably linoleic, but chicken, pork and fish also provide EFA including arachidonic acid which is a dietary need for the cat. The latter is also found in other animal tissues including liver, kidneys and egg yolk.

Supplementation

Pet owners supplement their pet's normal diet, occasionally, frequently, or on a daily basis. As a general rule supplementation of a 'complete and balanced' food is unnecessary.

Special situations, finicky feeders for example, may be catered for by addition of a balanced canned meat-based product to a balanced dry maintenance diet.

Often however owners will habitually feed varied assortments of table scraps constituting a mixed source of protein, carbohydrate and fat. Milk is frequently given to dogs and cats as part of their daily diet. Fresh meat is often offered with complete dry food types and fats and vegetable oils are also used to promote coat condition. Animals supplemented in this way but deriving their main nutritional support from a balanced basic diet generally remain in good health without untoward nutrient imbalance. A reasonable guideline to owners is that the supplementary food should not constitute more than 10% of the normal balanced diet on a weight or on a volume basis.

Difficulties arise however in getting the balance right when home-sourced ingredients constitute the total diet for the animal. Choosing the 'staples' such as fresh meat, chicken, fish and a carbohydrate source such as rice, pasta, bread or cereal is easy. However the fact that most of these table foods commonly fed to dogs and cats are calcium deficient constitutes a problem (Donoghue, 1992). It is not surprising then that low calcium is the most common problem with home-prepared diets. Phosphorus in table foods is usually present in greater amounts than calcium but less than the requirement for dogs and cats. The calcium:phosphorus ratio is as critical as the overall intake of both nutrients. The energy/nutrient balance is equally important in home-made diets as it is in the commercially available type.

Supplement	Measure	Calcium (mg)	Phosphorus (mg)
Bone meal	1 teaspoon (4g)	1200	630
Ground eggshell	1 teaspoon (5g)	1950	2
Dicalcium phosphate	1 teaspoon (4g)	1050	925
Calcium carbonate	1 teaspoon (4g)	2000	0

Table 2.9: *Calcium and phosphorus content of supplements used in home-made diets.*

Species	Dog		Cat	
Ingredient	**Measure**	**(weight, g)**	**Measure**	**(weight, g)**
White rice, raw	2/3 cup[1]	(140)	1/3 cup	(70)
Meat, lean	1/3 cup	(70)	2/3 cup	(140)
Liver	1/8 cup	(30)	1/8 cup	(30)
Bone meal	3 teasp.	(11)	3 teasp.	(11)
Corn oil	1 teasp.	(5)	1 teasp.	(5)
Iodised salt	1/2 teasp.	(2)	1/2 teasp.	(2)
Energy from recipe ≅ 800 kcal (3360kJ)†	**% ME from nutrients**		**% ME from nutrients**	
Storage Refrigerator for a few days or frozen	Protein Fat Carbohydrate	17% 31% 53%	Protein Fat Carbohydrate	31% 41% 28%
Cook rice, bone meal, salt and corn oil together in 2 volumes of water and simmer for 20 minutes. Add meat and liver, simmer for 10 minutes.				

Table 2.10: *Home-made diets for maintenance. (Adapted from Donoghue and Kronfeld (1994).)*

1 8 fl. oz or ≈ 240 ml cup.

† Enough for average 10kg dog for one day and for an average 3.8kg cat for 3 days.

NRC data indicate that the calcium requirement of dogs is 1.6mg calcium per kcal of dietary energy intake. The recommended calcium:phosphorus ratio in home-made diets should be between 1:1 and 2:1. The recommended minimum calcium intake for cats is not based on calorie intake but diet weight, being 8g calcium and 6g phosphorus per kg diet DM. Reference to Table 2.9 or to labels on purchased preparations will indicate the amounts of calcium and phosphorus in common mineral supplements. From the foregoing information it can be seen that the steps to determine appropriate supplementation for a dog fed a home-made diet are:

1) Assess the calorie intake appropriate to body weight from charts/tables.

2) Multiply this by 1.6 to give the calcium requirement in milligrams.

3) Determine the calcium contribution from the food intake (Table 2.7).

4) The shortfall must be supplied by the supplement, and the amount of supplement required can be determined by its calcium content (Table 2.9 or label).

Home-prepared diets having an acceptable calcium:phosphorus ratio may still have very low calcium and phosphorus levels overall. If a home-made diet does not have a calcium concentrate added it will almost certainly be deficient (Donoghue, 1992). Some dairy products are rich in calcium and may satisfy requirements but there may be limited tolerance due to lactose levels.

Home-Made Recipes

We can see from the foregoing discussion that 'getting the balance right' when formulating home-made rations for dogs and cats for use by owners or in the hospital, requires a methodical approach, particularly with respect to calcium and phosphorus levels and ratio. This involves reference to 'human food' charts to determine nutrient contribution from ingredients and to mineral supplement data or labels to ascertain their contribution of these minerals. However it is very useful and convenient to have recipes on hand which will cater for maintenance, special demand situations and disease status which can be used to prepare balanced diets in the home or hospital for dogs and cats.

Lest we 're-invent the wheel' we should refer to excellent work done by Kronfeld in the early 1980s, when he devised a system based on maintenance recipes for dog and cat which could be conveniently modified to meet special needs (Kronfeld, 1986). This has been further described in a recent publication (Donoghue and Kronfeld, 1994).

A single supplement is used, made from liver, bone meal, corn oil and iodised salt. The liver provides vitamins and trace elements, bone meal provides calcium and phosphorus in a palatable form, corn oil is a source of vitamin E, essential fatty acids and polyunsaturates, while the salt provides iodine. The liver may be conveniently frozen in blocks in ice cube trays.

The staples used are meat (medium fat minced beef), rice, and wheat bran (used in reducing and geriatric diets).

Further advantages of the system are quantities measured in breakfast cups (8 fluid oz or 240ml), minimal cooking and interchangeable ingredients to accommodate different needs. A cupful of dry (uncooked) rice supplies 720kcal (3024kJ) ME as does a cupful of medium fat minced beef, whilst a cupful of bran has only a quarter of this ME value.

Table 2.10 gives the recipes for maintenance diets for dog and cat, the level of nutrients provided from them, the cooking and feeding management.

Food Exchange Tables – Alternative Ingredients[1]

High Protein Low Fat Sources					
Food	**Weight (g)**	**Energy (kcal)[2]**	**Protein (% kcal)**	**Fat (% kcal)**	**CHO (% kcal)**
Beef can exchange with:	100	200	58	42	0
Lamb	100	200	50	40	0
Pork	90	200	50	47	0
Rabbit	100	200	50	44	0
Chicken flesh	100	200	45	55	0
3 Eggs	150	200	32	65	3
Cottage cheese, creamed	208	200	49	40	11
Plain yogurt	350	200	22	47	31

Table 2.11.

High Protein Low Fat Sources					
Food	**Weight (g)**	**Energy (kcal)[2]**	**Protein (% kcal)**	**Fat (% kcal)**	**CHO (% kcal)**
Chicken flesh can exchange with:	100	177	64	36	0
Turkey	112	176	80	20	0
White fish	227	177	96	4	0
Cottg. Cheese, low fat	226	164	71	13	16
Plain yogurt, low fat	280	178	33	22	45

Table 2.12.

Carbohydrate sources					
Food	**Weight (g)**	**Energy (kcal)[2]**	**Protein (% kcal)**	**Fat (% kcal)**	**CHO (% kcal)**
Rice cooked, long grain can exchange with:	100	110	8	1	91
Brown rice, cooked	93	110	9	5	86
Potato	145	110	11	1	88
Bread	45	110	15	15	70
Noodles	94	110	15	10	75

Table 2.13.

1 Adapted from Donoghue and Kronfeld (1994).
2 1kcal = 4.184kJ.

Tables 2.11 to 2.15 give interchangeable alternative foods for use in home-made diets.

Modification of Canine and Feline Home-Made Maintenance Diets for Extra-Demand Situations and Management of Disease Entities

Canine extra demand situation for growth, reproduction, lactation, work, stress, surgery and trauma – use the feline maintenance diet providing 31% protein, 41% fat and 28% carbohydrate on an ME basis.

Canine and feline low fat diets for weight control, malabsorption, pancreatitis, and non-specific gastrointestinal problems – use maintenance diet for dog or cat, but replacing the medium fat meat with very lean meat, lean poultry or white fish thus reducing the fat level by 50%. This may be further reduced by replacing the corn oil with safflower oil at 2.5g (half teaspoonful).

Canine and feline weight reducing diets for weight loss and fibre responsive gastrointestinal conditions – use maintenance diets for dog and cat but use 70g

Food Exchange Tables – Alternative Sources[1]

Oils			
Oil source	**Weight (g)**	**Energy (kcal)[2]**	**% Polyunsaturates**
Corn exchange with:	14	120	59
Sunflower	14	120	65
Soyabean	14	120	58
Wheatgerm	14	120	62
Safflower	14	120	74

Table 2.14

Macrominerals					
Source		**Calcium**		**Phosphorus**	
		(%)	(g)	(%)	(g)
Bone meal exchange with:	11g	24	2.6	12.6	1.4
Dicalcium phosphate	12g	21	2.5	18	2.2
Calcium carbonate	6.5g	40	2.6	0	0
Ground limestone	6.8g	38	2.6	0	0

Table 2.15.

1 *Adapted from Donoghue and Kronfeld (1994).*
2 *1kcal = 4.184kJ.*

(one third cupful) each of rice and of very lean meat and add 40g (two thirds cupful) of wheat bran. This recipe provides 600 kcal (2520kJ) with 24% protein calories. The cooking water must be increased by half to accommodate the bran. Commercially available cellulose preparations may replace the bran if it proves to be irritant to the bowel.

Feeding older animals - regimen and type of diet will vary with biological ageing, bodily condition and activity level. The majority of older dogs and cats will do well on the maintenance diets. If not well conditioned older dogs will enjoy and benefit from feline maintenance diet and substituting fatty meats for lean meat in the maintenance diet may add further advantage.

Hypoallergenic diets for dog and cat - eliminate suspect ingredients such as the meat type traditionally eaten by the animal. For example beef could be replaced by lamb, fish, rabbit or dairy produce. The liver in the supplement may have to be replaced by a human type vitamin/trace element mixture, corn oil with sunflower, bone meal with other supplements such as dicalcium phosphate.

Chronic renal failure diets for dietary management of chronic kidney disease in dogs and cats. A diet of moderate protein and reduced dietary phosphorus is achieved by initially introducing the respective maintenance diets and then replacing the bone meal with 3g of calcium carbonate, thus lowering the phosphorus to 0.3% from 1.1%. Protein is lowered by introducing fatty meat for the medium fat meat.

Feline lower urinary tract disease problems - use feline maintenance diet which will promote an acidic urine. Replace bone meal with 3g calcium carbonate or ground limestone thus lowering the magnesium from 0.15% to 0.08%. Increase the salt to 4g to promote water intake. If the urine pH does not prove to be clearly acid, the addition of $^1/_4$ to $^1/_2$ teaspoon of ammonium chloride to the recipe should be tried and assessed.

Chronic heart failure - use canine and feline maintenance diets and reduce salt to 1g which provides 0.25% sodium. In advanced cardiac failure eliminate the salt. If using potassium losing diuretics introduce 'lo salt' (half KCl, half NaCl) at a 1g level thus reducing sodium and increasing potassium.

REFERENCES

Adams CR (1981). The stability of vitamins in processed dog food. *Petfood Industry*, **23**(1).

Allard C (1988). Labelling and advertising pet foods. *Canadian Veterinary Journal* **29,** 403-405.

Brown SA (1994). Canine renal disease. In: *The*

Waltham Book of Clinical Nutrition of the Dog and Cat. Eds JM Wills and KW Simpson. Pergamon Press, Oxford pp 313-334.

Burger I and Thompson A (1994). Reading a pet food label. In: *The Waltham Book of Clinical Nutrition of the Dog and Cat.* Eds JM Wills and KW Simpson. Pergamon Press, Oxford pp 15-24.

Czarneki GL (1986). Bioavailability of nutrients in feed ingredients. *Petfood Industry* **28,** 18-20.

Donoghue S (1992). No bones about it: too little calcium is too common in home-made diets. *Veterinary Technician* **13**(6), 427-429.

Donoghue S and Kronfeld DS (1994). Home-made diets. In: *The Waltham Book of Clinical Nutrition of the Dog and Cat.* Eds JM Wills and KW Simpson. Pergamon Press, Oxford pp 445-449.

Dow SW, LeCouteur RA and Fettman MJ (1987). Potassium depletion in cats with hypokalemic polymyopathy. *Journal of the American Veterinary Medical Association* **191,** 1563-1568.

Hilton JW (1989). Potential nutrient deficiencies in pet foods. *Canadian Veterinary Journal* **30,** 599-601.

HMSO (1991). *The Feeding Stuffs Regulations 1991. SI No. 2840.* Her Majesty's Stationary Office, London, England.

Huber TL, Laflamme DP, Medleau L *et al* (1991). Comparison of procedures for assessing adequacy of dog foods. *Journal of the American Veterinary Medical Association* **199,** 731-734.

Huber TL, Wilson RC and McGarity SA (1986). Variations in digestibility of dry dog foods with identical label guaranteed analysis. *Journal of the American Animal Hospital Association* **22,** 571-575.

Kanarek RB (1975). Availability and caloric density of the diet as determinants of meal patterns in cats. *Physiology and Behaviour* **15,** 611.

Kronfeld DS (1986). Therapeutic diets for dogs and cats including a simple system of recipes. *Tijdschrift voor Diergeneeshkunde* **116**(Suppl. 1), 67S-70S.

Morris JG and Rogers QR (1991). Evaluation of commercial pet foods. *Tijdschrift voor Diergeneeshkunde.* **116 Suppl. 1:** 67S-70S.

NRC (1985). *Nutrient Requirements of Dogs.* National Academy of Sciences, Washington DC.

NRC (1986). *Nutrient Requirements of Cats.* National Academy of Sciences, Washington DC.

Pion PD, Kittleson MD, Rogers QR and Morris JG (1987). Myocardial failure in cats associated with low plasma taurine: a reversible cardiomyopathy. *Science* **237,** 764-768.

Remillard RL (1991). Providing dietary evaluations as a nutritional service in your clinic. *Veterinary Medicine* **July**: 734-742.

Sohail MA (1983). The ingestive behaviour of the domestic cat - review. *Nutrition Abstracts and Reviews – Series B* **53**(3), 177-186.

PART II

Feeding Healthy Animals – Dog and Cat

CHAPTER THREE

Adult Maintenance

Josephine M. Wills

HEALTHY ANIMALS

Within a home, pets are treated as individuals, and pet-owners develop feeding practices suitable for their own animal, taking account of the particular circumstances, likes and dislikes of the animal and their own view of convenience, cost, variety and suitability of foods. They must identify the particular needs of their animal and find a combination of food or foods to meet them.

The feeding recommendations in the following sections are intended only as **guides** for the average dog or cat in the usual range of environments found in European households. These guides can be used as a starting point to obtain an approximate estimate of a pet's needs, then by observation of the animal to decide whether to feed more or less, and by substitution of one food for another, the owner will arrive at a suitable regimen.

Adult Maintenance - Dog and Cat

Feeding Objectives

Most pet animals are healthy adults which live mostly indoors in a temperate climate. They are usually not pregnant or lactating, not involved in regular work or excessive exercise and are not subjected to extremes of temperature. In this situation, the animal is said to be *in maintenance*, nutritionally.

For an animal in maintenance, the diet must:

- provide the correct amount, balance and availability of nutrients to sustain physical and mental health and activity
- promote peak condition in the animal and hence reduce its susceptibility to disease
- be sufficiently concentrated to allow the animal to meet its requirements by eating an amount well within the limits set by appetite
- be sufficiently palatable to ensure an adequate intake, since an uneaten meal has no nutritive value.

The feeding occasion should be enjoyable, since this will help to reinforce the bond between a pet and its owner.

Requirements — Dogs

Energy: Adult dogs in peak condition vary in size from around 1.1kg up to 115kg (Burger and Johnson 1991). To make allowance for this wide range of body weights, and since energy needs are directly proportional to the weight of actively metabolising tissue rather than body weight, it is necessary to use an estimate for metabolic body size when calculating energy requirements in the dog (see Chapter 1). The most reliable estimates of metabolisable energy (ME) requirements of moderately active dogs can be obtained by using the formula:

$$\text{ME (kcal/day)} = 110W^{0.75}$$

where W is the body weight of the dog, measured in kilograms and $W^{0.75}$ is the metabolic body size of the dog (Burger, 1994). For more active dogs, this can be increased to $125W^{0.75}$.

The allometric relationship, however, assumes that neither shape nor body composition (ratio of lean body mass to fat) varies with size and this will not be the case for a range of breeds as widely disparate as those of the dog. As noted in Chapter 1, feeding studies have shown that Newfoundlands needed less energy than the predicted amounts whereas Great Danes needed more despite these two breeds being of comparable body weight.

Having calculated approximate energy needs of adults using this formula, the amount of food needed to meet these needs can be calculated from a knowledge of the energy values of the foods (See Chapter 2). These average amounts can then be rounded to a convenient unit for feeding, eg half a cup or can. In order to allow for variability between dogs and for differences in activity and environment, actual feeding recommendations are often quoted as a range which may cover from 25% below to 25% above the estimated average. Although this may seem a very approximate method of arriving at feeding recommendations, it does work very well in practice. It should not, however, surprise owners to find that their particular dog needs less than the amounts suggested, particularly if additional snacks, treats or table scraps are being added to the diet, or if the dog is relatively inactive. In addition, spaying may reduce the resting energy requirement of bitches by up to 10%.

Nutrients: Although the dog is a member of the order Carnivora, in a nutritional sense it is more accurately defined as omnivorous. Its long association with man has resulted in a degree of flexibility and adaptation in its nutritional requirements. Unlike the cat, the dog is able to survive on a diet composed entirely of vegetable material, although a diet based on animal tissue is likely to be preferred.

Diets for adult dogs in maintenance should be complete and balanced in respect of all the essential nutrients outlined in Chapter 1. The current recommendations for minimum nutrient requirements for adult dogs are given in the Appendix.

Requirements — Cats

Energy: The energy requirements of a cat can be calculated from a linear relationship, since domestic cats show a relatively narrow range of body weights (from around 2.5 to 6.5kg) and small adjustments for size are not considered important. In normal circumstances, an adult is known to require 70-90kcal/kg (293-377kJ/kg) body weight/day, depending on its level of activity.

Practical feeding studies have revealed that large, overweight cats and very inactive cats (such as those in a hospital situation) seem to require less food to maintain their body weight (Earle and Smith, 1991). This has led to the recommendation that maintenance rations for very inactive or caged, healthy cats should be based on an ME requirement of 50-70kcal/kg (209-293kJ/kg) body weight/day.

Cats have the ability to regulate their energy intake from day to day and unless they are fed an exceptionally palatable diet, or lead a particularly sedentary life, they will normally adjust the amount of food they eat to achieve the correct balance.

Nutrients: The cat exhibits a number of nutritional peculiarities which distinguish it from other Carnivora, such as the dog. These differences reflect the naturally predatory lifestyle of the cat and its ability to live on an almost entirely animal-based diet. Indeed, the cat is dependent on a supply of at least some animal-derived tissue in its diet and must, therefore, be regarded as an **obligate carnivore**.

The cat requires a higher level of dietary protein for maintenance than the dog, since the cat's ability to regulate amino acid catabolism is limited. It is unable to adapt to a diet which is extremely low in protein and indeed, such a diet is likely to be completely rejected by the cat since they find low protein diets rather unpalatable. Cats are particularly sensitive to a deficiency of the amino acid, arginine, and will exhibit severe adverse effects (hyperammonaemia) within 2-5 hours of eating a **single** arginine-free meal.

The cat has a particularly high requirement for the amino-sulphonic acid, taurine, partly because of its inability to conjugate bile salts with glycine (instead of taurine). Unlike the dog, the cat cannot meet its taurine requirement from dietary sulphur amino acids and so requires a dietary source of taurine. A deficiency of taurine causes central retinal degeneration, reproductive failure, developmental abnormalities in kittens and dilated cardiomyopathy. Taurine is found in significant quantities only in materials of animal origin.

Although cats have the necessary enzymes to convert tryptophan to niacin, an increased activity of the enzyme picolinic acid decarboxylase results in the diversion of tryptophan intermediate metabolites towards the synthesis of the alternative end product, glutamate. The cat cannot, therefore, synthesise sufficient niacin for its needs and has a greater dietary requirement for this vitamin.

A source of animal fat is required in the feline diet for two main reasons. The cat is unable to convert ß-carotene to retinol (vitamin A) and therefore requires a dietary source of pre-formed vitamin A. In addition, the cat cannot convert sufficient linoleic acid to meet its requirement for arachidonic acid. Neither pre-formed vitamin A nor arachidonic acid is found in plant tissues.

Finally, cats appear to be in a constant state of gluconeogenesis and they do not seem to be able to tolerate a high carbohydrate diet.

These characteristics are all consistent with the fact that a carnivorous diet is naturally high in protein and low in carbohydrate. The obligatory carnivorous nature of cats is emphasised by the fact that taurine, pre-formed vitamin A and arachidonic acid are only found in significant quantities in animal tissues. It is thus essential that the cat is supplied with at least some animal-derived materials in its diet. The current recommendations for minimum nutrient requirements for adult cats are given in the Appendix.

Food Types

Healthy adult dogs can be fed on one complete food (canned, dry or semi-moist) or with a number of varieties. Sudden changes in diet should be avoided as this may lead to diarrhoea. The simplest way to offer a varied diet without the risk of gastrointestinal upset is by making use of the different varieties available within a brand of dog food.

Adult cats may be fed entirely on canned or dry cat foods and a complete, balanced and interesting diet can be provided from the wide range of varieties available. Dry cat food also provides a change of taste and texture.

The need for at least some animal-derived tissue in the feline diet is again emphasised and it should be noted that long-term feeding of dog foods to cats is unacceptable as they may not meet the specific nutritional requirements of the latter.

Regimen — Dogs

Adult dogs in maintenance will usually have a good enough appetite to eat all they require in one meal per day and it is quite satisfactory to adopt a once-a-day feeding regimen. The advantages of a single meal are that it can usually be of sufficient size to satiate appetite; it is more controllable in that errors of dispensing occur only once a day, so under- or over-feeding is less likely; it can easily be fitted into the household routine at whatever is the most convenient time. It is usually best to avoid late evening meals since dogs may need to excrete faeces or urine within a few hours of feeding and this can be inconvenient in the middle of the night.

There is no disadvantage in feeding more frequently than once a day, provided that the total daily intake is limited to the dog's daily needs. Feeding two or three times a day after family meals is a common practice. The risk is that more food will be given and that overeating and obesity will result. The correct number of meals for any adult dog is that which the owner and dog find most convenient. It is desirable to establish a routine and stick to it. Meal times are the high spot of most days and dogs quickly become accustomed to being fed at the same time and place each day. Dogs which are unwell or have poor appetites, or very old dogs, may benefit from being fed two or more times daily with smaller meals.

Regimen — Cats

When allowed continuous access to food, cats tend to adopt a pattern of small, frequent (usually 8–16) meals throughout the whole 24 hour period. However, cats readily adapt to different feeding schedules imposed by their owners and are commonly fed two meals per day. Nevertheless, if feeding time is restricted then sufficient food must be provided to satisfy their daily nutrient and energy requirements.

Environmental factors are also known to affect the volume of food a particular animal will eat. Most cats do not relish cold food straight from the refrigerator and prefer to eat food that is close to their own body temperature and that of freshly killed prey. This response may reflect a behavioural strategy in the wild which ensures that only the freshest prey is eaten.

Cats do seek variety in their diet, as long as the new food is not **too** different from the familiar one, or the palatability too low. At times of stress, however, a familiar diet is preferred. Repeated exposure to fresh supplies of a new food which is not initially acceptable to the cat may encourage the cat to overcome its reticence. Furthermore, cats can often detect and may reject diets that are deficient in certain nutrients, so it is important that any diet offered is nutritionally complete.

Assessment of Feeding Regimen

The best criterion for judging the adequacy of a feeding regimen for maintenance is the health and appearance of the dog or cat. If the animal is in good condition with good skin and coat, alert, active, and neither too fat nor too thin, then it is on an adequate regimen. Regular weighing of the animal allows the owner to monitor its progress on a quantitative basis.

REFERENCES

Burger IH and Johnson JV (1991). Dogs large and small - the allometry of energy requirements within a single species. *Journal of Nutrition* **121,** S18-S21.

Burger IH (1994). Assessing the needs of companion animals. *Journal of Nutrition* **124,** S2584-S2593.

Earle KE and Smith P (1991). Digestible energy requirements of the adult cat at maintenance. *Journal of Nutrition* **121,** S45-S46.

CHAPTER FOUR

Reproduction and Lactation

Josephine M. Wills

REPRODUCTION AND LACTATION

Feeding Objectives

The reproductive life stage is a nutritionally demanding time for the bitch or queen. Lactation, in particular, places great stresses on the female and her energy and nutrient requirements may rise to up to four times the maintenance levels.

A suitable diet for the animal during this period must:

- supply all the energy and nutrients needed to meet the maintenance requirements of the bitch or queen **plus**
- supply all the energy and nutrients required to support fetal growth and development during pregnancy and milk production during lactation.

Because the requirements may be very high and therefore large amounts of food must be ingested, achieving a sufficient intake may be a problem. To remedy this, it is advantageous for the diet to be:

- concentrated in terms of its energy and nutrient density
- palatable to encourage feeding
- highly digestible to reduce bulk.

Requirements

Dog

Energy. The average duration of pregnancy in the bitch is 63 days, but it is not until the last third of the gestation period that most fetal weight gain occurs. Accordingly, the bitch's energy requirement will not increase until this time although there is considerable development of mammary and uterine tissues beforehand. Overfeeding early on in pregnancy should be avoided since this may lead to the deposition of unwanted fat and may predispose to problems at whelping.

Even during the last trimester, the need for extra energy and nutrients over and above maintenance requirements is relatively small. All that is required is gradually to increase the amount of food over the second half of gestation. A satisfactory regimen would be to provide weekly increments of 15% of the bitch's maintenance ration from the fifth week onwards. At the time of whelping, the bitch will be eating 60% more than when she was mated. The objective is to have a bitch at parturition which is not overfat and that has maintained her appetite.

Lactation presents the biggest test of nutritional adequacy of any feeding regimen. The bitch must eat, digest, absorb and use very large amounts of nutrients to produce sufficient milk of adequate composition to support the growth and development of several puppies. The extra energy needed is dependent on the normal energy intake of the bitch and the size and age of the litter.

Consider a Labrador Retriever bitch of 28kg with a litter of six 4-week-old puppies of 2.5kg each. At this stage each puppy will require an energy intake of about 500kcal/day (2090kJ/day) which is obtained from the bitch's milk. The bitch, therefore, has to supply 3000kcal (12550kJ) as milk each day. Bitch's milk contains about 1300 kcal/litre (5440kJ/litre) and so the amount of milk needed is at least 2.3 litres.

There are obviously some losses of energy in the production of milk by the bitch but if it is assumed that the process has an efficiency of 75% then in order to produce 3000kcal (12550kJ) as milk, the bitch must obtain 3000/0.75 (12550/0.75) or 4000kcal (16740kJ) from her food. In addition, to maintain her own body weight and condition, she will need her usual 1500kcal/day (6280kJ). The bitch's total energy requirement is therefore 5500kcal (23020kJ) or nearly four times her maintenance requirement. It is strongly recommended to feed such an amount of food in several small meals of a highly palatable and digestible diet.

Figures 4.1 and 4.2 show the body weight changes and the average energy intakes of a group of Labrador Retriever bitches during gestation and lactation studies at the WALTHAM Centre for Pet Nutrition (WCPN). If the bitch is unable to produce enough milk or to eat the amount of food she needs, then early supplementary feeding of puppies may be necessary if they are to do as well as they should.

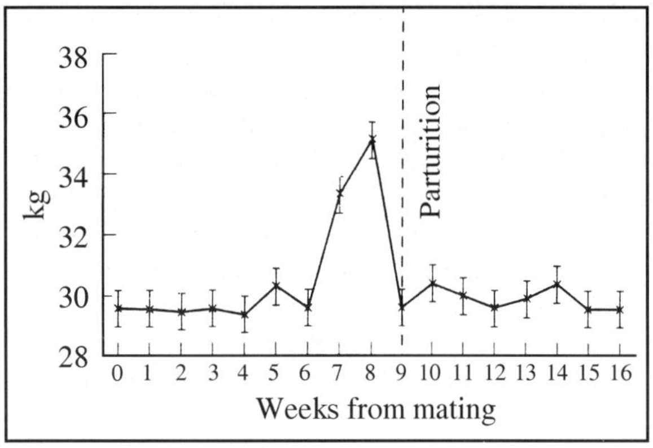

Figure 4.1: *Weight changes of Labrador Retriever during gestation/lactation. (Adapted from Burger, 1993.)*

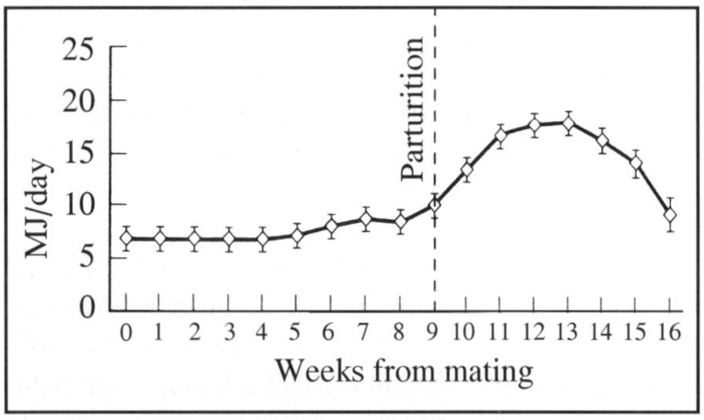

Figure 4.2: *Energy intake of Labrador Retriever during gestation/lactation (from Burger, 1993).*

Nutrients. Energy needs are increased during pregnancy and lactation, but requirements for other nutrients are similarly increased. Protein quantity and quality will affect milk production. It is therefore necessary to ensure that the extra food supplied is of good quality and is not made up only of high fat or high carbohydrate foods.

In 1981, Romsos *et al.* suggested that gestating/lactating bitches needed carbohydrate in order to whelp and rear healthy puppies. However, a later study conducted on Labrador Retriever and Beagle bitches (Blaza *et al.*, 1989) showed no differences in the reproductive performance of bitches fed either a diet in which there was no available carbohydrate or one where carbohydrate represented 11% of the estimated metabolisable energy. This is probably due to a higher protein content of the diet fed in the Blaza *et al.* study, which supplied sufficient gluconeogenic amino acids to allow the maintenance of the plasma glucose level. It was then concluded that, while carbohydrate is physiologically essential, it is not an indispensable component of the diet of gestating/lactating bitches.

The protein requirements for reproduction and lactation in the bitch have not been well defined. In one study, 12 out of 15 dogs maintained nitrogen balance and weight during gestation and lactation when fed diets containing approximately 25% protein (Visek *et al.*, 1976). Another study showed that bitches fed a carbohydrate-free diet required 30% protein compared with 16% in diets containing carbohydrate (Kienzle and Meyer, 1989).

Cats

Energy: The normal gestation period of the domestic cat is in the region of 64 days, although this is subject to considerable variation. Unlike most mammals, where most weight gain occurs in the last third of gestation, the cat gains weight at a steady rate throughout pregnancy. By the end of the third week of gestation, she has already gained almost 20% of the total amount of extra weight that she will carry. However, the **rate** of weight gain peaks towards the end of the second third of pregnancy and then slows down slightly.

At term, the total weight gain is dependent on litter size, but a queen with a single kitten will have gained about 32% of her pre-mating weight and a cat carrying four kittens will have increased her weight by about 39%. Following parturition, only 40% of this extra weight is lost (compared with almost 100% in the bitch) with the remaining 60% being lost during the course of lactation. Figure 4.3 illustrates the changes in weight gain seen in queens during pregnancy and lactation.

The fetal growth curves of puppies and kittens are not markedly different (with most fetal weight gain occurring in the last trimester), so it is thought that the queen lays down a supply of extra-uterine tissue early in pregnancy. This acts as an energy store which can be mobilised later on in pregnancy and lactation, when energy demands are at their greatest.

To parallel this steady increase in weight, the queen's food intake also rises continuously from mating and peaks at weeks seven and eight of gestation. Her energy requirements increase from around 60-90kcal/kg (250-380kJ/kg) body weight per day prior to mating, to around 100-110kcal/kg (420-460kJ/kg) body weight per day during gestation. For a short time before, and immediately after parturition, voluntary food intake is slightly reduced before the demands of lactation pro-

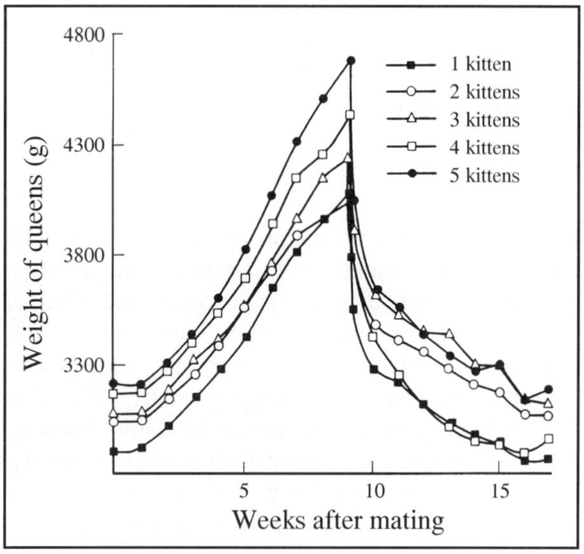

Figure 4.3: *Weight changes in queens during gestation/lactation (from Burger, 1993).*

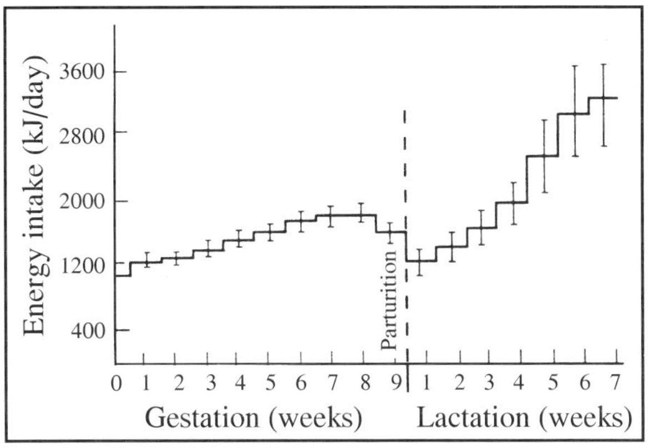

Figure 4.4: *Energy intakes of queens during gestation/ lactation (from Burger, 1993).*

mote a progressive increase in food consumption which varies according to litter size. The changes in energy intake during gestation and lactation are illustrated in Figure 4.4.

As with the bitch, the life stage of lactation in the queen proves to be the biggest test of nutritional adequacy, for not only is the queen having to obtain nutrients for herself but also for her many kittens through the milk she must provide. At birth the kittens weigh between 85g and 120g and there can be from one to eight kittens in a litter.

For the first 4 weeks of their life the kittens are entirely dependent on the milk supplied by the queen. The queen's energy requirements are thus far greater during lactation than through gestation as, by this time, the kittens are growing very rapidly. Although the kittens begin to take solid food from about 4 weeks of age, the queen's energy requirement remains elevated until after completion of weaning (at about seven or eight weeks of age). This is because the queen is still suckling (albeit to a lesser extent) and is also rebuilding her own body reserves.

The energy requirements of the lactating queen depend on the number of kittens she is rearing and their age, as both these factors will affect the amount of milk she needs to produce. Queen's milk has an energy density of 106kcal/100g (444kJ/100g) which is high compared with cow's milk at 65kcal/100g (272kJ/100g) (Baines 1981). The changes which occur in the queen's energy intake during lactation are illustrated in Table 4.1, although from week 4 onwards these figures represent the combined intake of both queen and kittens. These figures show that the queen's energy requirements during lactation are some three to four times that of her maintenance requirement.

Nutrients: The pregnant and lactating queen is more susceptible to nutrient deficiencies or excesses and so the diet should be carefully regulated at this time. For example, the calcium:phosphorus ratio must be more tightly controlled as this directly affects bone development in the kittens *in utero* and when suckling. The minimum protein requirement of the pregnant or lactating queen is higher than for maintenance.

Food types

During the period of pregnancy and lactation, the bitch or queen must eat sufficient food to satisfy her energy and nutrient requirements for maintenance **plus** an allowance for the additional demands of fetal growth or milk production. During pregnancy, the additional requirements are relatively small and it may be sufficient simply to increase the amount of the animal's normal food, provided that it is complete and nutritionally balanced. In late pregnancy and particularly if the litter is large, the gravid uterus may take up so much space in the abdomen that the physical capacity for food intake is limited. In this case, it may be useful to offer a more concentrated diet to ensure an adequate energy intake. Feeding of smaller, more frequent meals may also be beneficial.

During lactation, the nutritional demands on the female are very high. At peak lactation, the energy requirement may be between three and four times that of maintenance. In order to achieve an adequate food intake during this period, it is preferable to feed an energy- and nutrient-dense diet (such as puppy or kitten food) which is both highly digestible and highly

Week of lactation	Litter size					
	1	2	3	4	5	6
1	60	76	92	108	124	124
2	66	83	100	117	134	134
3	72	94	116	138	160	160
4	78	106	134	162	190	190
5	84	117	150	183	217	250
6	90	136	182	228	274	320

Table 4.1: *Daily energy intakes of queens during lactation.*

All figures as kcal/kg body weight (BW) (for kJ/kg BW multiply total by 4.184) and are based on the voluntary intake for queens of mean BW 3.8kg after parturition. Values from about week 4 include energy intake of kittens. (Data from National Research Council, 1986)

palatable. The extra food supplied should be of good quality (not simply high fat or high carbohydrate) because protein quantity and quality in the diet will affect milk production.

Many diets are suitable for lactating bitches. If canned food and a good quality mixer is the usual diet, it may be necessary to increase the proportion of biscuit used to achieve satisfactory energy intakes. The use of more concentrated foods, such as puppy food, semi-moist or complete dry foods, is another means of achieving higher energy intakes. If the dog is willing to eat different kinds of food this makes it easier, although it is quite satisfactory to keep to one or two foods if this is the normal regimen. Similarly, the increased requirements of lactating queens may be met by feeding concentrated canned (such as kitten food), semi-moist or dry nutritionally complete diets.

The breeding bitch or queen does not require special vitamin/mineral supplements if a balanced diet is used. Indeed this could actually cause an imbalance in the food. Supplements of calcium and vitamin D are sometimes given to bitches in late pregnancy or lactation, but these do not prevent eclampsia and may produce calcinosis in the bitch and developmental abnormalities in the puppy.

Regimen

Dogs

During the early stages of pregnancy, the bitch does not require any additional feeding. From the fifth week on, the ration may be gradually increased by 15% of her maintenance allowance per week until whelping, when she should be eating approximately 60% more than she was pre-mating. In many cases, it is sufficient simply to feed more of her normal diet (provided it is well balanced). However, a bitch with a large litter may have such an enlarged abdomen and reduced activity that her appetite falls during the last week or 10 days of pregnancy. In such cases, it is sensible to feed several smaller meals during the day to achieve a satisfactory intake.

During the period of lactation, the nutritional demands on the bitch are very high. The amount of extra food she requires varies according to the size of the litter, but at peak lactation (some three or four weeks after whelping) her food intake may be as much as three or four times the normal amount. Because the amounts needed are very large, it is usually necessary to feed a concentrated, highly palatable food in several small meals per day or *ad libitum* and food should be made available throughout the night. An unlimited supply of drinking water will also be necessary.

Weaning should be a gradual process. An abrupt separation of bitch and puppies may lead to mastitis in the bitch and a check in growth of the puppies. Puppies may be offered small amounts of soft foods from as early as two weeks of age, but only if they show an interest. Much will depend on the size of the litter and the milk supply of the bitch. However early the puppies take alternative foods, the bitch's milk should remain the prime source of nutrients until the puppies are at least four weeks old. Gradual separation and withdrawal of the bitch will allow her milk supply to dry up without the use of medicaments and allow the puppies to adapt to their new food naturally. It may be advisable to cut the bitch's food down to half the maintenance level immediately after total separation. Nevertheless, if the bitch has lost condition during lactation, she will need additional food to bring her body weight back up to normal as soon as her milk supply has diminished and weaning is completed.

Cats

It can be expected that pregnant queens will start to eat more and gain weight within a week of a successful mating and that sufficient food should be available throughout the whole period of gestation and lactation. On a practical note, cats rarely overeat and so *ad libitum* feeding is quite acceptable. In this way the queen will be able to take exactly the amount of energy she needs and the owner simply needs to offer slightly more than they would to the non-pregnant queen.

As with the bitch, energy requirements of the lactating queen may be up to four times her maintenance requirement. Thus the queen needs to be offered a highly palatable and digestible food which is high in energy (such as kitten food). She also will need to take frequent small meals to ingest the required amount and again, *ad libitum* feeding is highly appropriate as the queen will be able to control her energy intake very successfully. Food should be available throughout the night as well as during the day. Fresh water should be available at all times as a great deal will be lost from the queen's metabolism through the production of milk.

After weaning, the additional food can be gradually cut back until the queen is eating her normal amount. Observation of the general health and condition of the queen is essential. If any signs of weight loss or gain are apparent, the meals should be adjusted accordingly.

Assessment of feeding regimen

Assessment of the suitability of the diet may be carried out by observation of the health and body condition of the bitch or queen and of the offspring. It should be noted that overfeeding of the pregnant bitch is undesirable since this may lead to problems at whelping. Cats, however, are more efficient at regulating their energy intake and problems are less likely to be encountered in ensuring a sufficient intake. Throughout lactation, it is normal for the queen to lose weight as her body reserves are utilised, but her pre-mating weight should be achieved by the time the kittens are weaned. The bitch, on the other hand, normally returns to her pre-mating weight following parturition and her body weight should remain relatively stable throughout lactation. The nutritional adequacy of the mother's diet will also be reflected in the health and development of the kittens or puppies.

REFERENCES

Baines FM (1981). Milk substitutes and the hand rearing of orphaned puppies and kittens. *Journal of Small Animal Practice* **22,** 555-578.

Blaza SE, Booles D and Burger IH (1989). Is carbohydrate essential for pregnancy and lactation in dogs? In: *Nutrition of the Dog and Cat.* Eds IH Burger and JPW Rivers. Cambridge University Press, Cambridge. pp 229-242.

Burger IM (1993). *The Waltham Book of Companion Animal Nutrition.* Pergamon Press, Oxford.

Kienzle E and Meyer H (1989). The effects of carbohydrate-free diets containing different levels of protein on reproduction in the bitch. In: *Nutrition of the Dog and Cat.* Eds IH Burger and JPW Rivers. Cambridge University Press, Cambridge. pp 243-258.

National Research Council (1986). *Nutrient Requirements of Cats.* National Academy Press, Washington D.C.

Romsos DR, Palmer HJ, Muiruri KL and Bennink MR (1981). Influence of a low carbohydrate diet on performance of pregnant and lactating dogs. *Journal of Nutrition* **111,** 678-689.

Visek WJ, Robertson JB, Gagnon JP, Clinton SK and Ulman EA (1976). Dried brewers grains for mature and growing dogs. *Journal of Animal Science* **43,** 442.

CHAPTER FIVE

Feeding Puppies and Kittens

Josephine M. Wills and James G. Morris

FEEDING PUPPIES — *J.M. WILLS*

In relation to body weight, the energy and nutrient requirements of growing animals are far greater than those of adults. The young growing animal needs a higher plane of nutrition to fuel its rapid growth and to provide the boundless energy which is so characteristic of puppies.

Feeding Objectives

Growth is a complex, highly integrated process involving interactions between nutrients, genotype, environment and a host of different hormones and their receptors. In formulating a diet suitable for growth in puppies, the following objectives should be considered:

- The diet must contain the correct amount and balance of nutrients to support normal body functions (maintenance).
- The diet should permit normal development in the puppy and prepare it for a long, active and healthy life.
- Growth should be achieved at a rate which will allow the puppy to fulfil its genetic potential while its long bones are still capable of lengthwise growth (i.e. before closure of the growth plates), but not so rapidly as to produce abnormalities of growth.
- The diet must be balanced in respect of all the nutrients required to achieve these objectives.
- The diet should be palatable to encourage adequate intake and to give enjoyment.

The rapid growth phase of puppies is a nutritionally demanding time and errors in the diet at this stage can have long lasting and often irreversible consequences. Generalised undernutrition in the young dog can lead at best to poor growth and condition, but this can be reversed if the diet is corrected while the puppy is still growing. Deficiencies or imbalances of specific nutrients can have more serious effects.

Nutritional secondary hyperparathyroidism is caused by a deficiency of calcium (absolute or relative) and is typically produced by feeding an 'all-meat' diet, which is a poor source of calcium. **Rickets**, although rarely seen in clinical practice, is caused by a vitamin D deficiency and is often compounded by a low calcium intake. Both of these conditions give rise to serious disturbances in bone growth and development (see Chapter 20).

Overnutrition in young dogs is more commonly seen, particularly as there is a tendency among some owners to overfeed (to produce rapid growth rates) or to oversupplement the diet (to avoid the classic deficiency diseases). Excessive energy intake in the growing dog, however, is likely to cause obesity in small breeds and rapid growth rates in large and giant breeds. A rapid growth rate is not necessarily beneficial to the animal and the premature increase in body weight places undue stresses on the juvenile skeleton. This can lead to a variety of multi-factorial diseases characterised by abnormalities in bone development and growth, including **osteochondrosis syndrome, hip dysplasia, wobbler syndrome and enostosis (panosteitis)**. Excessive dietary calcium is also thought to play a major contributory role in a number of these conditions (see Chapter 20).

Oversupplementation with fat-soluble vitamins, especially vitamins A and D, are also particularly harmful (see Chapter 1). Care must therefore be exercised if using a supplement such as cod liver oil, which is a rich source of both these vitamins. Such additions to the diet are unnecessary if a balanced diet is fed, particularly if the product is specifically formulated for growth.

Requirements

Energy

The dog is unique in that it has the widest range of normal adult body weights within any single species. The rate of growth in the early stages is very rapid and, in general, most breeds of dog will attain 50% of their mature adult weight at a similar age, that is 5–6 months. However, because of the wide variation in adult body weight, different breeds continue to mature at different relative rates and, in general, larger breeds take longer to reach their adult body weight than smaller breeds of dog (Figure 5.1). For example, a miniature Dachshund

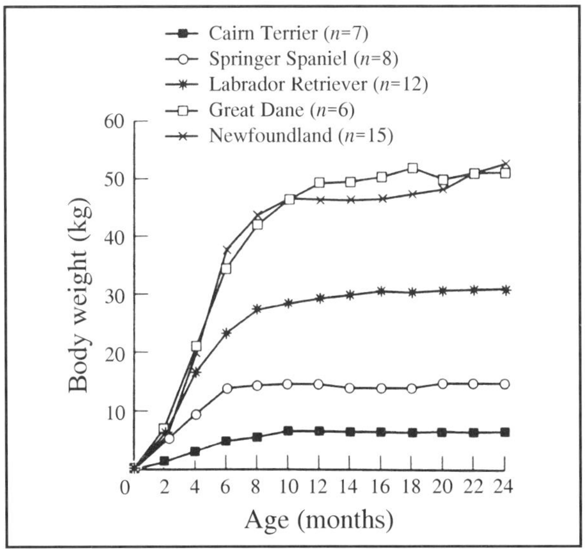

Figure 5.1: Growth curve of different breeds of dog (from Burger, 1993).

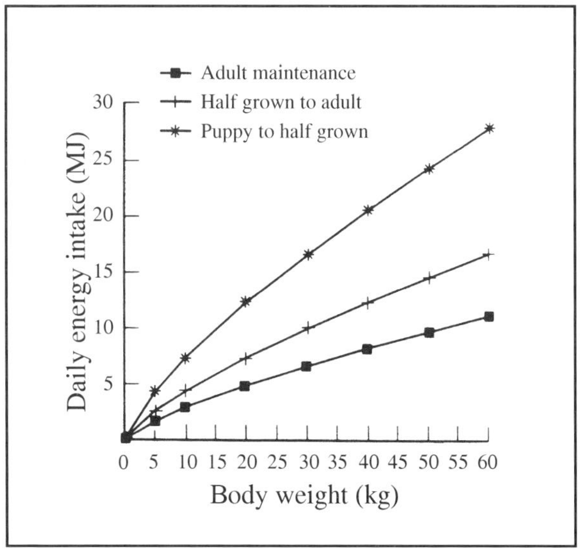

Figure 5.2: Energy requirement of dogs at different life stages (from Burger, 1993).

may reach maturity at around 9 months old, whereas a Labrador Retriever and Newfoundland are likely to attain their adult body weights at about 15 months and 18 months, respectively. Individual variations occur due to a variety of factors, either intrinsic (for example, male dogs are usually heavier than females of the same breed) or extrinsic (that is, husbandry and nutrition).

The feeding regimen is of primary importance in determining the growth rates of large and giant breeds in particular. Individuals of certain of these breeds that have the most rapid growth rates are more prone to disturbances in their skeletal development. Maximum growth is not, therefore, necessarily compatible with optimal growth and provided that skeletal and muscle development are not ultimately impaired, then an elongated period of growth is likely to be advantageous to such puppies.

At weaning (between 6 and 8 weeks of age), the energy requirement per unit body weight of puppies is about double that of an adult of the same breed. As they grow, this requirement declines progressively and by the time they have attained 40% of their adult weight, it is only 1.6 times that required for adult maintenance. When they have reached 80% of their mature weight, they need only 1.2 times as much energy as an adult per unit of body weight. Table 5.1 and Figure 5.2 illustrate the energy needed by puppies of different sizes as their weight increases.

Nutrients

Growing dogs not only need more energy than adult dogs, but also larger amounts of other essential nutrients. In particular, the protein requirements of growing puppies are much greater than those of adult dogs. In addition to the requirement for protein to replace that which is broken down and lost from the body every day, growing puppies also need protein to synthesise tissue for growth.

The following amino acids are required by the immature dog for optimum growth and nitrogen balance:

- Arginine
- Methionine
- Histidine
- Phenylalanine
- Isoleucine
- Threonine
- Leucine
- Tryptophan
- Lysine
- Valine

It is important that a diet for a growing dog supplies all these amino acids at the appropriate levels, as well as supplying extra nitrogen to allow the dog to synthesise dispensable amino acids and other nitrogen-containing compounds.

The **minimum** level of protein recommended for growth in dogs varies between 11% and 22% of energy intake (Johnson, 1993), depending on variables such as environmental factors, breed of dog and dietary source of protein and decreases with age after weaning. The dietary requirements of a particular protein or a mixture of proteins are determined by the ability of the protein(s) to meet the dog's metabolic requirements for amino acids and nitrogen. The closer the supply of the complement of amino acids to the requirement, the lower the percentage of protein required in the dog's diet.

Based on the results of a number of studies, the National Research Council concluded that 12% protein from lactalbumin or a similar high quality source should support growth (National Research Council 1985). However, a recent study by Nap *et al.* (1991) suggests that a protein level of 15% is marginal for giant breeds, such as the Great Dane. Moreover, they found that a high protein diet (33%) does **not** have a causative role in the development of osteochondrosis in dogs.

Body weight	Age in months				
kg	2	3	6	12	24
1	250	225	150	125	125
2	495	390	260	210	210
5	1090	795	545	415	415
10	1760	1690	985	700	700
15		2380	1525	950	950
20		3075	2010	1300	1180
30			3205	1925	1600
50			5875	3055	2350
60				3505	2695

Table 5.1: *Energy requirements of puppies throughout growth (kcal[1]/day).*

[1] *For kJ/day multiply result by 4.184*

The amino acid profile of the diet must therefore be suitable to support growth in the young dog. In addition, the protein must be in a digestible form.

Some breeders believe that the inclusion of large amounts of additional protein in a puppy diet will aid the development of good condition and muscle. Unfortunately, this is not the case and protein which is consumed in excess of requirement is, rather, metabolised to produce energy or stored as fat.

Fat is a useful dietary source of energy in growth formulations since it is a concentrated source of energy (without adding bulk) and it enhances the palatability of the food.

Carbohydrate is not an essential component of the puppy's diet, provided that sufficient protein is available for glucose synthesis. However, carbohydrates form a useful and economical source of energy in the dog's diet. Once weaning has taken place, young animals become less efficient at digesting lactose and some individuals become totally intolerant of this particular nutrient. Even if some ability to digest lactose is retained, the animal may not be able to cope with large amounts. Contrary to popular belief, milk is not an essential part of a puppy's diet after weaning, but it remains a useful source of nutrients for individuals that can tolerate it, if fed in restricted amounts.

The requirements for vitamins in the growing dog do not differ markedly from those of adult dogs. However, the supply of fat-soluble vitamins, which can be stored in the body, is more critical in the growing dog than in the adult and care should be taken to ensure that toxicities do not occur through injudicious supplementation. The vitamin E requirement of growing puppies is approximately double that of an adult. Unlike other species, puppies do not synthesise sufficient vitamin D through UV irradiation to match their requirements, hence a dietary source of this vitamin is required.

The demand for minerals required for bone formation (especially calcium) is higher in the growing dog than in the adult, particularly in the fast-growing large and giant breeds. It is essential that these nutrients are provided not only in the correct amounts but also in the correct ratio to each other. In particular, the requirement for calcium is closely linked to the phosphorus content of the diet, and a relative deficiency of calcium may arise in a diet which is apparently sufficient in calcium if the phosphorus content is too high.

The optimal absolute amount of calcium in the diet of growing puppies needs to be strictly controlled and should be in the range 0.8g to 1.5g on a dry matter basis. Furthermore, the amount of phosphorus in the diet should be adjusted to ensure the ratio of Ca:P is not lower than 1:1 or greater than 1.5:1. However, a certain amount of regulation of calcium absorption and retention does occur, and it would seem that unless the Ca:P deviates vastly from the normal, the calcium content *per se* is more important than the Ca:P ratio (Hazewinkel *et al.*, 1991).

Puppies of the fast-growing large and giant breeds are particularly susceptible to nutrient imbalances, which can give rise to a variety of skeletal deformities, some of which may be irreversible (see Chapter 20). Since animals eat to meet their energy requirements, all nutrients must be balanced in respect of the energy content of the diet. A properly balanced diet which is formulated for growth does **not** require supplementation and injudicious use of additives can have serious deleterious effects. This is true even of large breeds since their extra needs are catered for by their increased food intake.

Food Types

Diets for puppies may be moist (canned), semi-moist or dry, but in younger animals (under two months, depending on breed), it is recommended that dry foods are softened with water, gravy or milk, and that food is finely divided (chopped or minced) to make it easier for the young animal to eat. Soft, wet foods are easy to digest and can be more palatable.

It is possible to feed an adult formulation, but the young animal has very high requirements and will need to eat proportionately more of the diet. A young puppy has a limited stomach capacity and may not be physically capable of ingesting enough to meet its requirements. A suitable diet for weaning and growing puppies, therefore, should be concentrated, highly digestible and very palatable. Many products are commercially available that have been specifically formulated for puppies. A typical canned dog food designed for adults will have an energy density of approximately 80kcal/100g (335kJ/100g), whereas one formulated for puppy growth will provide 120kcal/100g (500kJ/100g).

It is unnecessary to supplement growth formulations with other foods but some owners may like to offer alternative foods from time to time. If so, only a few different foods should be introduced gradually at any time to allow the digestive system to adapt to the new food. Meat, offal, eggs, cheese and bread are some of the foods which are commonly fed to dogs. If these foods are to form the major part of the diet, then careful supplementation with vitamins and minerals will almost certainly be required. In order to provide the correct balance of nutrients, food composition tables should be consulted when formulating a home-prepared diet.

Care of motherless puppies

- Ideally, the environment should be controlled by an incubator (0–7 days old 32–30°C; 7–14 days old 30–28°C; 14–21 days old 28–26°C; 21–28 days old 26–24°C)
- Alternatively, a heating pad with adequate insulation of the pen can be used
- After the puppies have been fed, a vital aspect of tending motherless pups is to stimulate the mother's tongue action on the ano-genital area which provokes reflex defaecation and urination
- The necessary result can be achieved by applying a piece of damp cotton wool at the ano-genital area or simply by running a dampened forefinger along the abdominal wall
- Between 16 and 21 days, puppies no longer require stimulation to urinate and defecate and from 28 days, when they completely control their body temperature, they begin to explore their surroundings and become more independent

Figure 5.3: *Care of orphaned puppies.*

Feeding Regimen

The first two weeks of a puppy's life are spent eating and sleeping and its energy needs are catered for by its mother. Clearly during this period there is no need for any external source of food. Naturally if the bitch cannot produce enough milk, for example if it is a big litter, or of course if the puppies are orphaned, then they must be hand-reared.

The most obvious alternative to a bitch rearing her puppies is for another bitch to act as a foster mother. However, the chances of a bitch at the right stage of lactation and with sufficient resource to rear a litter being available at the right time are poor. It can, however, be done and good communications within a breed club, for example, obviously improve the chances of finding a suitable foster mother. Motherless puppies have vital requirements in two main areas: provision of a suitable environment and nutrition. Important aspects of the husbandry of orphaned puppies are summarised in Figure 5.3.

Puppies grow at a rapid rate and will double their birth weight in a matter of days. Because of this, puppies require large quantities of their mother's milk or a food which can substitute for it. The food has to be a concentrated source of nutrients based on the composition of normal bitch's milk. Table 5.2 shows the average composition of milk from bitches, cows, goats and queens. It is clear that cow's and goat's milks are inadequate as a substitute for rearing puppies since the protein, fat and calcium levels are too low. Many commercially available bitch's milk substitutes are now available. They are usually based on cow's milk which has been modified to resemble bitch's milk more closely. They can be administered by means of a small syringe or a puppy feeding bottle.

Dried milk feeds should be reconstituted daily and fed warm (38°C). Food must be given slowly and must not be forced into the puppy. When feeding from a miniature bottle, the hole in the teat may need to be enlarged so that the flow is improved and the puppy does not suck in air. When puppies begin to explore their surroundings (at 3–4 weeks), a high quality puppy food can be introduced. This can be mixed with a milk substitute to begin with and then offered separately.

In the early stages of weaning, (3–4 weeks after parturition) the bitch's milk is still the most important source of nutrients and the puppy's digestive system is learning to handle new sources of nutrients. At this stage, puppies should be encouraged to take soft, wet food or even small kibbles of dry food moistened with warm gravy or water. Although many people assume that milk and milky feeds should figure prominently in a weaning regimen, they are not essential. The litter should be fed together from one or two trays depending on the litter size to encourage competition between puppies, although meal times should be supervised to ensure that each puppy receives enough food.

	Bitch	Cow	Goat	Cat
Moisture %	77.2	87.6	87.0	81.5
Dry matter %	22.8	12.4	13.0	18.5
Protein %	8.1	3.3	3.3	8.1
Fat %	9.8	3.8	4.5	5.1
Ash %	4.9	5.3	6.2	3.5
Lactose %	3.5	4.7	4.0	6.9
Calcium %	0.28	0.12	0.13	0.04
Phosphorus %	0.22	0.10	0.11	0.07
Energy[1] kcal/100g	135	66	70	106

Table 5.2: *Average analyses of milk of various species.*

[1] *Calculated using protein 4kcal/g; fat 9kcal/g and lactose 4kcal/g (from Baines, 1981)*
For energy in kJ multiply by 4.184

Highly palatable, energy- and nutrient-dense foods are the most suitable for weaning. Most puppies can be fully weaned on to a varied diet or a single complete food between 6 and 8 weeks of age, after which they are ready to leave their mother's side. At this stage, it is better to feed them four small meals a day rather than allow them continuous access to food.

Assuming canned puppy foods are around 120kcal/100g (500kJ/100g), a 12-week-old puppy weighing 10kg would have to eat 1.45kg/day (6kJ/day) to cover its energy requirement. Because the puppy must take in such large quantities of food, despite its small physical capacity, the food on offer should be, ideally:

- concentrated in terms of its energy and nutrient content
- highly digestible
- palatable
- totally balanced for growth in its nutrient content.

Commercial diets prepared specifically for growth are ideal. It is recommended that a growth diet is fed until the puppy attains at least 75% of its adult weight.

To accommodate their high requirements, puppies should have their food allowance divided into four or five meals a day until around 10 weeks and then three meals a day until 50% of adult body weight is reached. At this stage (about 5-6 months), the frequency of feeds can be reduced to twice daily. As the puppy approaches its adult weight, the total food allowance can gradually become incorporated in a single meal as in the adult. It is not recommended to feed puppies *ad libitum* since they will tend to overeat and could become obese or subject to skeletal developmental abnormalities.

In assessing the requirements of the growing puppy, it is very difficult to give precise amounts. Different foods have different calorie densities and the puppies themselves are subject to individual variation. Apart from breed size, variations in levels of activity, environmental factors, body type and gender will all affect the puppies' requirements. It is important therefore that the growing dog is regularly assessed 'by hand and eye' to ensure that it is making satisfactory progress and to allow any necessary alterations in the diet to be made.

Assessment of Feeding Regimen

A puppy should be fed to put on weight and grow at a rate which is neither too slow nor too fast. The weight, size and state of maturation should be compared with littermates or other dogs of the same age and breed. However, established standards of size and weight for growing dogs of many breeds (and crossbreeds) are not available. As previously noted, the health and condition of the animal should be regularly assessed 'by hand and eye' and the puppy's progress monitored in this way.

FEEDING KITTENS — *J.G. MORRIS*

Maternal nutrition is an important element contributing to a successful pregnancy and birth of healthy kittens. Nutritional deficiencies in the diet of queens during pregnancy lead to kittens born with depleted nutrient reserves, sub-normal birth weights, reduced vigour, and malformations. Almost immediately after conception queens prepare for the demand of pregnancy and lactation by increasing their intake of food and building body reserves that can be mobilised during lactation. Diets that do not supply sufficient nutrients result in sub-optimal lactation by the queen, and compromise the kittens.

The average body weight of kittens at birth is about 100g, but is dependent on the number of kittens in the litter. Large litters tend to have kittens of lower birth weight than small litters. Growth rate during the suckling period is entirely dependent on milk production of the queen and litter size. Generally queens have sufficient milk for all kittens for the first few days of life and growth rate is independent of litter size. However, after about the first week of lactation the demand of large litters exceeds the queens's milk supply and growth rate is less than that in small litters.

Feeding Objectives

While early postnatal nutrition of kittens is largely determined by the queen, this nutritional support is rapidly supplanted by the diet the kitten receives. The choice of this diet will be dependent on our objectives for the kitten. Some of the nutritional considerations important in selecting a diet are as follows:

- Sufficiently palatable such that kittens consume adequate quantities of the diet.
- Concentrations of all essential nutrients high enough to allow kittens to have nutrient intakes in excess of their minimal requirements.
- Should not contain excessive levels of any nutrient that may pose a hazard to the kitten, or interfere with the utilisation of other nutrients.
- Should not only prevent nutritional deficiencies, but provide nutrients that promote longevity and freedom from disease.
- Promote desirable aesthetic and behavioural characteristics in the kitten.

Requirements

Energy

The term 'energy' is used to indicate the sum of the nutrients in the diet that are oxidised to yield energy. These nutrients in the diet are fat, carbohydrate and protein, so the energy intake of a kitten is the sum of these nutrients that are available from the diet. While these nutrients can substitute for one another in their contribution to the total energy requirement of kittens, protein and some of the fatty acids in fats have functions distinct from their contribution to energy. Growing kittens need higher energy intakes per unit body weight than adult cats, as they have to synthesise new tissue as well as sustain the normal maintenance of the body. Little is known in quantitative terms of the actual intakes or requirements of energy by kittens while suckling, but because kittens have relatively high growth rates the energy intake per unit body weight must also be high.

Protocol testing of pet foods has resulted in the generation of a large amount of information on the growth rates of kittens from 10 to 18 weeks of age. Kittens given good quality diets grow rapidly in this post weaning period and body weight gains exceeding 30g/day are often recorded in individual male kittens. However, mean body weight gains of male and female kittens of 18–20g/day are more usual, gains of male kittens being greater than females.

Kittens should have food available at all times, as cats eat many small meals (about 16 a day) rather than one large meal. Restricting the availability of food reduces total daily food intake and can be a reason for some kittens doing poorly.

The energy intake of kittens is the highest of all physiological stages other than lactation. Kittens need about 160kcal/kg (670kJ/kg) body weight/day.

Protein

Cats of all ages require higher protein intakes than most other mammals including dogs. The higher protein requirement of cats is probably a reflection of their evolution as strict carnivores. The higher protein need arises from an inability of cats to conserve nitrogen from dispensable amino acids. Thus the higher protein requirement of kittens is actually a higher requirement for nitrogen rather than a higher requirement for all the essential amino acids. Once the minimal nitrogen requirement of cats has been met, the amount of protein required in the diet depends on the amino acid composition of the protein. Kittens require ten essential amino acids in the diet, which are:

- Arginine
- Leucine
- Phenylalanine
- Valine
- Histidine
- Lysine
- Threonine
- Isoleucine
- Methionine
- Tryptophan

Methionine is the amino acid most likely to be deficient in kitten diets because cats have a relatively high requirement for this amino acid, and methionine is the first limiting amino acid for cats in some of the major protein sources in cat food.

The amino acid requirements for weaned kittens for maximal growth have been determined and are available in the publication *Nutrient Requirements of Cats* by the National Research Council (1986). As proteins have distinct amino acid patterns the minimal protein requirement depends on the source of protein in the diet to satisfy the amino acid and nitrogen needs of kittens. For most good quality proteins such as meat, 30 to 35% protein in dry matter of the diet will supply all the nitrogen and essential amino acids for the growing kitten.

Carbohydrates and Fats

Even though cats evolved as strict carnivores they are quite efficient in their digestion of cereal starch, especially after the starch is cooked. Starch from grains in dry (expanded) diets provides a useful source of energy for kittens. Some other carbohydrates are not well utilised by cats, especially after weaning. Cats along with most other mammals lose, to a variable extent, their ability to digest lactose (milk sugar) with age, because the activity of the brush border enzyme lactase declines with age. Lactase splits the disaccharide lactose into the two monosaccharides glucose and galactose. Milk fed to individuals that have reduced ability to digest lactose induces diarrhoea and flatulence due to microbial degradation of lactose in the large intestine. Milk is not an essential part of the diet of kittens after weaning, but provides useful nutrients for those kittens that can tolerate lactose.

Sucrose, another disaccharide, is not well utilised by cats if too much is present in the diet. The problem here is not a reduced activity of an enzyme in the intestine to split the disaccharide to two monosaccharides glucose and fructose, but in the metabolism of fructose. Large amounts of sucrose in the diet induces fructosuria.

Fats are important sources of energy in the diet of kittens and generally increase the acceptance of dry diets by kittens. Fat provides about 2.25 times the energy of an equal weight of carbohydrate or protein. One way to increase the energy intake of kittens is to increase the level of fat in the diet. Many of the high energy canned foods contain more than 40% fat on a dry matter basis. These diets often contain very little carbohydrate, so the energy is coming predominantly from fat. Most expanded dry diets contain about 10% fat, but some of the higher energy dry diets contain closer to 20% fat.

Fats are the source of essential fatty acids in the diet of kittens. All animals need a source of essential fatty acids in the diet but kittens need preformed arachidonic acid. Arachidonic acid occurs only in animals so some animal fat is required in the diet of cats to provide this essential fatty acid.

Polyunsaturated fats, especially those in fish oils, rapidly become rancid on exposure to oxygen in the air. Rancidity is accelerated by the presence of catalysts such as iron and copper compounds. These polyunsaturated fats also become oxidised in the body leading to the production of ceroid pigment and yellow fat producing the condition known as steatitis. Steatitis can be prevented if the diet contains sufficient vitamin E, but in the case of some fish fats, the level has to be very high in order to prevent the disease.

Minerals

Kittens need all the essential minerals in the diet required by other animals. However, as growing kittens are laying down bone, the quantitative requirements for calcium and phosphorus exceed those of all other minerals. Cats in the wild state obtained their calcium and phosphorus by eating the whole body including the skeleton of small animals such as mice, rats and birds. In whole rats about 2% of the dry matter is composed of calcium. Organ and muscle meats are particularly poor sources of calcium and are also deficient (but to a lesser degree) in phosphorus. Kittens consuming a diet of organ or muscle meat alone, develop chronic calcium deficiency leading to nutritional secondary hyperparathyroidism. Affected kittens have poorly calcified bones, develop spontaneous fractures of the long bones and compression fractures of the vertebrae. The calcium requirement range for growing kittens is 0.5–2.0g/400kcal (0.3–1.2g/MJ). Growing kittens unlike growing puppies are less demanding in regard to their calcium and phosphorus requirements.

Most commercial pet foods contain adequate quantities of calcium and phosphorus and should not be supplemented with these minerals.

The amount of potassium needed in the diet of kittens is only slightly less than that of calcium, as potassium is the major ion inside cells. Potassium deficiency has occurred in kittens given both commercial and home-prepared diets. Kittens with potassium deficiency are reluctant to move, and assume a sitting position on the hind limbs with ventroflexion of the head.

The amount of sodium required in the diet of kittens is only about a third that of potassium. Chronic sodium deficiency in kittens produces polydypsia, polyuria, low urine specific gravity and an increase in the concentration of aldosterone in plasma and urine.

While magnesium is an essential mineral for kittens, naturally occurring cases of magnesium deficiency have not been recorded. High levels of magnesium in the diet increase urinary excretion of magnesium and the probability of formation of struvite uroliths, and eventual obstruction. Other factors involved in urolith formation include urine pH, urinary concentration of other ions and total water intake (see Chapter 19).

Kittens probably need all the 14 trace elements shown to be essential for other animals, but naturally occurring trace element deficiencies are relatively rare

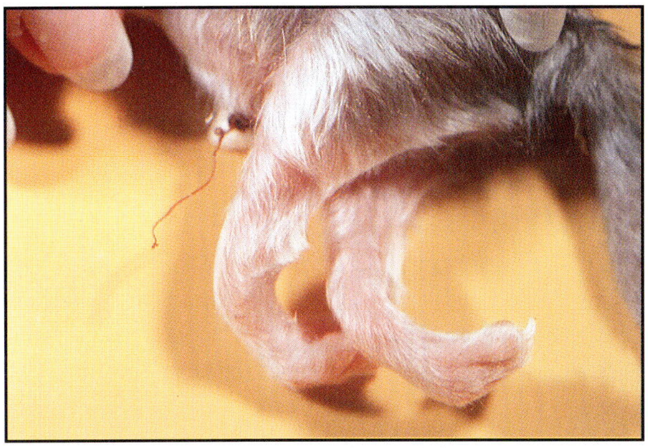

Figure 5.4: Leg deformities in a kitten fed a copper-deficient diet.

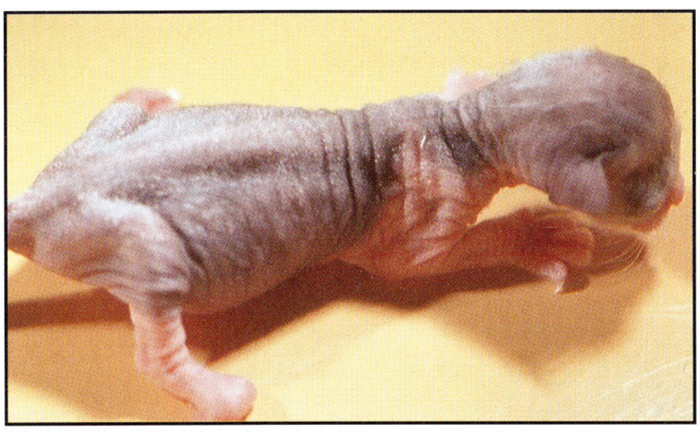

Figure 5.5: Hairless kitten fed a copper-deficient diet.

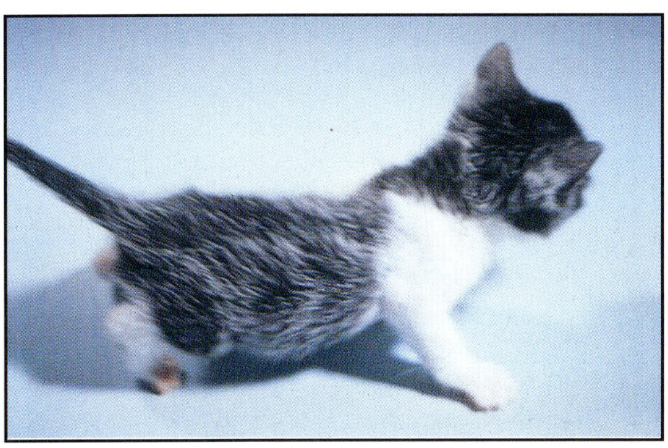

Figure 5.6: Grey coat colour in a kitten fed a copper-deficient diet.

in kittens with the possible exceptions of copper and zinc deficiencies. These deficiencies have been observed mainly in newborn and suckling kittens. The copper requirement of growing kittens is comparable to other animals, but the requirement of the queen for pregnancy may be higher. Copper deficiency has occurred in queens given commercial diets containing copper oxide as a source of copper. Queens frequently aborted and kittens born to these queens had low birth weights, poor survival rate and a high incidence of deformed limbs (Figure 5.4) and hypochromatricia (Figures 5.5 and 5.6).

In zinc deficiency small circumscribed areas of roughened skin are found on the ventral surface of kittens particularly in the axillary region. Kittens do not exhibit as pronounced parakeratotic lesions as found in dogs given diets low in zinc.

Studies on animals other than cats have shown that excessive levels of minerals can be deleterious. Little is known about excessive levels of minerals in the diet of kittens. Some fish products are known to contain high levels of mercury and selenium which may be deleterious.

Vitamins

Kittens need a special array of vitamins in their diet because they cannot synthesise certain vitamins from precursors and require higher levels of some of the other vitamins. Animal tissues provide all the essential vitamins needed by cats in the preformed state. Most animals, while they need certain vitamins, can synthesise them from precursors or pro-vitamins in the diet. Dogs and most other mammals can synthesise vitamin A from the yellow pigment carotene in the diet. Cats are unable to make this coversion and need the vitamin A to be pre-formed. Very little carotene occurs in animal tissue as it is mostly converted to vitamin A.

Cats do not synthesise adequate vitamin D on exposure to sunlight or ultraviolet light. So when a kitten lies in the sun it is just enjoying warmth, and does not do it to get its vitamin D. Vitamins A and D are present in animal tissues, cats being strict carnivores obtain sufficient of these vitamins from the bodies of their prey.

Kittens also require higher levels of some of the water-soluble vitamins than other animals, including dogs. Niacin, one of the water-soluble vitamins of the B group, must also be present pre-formed in the diet as cats, unlike dogs, are unable to make it from the amino acid tryptophan.

While vitamins are essential in the diet, too great an intake of certain vitamins, particularly vitamins A and D, can be toxic. Vitamin A is stored in the liver of all animals and prolonged feeding of liver to cats induces hypervitaminosis A, which leads to thinning of the long bones and formation of exostoses on the cervical vertebrae. Similarly excess intake of vitamin D produces hypercalcaemia, calcification of soft tissues and renal damage. Some commercial cat foods, especially canned cat foods containing fish produced in the United States, have been reported to contain excessive levels of vitamin D.

As cats are often fed diets based on fish products which contain large amounts of polyunsaturated fatty acids, the intake of vitamin E is critical for cats. Polyunsaturated fatty acids in foods undergo auto-oxidation to produce peroxides which are deleterious to animals. Vitamin E is a powerful antioxidant preventing formation of lipid peroxides. Kittens given diets high in polyunsaturated fatty acids need higher dietary levels of vitamin E than when fed lower levels of fatty acids.

Amongst the water-soluble vitamins, thiamin is the vitamin most likely to be deficient in the diet. Unlike the fat-soluble vitamins, the body's ability to store thiamin is limited, so it is unable to buffer a deficiency in the diet. Thiamin is also destroyed in canned foods by heat processing, and manufacturers add sufficient thiamine to ensure adequate availability in the processed product. Kittens deficient in thiamin develop neurological deficits, involving positional and righting reflex deficits. While deficiencies of the other water-soluble vitamins have been produced in kittens, in practice they are not often encountered as single vitamin deficiencies but as multiple vitamin deficiencies.

Adequate levels of vitamins occur in most commercial pet foods and one should be particularly careful not to be over liberal in giving vitamin supplements to kittens. Vitamin supplementation will not compensate for poor food quality. The best assurance of good nutrition is to feed a good quality commercial diet.

Taurine

The sulphur amino acid taurine occurs as free amino acid in all animal tissues, its concentration generally being highest of all the free amino acids. For most mammals, taurine is not an essential dietary nutrient, sufficient taurine being synthesised from the degradation of the sulphur amino acids methionine and cystine. Cats, and apparently all other felids, do not synthesise adequate amounts of taurine to meet their body needs and coupled with this they are unable to reduce the loss of taurine in bile. Cats, unlike most other mammals, are unable to conjugate bile salts with glycine when taurine is limited . This obligate loss of taurine for conjugation results in a deficiency when inadequate amounts of taurine are supplied in the diet. A deficiency of taurine in the diet of kittens leads to a number of clinical problems including loss of visual elements of the eye, producing central retinal degeneration, and delayed development of hearing. In breeding queens, inadequate taurine in the diet leads to reproductive disorders including fetal resorptions and abortions and developmental abnormalities involving all major organ systems of the fetus.

The requirement for taurine depends on the type of diet; canned diets require higher levels of taurine per unit dry matter than dry or expanded diets. The reason for this difference lies in the degree of degradation of taurine in the enterohepatic circulation of cats. Taurocholic acid is deconjugated by bacteria in the gut, and the taurine is then degraded by the microflora. In canned diets the extent of deconjugation is higher, and the degradation of taurine greater, than in dry or expanded diets. Canned diets have to contain about twice as much taurine on a dry matter basis than expanded diets to compensate for the greater loss in the gut.

A diet high in animal products generally supplies sufficient taurine, provided the taurine which is water soluble has not been leached out from the meat product. Taurine, unlike most of the other common amino acids, does not form a polypeptide, so the amount of protein is not an indication of the taurine content. Pet food manufacturers often add synthetic taurine to the diet to assure adequacy. Synthetic taurine is utilised at the same efficiency as naturally occurring taurine.

Essential Fatty Acids

Certain long chain polyunsaturated fatty acids are required in the diet of all animals, for the maintenance of healthy skin, reproduction and as precursors for the body to synthesise biologically active substances including prostaglandin, thromboxanes and leucotrienes. Felids have more stringent requirements for these essential fatty acids than dogs and other mammals. There are two families of essential fatty acids designated according to the position of the first double bond as either *n*-3 and *n*-6 or omega-3 and omega-6. More of the *n*-6 than the *n*-3 fatty acids are needed in the diet, as the *n*-6 fatty acid linoleate is required to prevent water loss from the body. The requirement for *n*-6 fatty acids of dogs can be met solely by linoleic acid which, by chain elongation and desaturation, can be converted to arachidonic acid. Cats also require linoleate, but in addition also need arachidonic acid in the diet. Cats are able to elongate fatty acids, but cannot undertake the critical desaturation step for the production of arachidonate. Arachidonic acid occurs only in animal tissue and is absent from plants. This is another example of the cats need for animal products in the diet, and supports the thesis that cats have evolved as strict carnivores.

Food Types

Commercial foods for kittens are prepared as canned, semi-moist and dry or expanded diets. Semi-moist diets preserved with propylene glycol are not recommended as this compound leads to the formation of Heinz bodies in the kitten's erythrocytes. Kittens will eat expanded diets prepared for adult cats as they have quite well developed dentition, but the smaller kibble size of kitten expanded foods makes them easier to eat. The acceptability of expanded diets for kittens can be improved by moistening especially by adding some warm water to a canned diet and pouring it over the dry food.

While there are specially formulated diets for kittens, adult diets (other than special low calorie or veterinary diets) with an all life stage claim are capable of giving excellent growth in kittens.

Feeding Regimen

Kittens do not open their eyes until about 10 days old and start to explore beyond the nest when they are about 3 weeks of age. Up until this time they are dependent entirely on the milk of the queen and have no need for external sources of food or water. Kittens when suckling should increase their body weight by about 10g per day so by 10 days of age they should have doubled their body weight (Figures 5.7 and 5.8).

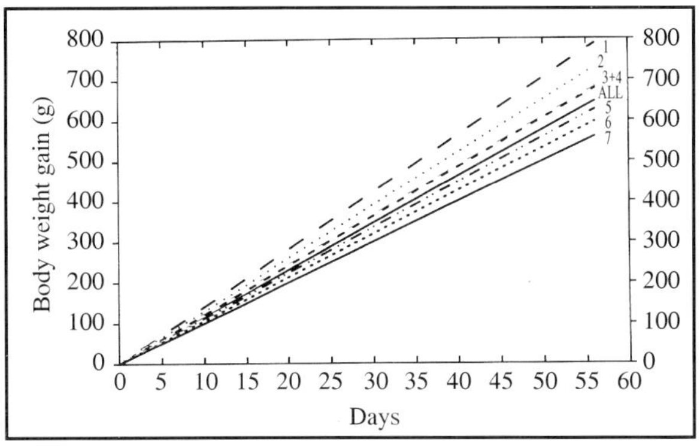

Figure 5.7: *Weight gain of kittens from queens fed canned diets (linear).*

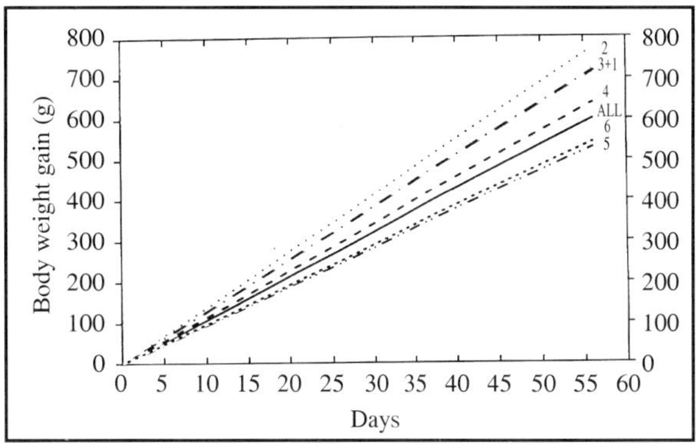

Figure 5.8: *Weight gain of kittens from queens fed expanded diets (linear).*

Once kittens begin taking food beyond queen's milk, the food should be available to the kittens at all times. If canned food or moistened expanded food is fed, the uneaten residue should be discarded at least twice daily and replaced with fresh food. The intake of solid food increases with age such that by 6 weeks of age kittens may be weaned. Some post-weaning growth depression is likely to occur at this age in large litters, whereas if weaning is delayed to 8 weeks there is generally no growth depression at weaning. Queens if not separated from their kittens will often allow them to suckle after 8 weeks of age. Unlike puppies, where overfeeding in the growing phase can predispose to adult obesity, kittens can have unrestricted access to food, as cats do not have the same tendency for development of obesity as dogs.

Kittens generally have difficulty eating from food bowls used for adult cats. Food for kittens should be given in shallow dishes that do not readily tip over when the kitten walks on them. Water should also be available in a shallow dish at all times especially if an expanded food is being given to the kittens or they are to be weaned on to an expanded diet.

Orphaned Kittens

The most satisfactory method of rearing orphaned kittens is to cross foster them to a lactating queen. The lactating queen not only supplies milk for the kittens, but also warmth and takes care of their toilet needs. Queens lick the perineal region of kittens to stimulate urination and defecation. In the absence of a queen this stimulus can be provided by stroking the perineal region with a soft moistened cloth or paper towel. While queens readily accept kittens born to another queen, unless the fostered kittens and the lactating queen's kittens are approximately the same size, there will be unequal competition for milk. Cross fostering of newborn kittens generally has a higher success rate if the queen is in early lactation and her kittens are old enough to be weaned and taken away from the queen to some place where she cannot have access to them.

A number of commercial queen milk substitutes based on modified cow's milk are available for the hand rearing of kittens. Cow's milk is a poor substitute for queen's milk as it is much lower in protein, fat and calories than queen's milk. The composition of queen's milk changes with lactation; colostrum has a higher content of protein and fat and lower lactose content than in the first week of lactation. From the first week of lactation, the protein and fat contents of queen's milk increases from about 6% to over 8% protein and from 7% to over 12% fat. In contrast, cow's milk contains about 3.3% protein and 3.8% fat. A substitute for queen's milk can be made by preparing full cream powdered milk at twice normal concentration. However, this milk contains about twice the lactose content of queen's milk and tends to promote diarrhoea.

Hand rearing of kittens requires keeping the kittens warm, feeding small meals frequently during the day, and stimulating defecation and urination. Newborn kittens should be fed warm milk from a special kitten bottle and teat at least four times daily. If diarrhoea develops, continue feeding, but reduce the concentration of milk solids while maintaining the same amount of water. At about 3 weeks of age kittens can be taught to lap warm milk from a shallow dish and introduced to commercial canned cat food. Smearing a small amount of food around the mouth of the kitten with a finger will often stimulate them to begin eating the food.

REFERENCES

Baines FM (1981). Milk substitutes and the hand rearing of orphaned puppies and kittens. *Journal of Small Animal Practice* **22,** 555-578.

Burger IM (1993). *The Waltham Book of Companion Animal Nutrition.* Pergamon Press, Oxford.

Hazewinkel HAW, Van den Brom WE, Van T'Klooster ATh, Voorhout G and Van Wees A (1991). Calcium metabolism in Great Dane dogs fed diets with various calcium and phosphorus levels. *Journal of Nutrition* **121,** S99-S106.

Johnson JV (1993). Protein requirements of dogs. *WALTHAM International Focus* **3**(1), 9-14.

Morris JG and Rogers QR (1994). Assessment of the nutritional adequacy of pet foods through the life cycle. *Journal of Nutrition* **124,** 2520S-2534S.

Nap RC, Hazewinkel HAW, Voorhout G, Van den Brom WE, Goedegebuure SA and Van'T Klooster ATh (1991). Growth and skeletal development in Great Dane pups fed different levels of protein intake. *Journal of Nutrition* **121,** S107-S113.

National Research Council (1985). *Nutrient Requirements of Dogs.* National Academy Press, Washington, DC.

National Research Council (1986). *Nutrient Requirements of Cats.* National Academy Press, Washington D.C.

CHAPTER SIX

Nutrition of Racing and Working Dogs

Dominique Grandjean

INTRODUCTION

Heavy work and competition induce both physiological and psychological stress in dogs, just as in men and horses. Accordingly, nutritional adaptation must take into account not only the specific energy requirement for muscular effort itself but also the nutritional needs of the animal's state of stress.

Thus, along with genetics, training and psychology, diet is one of the basic foundations of sporting performance. Of these four areas, diet is undoubtedly the one which has given rise to the greatest amount of scientific work in view of its potential economic and industrial repercussions.

The racing dog is a prime athlete and an understanding of it as a nutritional model has considerable potential implications for dogs who are pets.

In practice, food for racing and working dogs should meet the following criteria:

- provide a good source of energy in adequate amounts
- minimise the weight and volume of the intestinal bolus insofar as possible
- help to maintain a suitable state of hydration in the animal
- have a possible buffer effect on any metabolic acidification induced by running
- aid in optimising the result of other ergogenic actions (training etc.)
- make up for any physiological shortages brought about by stress.

METABOLIC BASES

In addition to having a direct effect on the nature and amount of energy requirements, muscle work also has a great influence on the nutritional balance of food intake via induced stress. We will restrict ourselves however, to fundamental or novel aspects of knowledge concerning the physiological bases of exercise in the dog.

Energy Mechanisms during Exercise

The chemical energy released during muscle contractions is derived solely from the high-energy bonds in adenosine triphosphate (ATP). Intracellular ATP is, or tends to be, decreased during exercise, and is then reconstituted instantaneously *in situ* by means of four processes:

1) transfer from phosphocreatine (PCr)
2) destruction of glycogen
3) oxidation of glucose
4) oxidation of fatty acids (Table 6.1).

The metabolic specificity of each type of exercise is determined by the relative contribution of each process in reconstituting the store of ATP.

Phosphagens

Phosphocreatine allows such rapid reconstitution of ATP within the muscle cell itself that ATP and phosphocreatine form an indissociable system known as the phosphagen system. This energy system predominates during supramaximal exercise not lasting more than a few seconds (jumping, start of a race). The bioavailability of muscle phosphagens is in no way affected by training or diet.

Glycogenolysis

ATP can also be regenerated by anaerobic glycogenolysis, which leads to the release of lactic acid. The rate of ATP renewal by anaerobic glycogenolysis represents only a third to one half of that generated by the phosphagen system. Consequently, the lactic anaerobic system can only create half the maximum power (work/time) generated by the alactic anaerobic system (phosphagens). The power induced by lactic anaerobiosis is probably at its peak after 3–10 seconds and remains predominant for 30 or so seconds at the most.

Oxidation of Glucose

Glucose is transported in the blood and then penetrates the muscle cells where it undergoes oxidation in the mitochondria. Its degree of oxidation depends largely on its ability to enter muscle cells, which is linked to the

Reaction		ATP / mol.		Respiratory Quotient
		Substrate	O_2	
Glycogen	→ Lactate	3	–	–
Glucose	→ Lactate	2	–	–
Lactate	→ $CO_2 + H_2O$	17	5.7	1.00
Glycogen	→ $CO_2 + H_2O$	37	6.2	1.00
Glucose	→ $CO_2 + H_2O$	36	6.0	1.00
FFA	→ $CO_2 + H_2O$	138	5.6	0.71
Acetoacetate	→ $CO_2 + H_2O$	23	5.7	0.73
ß hydroxybutyrate	→ $CO_2 + H_2O$	26	5.8	0.80

Table 6.1: *Production of ATP per unit of substrate consumed, depending on the metabolic pathway concerned.*

blood glucose level and corresponding regulatory hormones such as insulin, glucagon, growth hormone and cortisol. The rate of ATP renewal from the oxidation of glucose is approximately 50% of that obtained via anaerobic glycolysis, with consequently an equivalent power ratio.

The anaerobic metabolism of glucose, like that of glycogen, produces lactic acid; both have one important point in common, i.e. the conversion of pyruvate to lactate or acetyl-CoA. (This conversion is catalysed by a pyruvate dehydrogenase complex, an enzyme which is controlled by cofactors derived from thiamin, lipoic acid, pantothenic acid, pyridoxine and niacin.)

Glucose oxidation is probably the main source of muscle energy during any exercise lasting 60 seconds to a few minutes; it is enhanced by the ingestion of slowly metabolised carbohydrates and can be decreased by an intake with an excessive fat content or by fasting.

Lipid Oxidation

The fatty acids oxidised in the muscle cell are derived from long chain free fatty acids circulating in the plasma (free fatty acids or FFA). FFA enter the cells by a process of diffusion and consequently their entry is increased when their plasma concentration rises.

Once inside the muscle cells, carnitine plays a very important role in their transportation (linked to acylCoA) across the mitochondrial membrane. Intramitochondrial enzyme activity constitutes the final step prior to the beta-oxidation of fatty acids.

At the same time, FFA can be removed by the liver, converted into ketone bodies and released into the blood, with acetoacetate and ß-hydroxybutyrate subsequently being oxidised in muscle.

The oxidation of FFA acts as the principal energy source for muscle during lasting exercise which is low to moderate in intensity, i.e. approximately semimaximal. As with the oxidation of ketone bodies, the FFA oxidation is augmented by fasting, undernourishment and training, especially when the latter is conducted using nutrition with a high fat content.

Protein Catabolism

Branched-chain amino acids (leucine, isoleucine and valine) can supply 5–10% of oxidative energy to the muscles. Their amino groups are transferred to the pyruvate, forming alanine, and to glutamic acid, forming glutamine. Alanine and glutamine are released into the blood and then removed by the liver and used for glucose synthesis. In its turn, glucose is released into the blood and becomes available for intramuscular oxidation.

Roles of the Lactic Anaerobic Energy System

Lactates during Supramaximal Exercise

Supramaximal exercise implies the development of power exceeding that possible using oxidative systems (aerobiosis) during intense muscular exercise (as in racing greyhounds). In this case, anaerobic hypercatabolism of glycogen in muscle gives rise to the sudden, massive release of lactic acid which accumulates in muscle before passing into the blood.

In the greyhound, for example, hyperlactacidaemia occurs and can attain or exceed 14 (Wolter, 1986) or even 22mmol/litre (Grandjean, 1987). Under such conditions, lactic anaerobiosis is obviously largely predominant in supplying energy requirements to the muscle (Figure 6.1).

By evaluating the lactic acid produced and oxygen spared by anaerobic glycolysis, an energy equivalent of the lactates formed *in vivo* was determined in man (Margaria *et al.*, 1963) and found to be approximately 920kJ (220kcal) per gram of lactates formed.

The only available datum of this type relating to the dog was obtained in isolated gastrocnemius muscle perfused using the 'stop-flow' technique. The forma-

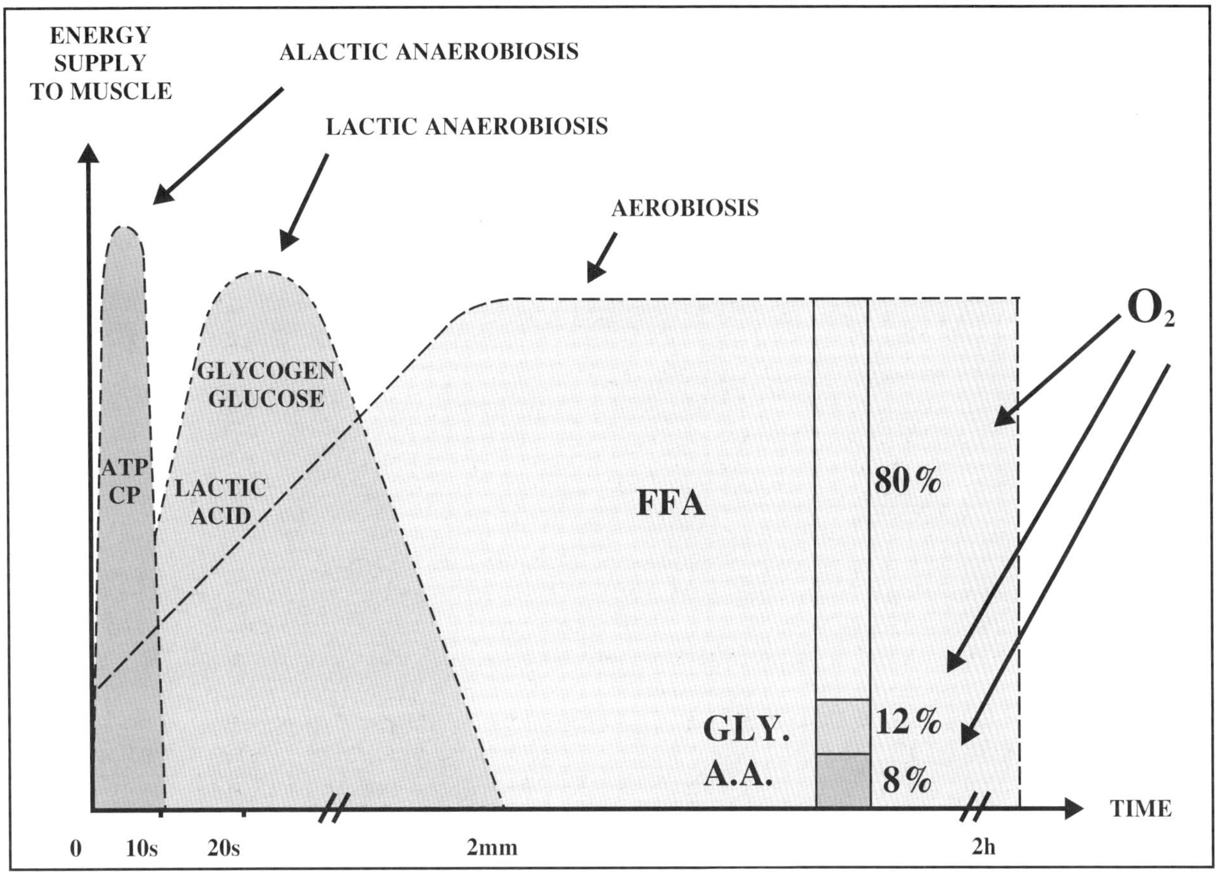

Figure 6.1: *Different sources of energy for muscle work.*

GLY. = glycogen; A.A. = amino acids.

tion of 1g of lactates in such a case corresponds to the release of 1038kJ (248kcal) (Cerretelli *et al.,* 1969), which is very similar to the result obtained in man.

This approach might prove to be of basic interest for the improved determination of quantitative energy requirements in dogs such as greyhounds. However, it has certain limitations:

- lactates generally reach their peak in the blood several minutes after the effort has been made and then drop exponentially, with a half-life of 15 minutes (Freminet, 1986) (Figure 6.1)
- during this type of exercise, there is a concentration gradient of lactates in the blood which cannot be considered as totally representative of the lactates produced by the system (Grandjean *et al.*, 1987; Freund and Zouloumian, 1981a, b).

Be that as it may, the accumulation of lactic acid has numerous adverse effects (Sahlin, 1983), including the following:

- inhibition of glycogenolysis and glycolysis
- inhibition of lipolysis
- induction of osmotic muscle oedema
- reduction of lactic acid influx into the muscle cells.

Concept of an Oxygen Debt

Muscles employ more energy than the aerobic system can provide during any intense, brief effort. During this period, it therefore builds up an energy debt which is known as the 'oxygen debt'. During the recovery phase, any oxygen supplied over and above maintenance needs is used to pay back the oxygen debt. It allows glycogen to be re-synthesised from lactates, including the energy lost during the process, the yields being less than one.

Nevertheless, it should be remembered that a considerable portion of the lactates is oxidised for energy production during recovery and thus is not taken into account during evaluation of the oxygen debt, which is consequently underestimated. In overall terms, the two processes compensate for one another so that the debt repaid is usually identical to the debt incurred.

More recently, the lactic oxygen debt was evaluated on the basis of lactates accumulated in the blood and the oxidative energy thereby spared (Rieu, 1988). Analysis showed that, disregarding the theory of multiple distribution, blood lactates accounted for the sparing of 3.3ml of oxygen per kilogram of body weight.

Using the maximal lactacidaemias observed in Greyhounds as a basis (15-20mmol/litre), the lactic oxygen debt can be estimated at between 1.7 and 2.2 litres of oxygen in a Greyhound weighing 30 kg. Consequently, if a mean thermal coefficient of

20.9kJ(5 kcal)/litre of oxygen and a mean muscle energy yield of 22% are accepted, the lactic anaerobic energy expenditure (LAEE) of a 30kg Greyhound during a race can be estimated as follows:

$$\text{LAEE} = \frac{2\ (1\ O_2) \times 20.9\ \text{kJ}(5\text{kcal}) \times 100}{22} = 190\text{kJ}\ (46\text{kcal})$$

This would correspond to approximately 2.7% of the maintenance energy requirement of such a dog.

Fate of Lactic Acid following Exercise

As we have seen, after exercise, the body can recover the energy used in oxidising lactates by subtracting it from the utilisation of other energy molecules (glucose, lipids etc.); the energy required for the re-synthesis of glycogen from lactates is an additional metabolic load. It seems that lactic acid is oxidised following exertion when there is little accumulation and when the metabolic level during the recovery phase remains greater than during maintenance (Cerretelli, 1980).

In such a case, the body has no oxygen debt to repay (Haralambie, 1981); this includes cases where mixed aerobic-anaerobic effort is involved, as in dogs which perform in the ring and trials of agility. Conversely, when there is considerable accumulation of lactic acid (as with racing greyhounds) and recovery is passive, an appreciable portion of the lactates is removed for re-synthesis into glycogen, and the oxygen debt is relatively high.

Greyhounds: Respective Contributions of the Various Metabolisms

We have seen that three distinct metabolic pathways are closely interwoven during any expenditure of effort, with one type becoming predominant, depending on the type of exertion involved (Table 6.2). The racing Greyhound is a model sprinter worthy of study since it demonstrates the differences between the three pathways.

Of the total capacity of the phosphagen system (alactic anaerobiosis) 50% is used in Greyhound racers, thereby supplying approximately 8.4kJ (2kcal), whereas the lactic anaerobic route provides almost 209kJ (50kcal). Recent work (Meyer *et al.*, 1980; Serresse *et al.*, 1988) showed that 28-30% of the energy was derived from the aerobic pathway (Figure 6.2), even during very brief exercise lasting 30 seconds.

By integrating this fact into the case under discussion, aerobiosis is thus seen to contribute 96kJ (23kcal) to a global expenditure of energy related to running of close to 314kJ (75kcal), i.e. 4.5% of the maintenance energy needs of a Greyhound (Figure 6.3). Due to the lack of specific data, this must of course be considered as an approximation.

Roles of the Aerobic Energy System

When exercise is prolonged (more than a few minutes) and of moderate intensity (50 to 70% of the maximum oxygen consumption, still poorly quantified in the dog), aerobiosis becomes the system used in covering muscular energy requirements (Figure 6.1) (Grandjean and Paragon, 1986; Grandjean, 1987; Wolter, 1989). During an endurance test, fatty acids, derived from tissue lipolysis in considerable amounts (Gazzola *et al.*, 1984), form the principal energy source of muscle cells when:

- the animal undergoes suitable basic training
- food intake has a high fat content
- the free plasma fatty acid level is high.

Prolonged muscle work is therefore responsible for a marked increase in FFA (Brezezinska *et al.*, 1980; Issekutz *et al.*, 1965; Issekutz, 1979; Rodahl, 1964), the increase occurring earlier and more effectively during cold weather. In fact, adipose

Sporting type	Alactic anaerobiosis	Lactic aerobiosis	Aerobiosis
Jumping	+++	+	#0
Short attack	++	++	+
Greyhound racing	+	+++++	++
Agility	≈0	++++	++
Ring competition	≈0	+++	+++
Field trial	≈0	++	+++
Newfoundland	≈0	+	++++
Tracking/Campaign	≈0	≈0	++++
Flock	≈0	≈0	+++
Hunting	≈0	≈0	++++
Sled dog racing	≈0	≈0[1]	+++++

Table 6.2: *Relative intensities of various energy metabolic pathways called into play during exercise in dogs.*

1 *apart from speed racing: + to ++*

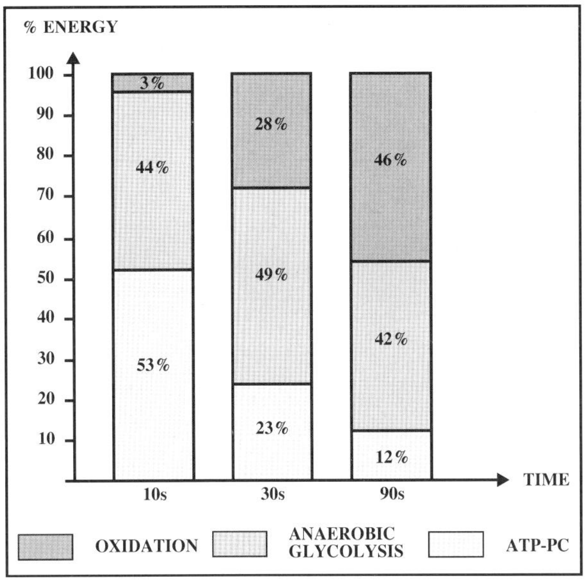

Figure 6.2: Estimated respective contribution of the three energy metabolic pathways during three short-term exercise tests (expressed as per cent of the total work provided) (Segers, 1969).

tissue supplies the dog with the major part of its energy for combating the cold. At low temperatures, blood levels of FFA can be multiplied by 1.88 (Vincent Falquet *et al.*, 1972): the renewal of these acids and their rate of oxidation are increased 4.5 and 8.3 times, respectively, whilst at the same time the relative participation of FFA in carbon dioxide formation rises from 36 to 64%. This observation is confirmed in Huskies where an increase of close to 50% is noted in blood concentrations of lipids during winter (Wolter *et al.*, 1983).

Apart from supplying energy to muscle cells, the aerobic system thus makes it possible for full advantage to be taken of the pre-existing metabolic adaptation and above all to spare the animal's glycogen reserves. The exhaustion of glycogen reserves is the chief factor limiting any continued effort.

Metabolic Fatigue

The following metabolic considerations are among those which determine fatigue:

- substances whose concentrations drop as a result of exercise (ATP, glycogen)
- substances which accumulate during exercise (lactates, hydrogen ions).

The transition of lactic acid from muscle into blood is enhanced by the rapid circulation of blood and by the presence of bicarbonates in the blood. The accumulation of lactates in the blood (hyperlactataemia) is traditionally associated with anaerobic metabolism and an oxygen debt. It is not restricted to dogs making short, intensive efforts.

In fact, hyperlactataemia associated with hyperglycaemia can be found in Huskies, the combination of the two indicating the animal's excitement and the fatigue that it induces by encouraging anaerobic glucose metabolism. On the basis of such observations, it is therefore recommended that Huskies (and any other dogs which have to contribute a relatively prolonged effort - such as ring, tracking, field and hunting dogs) should be kept under quiet conditions before competing. This is, in fact, the opposite of what usually occurs.

Muscle glycogen is another major determining factor in fatigue. Its concentration may be appreciably increased before a competition by loading with carbohydrate (Blom, 1982; Lacour, 1983), or even by the implementation of dissociated diets (3 days without carbohydrates in the diet to lower glycogen stores, then 2 days with carbohydrates). These are of no value in the dog since they increase the risk of muscle disease (Grandjean and Paragon, 1987).

At the same time, it is known that the oxidation of fatty acids spares muscle glycogen, especially after long metabolic adaptation to fatty acids. Consequently, rival nutritional strategies which consist of

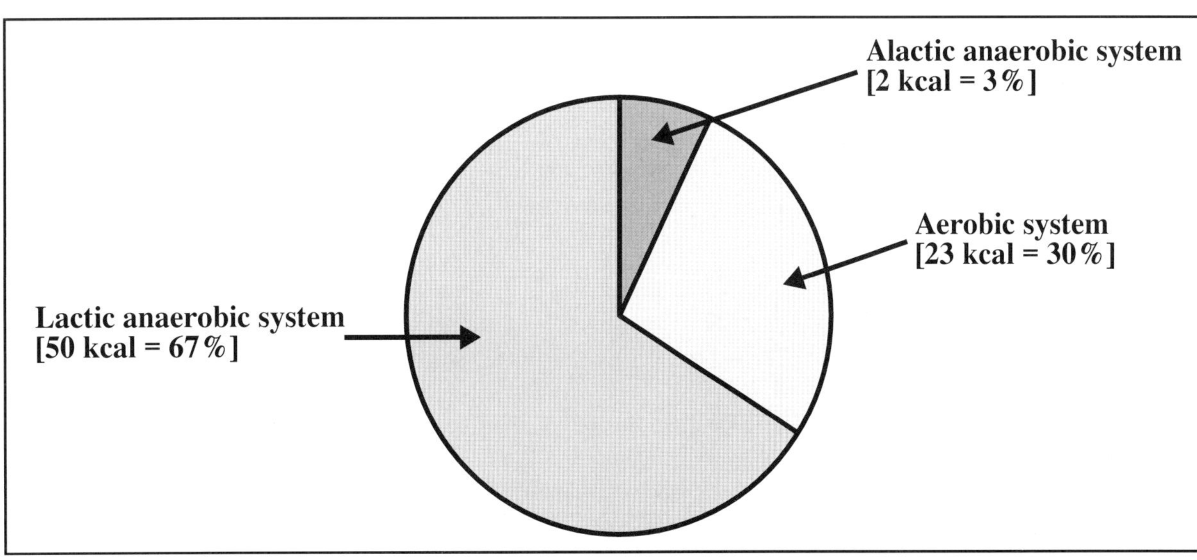

Figure 6.3: Estimated respective contribution of the three energy systems during Greyhound racing.

carbohydrate loading and fat adaptation must be adjusted (in terms of their respective intake) to the various intensity levels and duration of the exercise concerned.

Power *versus* Speed

As in men and horses, a balance is created between power and speed during exercise in dogs and affects the choice of nutrition. The relationship between power and speed varies as a function of a certain number of external factors related to the nature of the ground, the corresponding tractive force, speed and air resistance.

In the case of dogs which exceed 50km/h, their speed varies in proportion to the square root of the power (Kronfeld and Ferrante, 1990) and this corresponds to the metabolic considerations previously discussed. Thus, if the power developed is doubled, the speed is multiplied by 1.4 (approximately the square root of 2); when there is a three-fold increase in power, the speed is multiplied by a factor of 1.7. The power developed - and hence the type of metabolism involved - can be assessed from an analysis of an animal's racing speed.

Given the various types of competition available (speed, middle distance, long distance), the dog sled gives a typical illustration of these theoretical concepts.

Sled dogs trained for endurance can keep up an 'Iditarod' type of trot (approximately 16km/h) for 10-14 hours per day for several days running; this is only possible when their diet consists predominantly of lipids. It is therefore reasonable to assume that the preferred energy source in such dogs is the oxidation of fatty acids and to assign it a power factor of 1 (compared to muscle in man, this is equivalent to approximately 0.25mmol of ATP/kg/s).

Glucose can in turn be oxidised and, as previously described, generate twice as much developed power (power factor 2), and consequently increase the speed by a factor of 1.4, i.e. approximately 23km/h. This speed corresponds to a moderate gallop or a rapid trot which good dogs can keep up for several hours per day for several days (middle distance races of the 'Alpirod' type).

As for glycogen utilisation, it ensures a yield twice that obtained from the oxidation of glucose in terms of developed power. It is used by sled dogs when racing at speeds above 30km/h (32-34km/h for the best teams). This speed is maintained by good teams in speed trials carried out over two or three legs of 25-35km.

Finally, the phosphagens can come into play and generate two to three times as much power as that released by anaerobic glycolysis. This enables sled dogs to attain maximum speeds close to 45km/h for 30 seconds, or even peaks of 50-55km/h for a few seconds.

This highlights the fact that, in practice, the three clearly distinct theoretical energy metabolic pathways are superimposed on one another and this must be taken into account when deciding on nutritional requirements. Strictly aerobic metabolism under pure endurance conditions can give way to aerobic -anaerobic metabolism once the trial decreases in length (but the zone of aerobic-anaerobic transition, corresponding to the appearance of the anaerobic threshold, is still ill-defined in the dog), or even to the enhancement of lactic (glycogen) or alactic (phosphagen) anaerobic catabolism during peaks in speed in so-called sprint racing.

Accordingly, it becomes possible to feed and train canine athletes so as to improve oxidative yields and the required balance between the use of fatty acids or glucose as energy fuels. Various similar methods can be used to increase the storage of glycogen in muscle and anaerobic glycolysis. But there is currently no known method of modifying the metabolic behaviour and stores of phosphagen.

SPECIFIC NUTRITIONAL APPROACH

In outline, there are three groups of factors which affect the nutritional needs of racing dogs:

- the provoked energy expenditure which must be envisaged: this is highly variable in quantitative terms but basic in qualitative terms
- stress, when this is induced by training and competition and thus gives rise to the requisite nutritional adaptation
- dehydration, which can be avoided to an appreciable extent by suitable nutrition.

Specific nutritional recommendations can be defined on the basis of such data, whilst bearing in mind that the only scientific data currently available relate to Greyhounds (sprinter prototype) and Huskies (prolonged effort prototype).

Quantitative Change in Energy Requirements

The daily energy requirements of racing dogs depend on numerous variables and are still sometimes difficult to predict; each owner's aim must primarily be to sustain the dog's in-form weight by weighing each dog every week where possible and consequently adjusting the amount of food provided. However, there is a wide difference between racing Greyhounds and Huskies and an approach can be made on the basis of a certain amount of data.

Racing Greyhounds

We have already seen that the strict energy requirements for a race lasting 30 seconds can be calculated by estimating the oxygen debt incurred (approximately 314kJ, 75kcal).

For any given muscle effort, the energy expenditure related to movement is independent of speed for non-aerodynamic forces, and dependent on the square of the speed for air resistance; it includes the energy required for the body's initial acceleration from zero to racing speed.

Insofar as a 30kg Greyhound measuring 72cm and a reference male human of 70kg and 175cm in this model have an equivalent weight:height ratio (close to 0.4kg/cm), the proposed equation would, by extrapolation, give an energy expenditure for a 480m race of approximately 293kJ (70kcal).

In other words, a Greyhound taking part in a race over a distance of 480m at a speed of 17m/s would correspond to an expenditure of energy of approximately 293kJ (70kcal) in this model: this is very similar to the evaluation that we made and represents 4.1% of the ME requirement.

However, the following factors which affect the animal's energy requirements must be incorporated into this theoretical approach:

- number of races during the day (Griess, 1987); if each race represents 4-5% of the ME requirements (approximately 7537kJ (1800kcal) on the basis of 552kJ (132kcal) ME/kg$^{0.75}$), energy needs will obviously be increased if there are two or even three races per day, together with placement in the starting box. Such needs should not exceed 110-120% of the strict maintenance requirements during periods of competition;
- climatic conditions; a drop from 15°C to 8°C in room temperature causes a 25% increase in metabolisable energy (ME) requirements in the dog (Blaza, 1982). In hot climates, stores of glycogen appear to be more rapidly depleted when the body is at work (Costill, 1981); this is accounted for by the appreciable energy cost entailed in thermoregulation (Manore and Leklem, 1988).

Thus, the energy requirements for a given dog and a given effort (racing Greyhound) range from 628 to 796kJ (150 to 190kcal) ME/kg$^{0.75}$.

Sled Dogs

Huskies tend to be distinctly different from other types of racing dogs as far as changes in their energy requirements are concerned. Firstly, these needs are lower for any given weight under maintenance conditions, and this is especially true in the case of Siberian Huskies (418 to 461kJ (100 to 110kcal) ME/kg$^{0.75}$ weight compared with 561kJ (132 kcal) for other breeds). This is undoubtedly due to an improved metabolic energy yield and also to decreased expenditure on thermoregulation because of thermal insulation by the animal's fur and a body temperature slightly lower than normal.

Period	Energy Requirements (in kcal ME)
Maintenance	1000-1200
Training (5 to 8 km/day)	1300-1400
Training (10 to 20 km/day)	1700-1800
Training (30 km/day)	2000-2400
Speed racing	1400-1800
Long distance race (Alpirod)	2500-3000
Iditarod	7000-8000

Table 6.3: *Changes in energy requirements of a Husky in harness (a dog weighing 20kg).*

During training and racing, energy requirements alter in accordance with the type and length of exercise involved, and the external temperature. Examples of such changes are shown in Table 6.3.

A more precise approach should consider that the total daily energy requirement is the total of: maintenance energy requirement (MER) + thermoregulation energy requirement (TER) + racing energy requirement (RER) (Grandjean and Paragon, 1992; 1993a, b).

Depending on the type of race, temperature and distance, the daily energy requirement of a racing sled dog might change from 12560 to over 37680kJ ME (3000 to 9000kcal).

Other Dogs

One hour of work leads to approximately 10% increase in maintenance energy requirements, and this may give rise to a 40 to 50% increase in energy intake for one day of work or sport. Variations in external temperature seem to have a greater impact on energy requirements in these other dogs compared to the Husky, which appears to have a broader area of thermal neutrality. This is illustrated in Figure 6.4.

Qualitative Aspects of Energy Requirements

The quality of the energy supplied to dogs during a work period is of primary importance, and hence **optimum energy** criteria have been defined for racing dogs. Apart from the very nature of the nutrients employed, the following two qualitative considerations must be borne in mind:

1) The energy must be readily and rapidly available at the site of use (muscle cells);
2) The balance of the energy components must be such that their combustion is accomplished with maximum efficiency, minimum waste, and without risk of metabolic blockade.

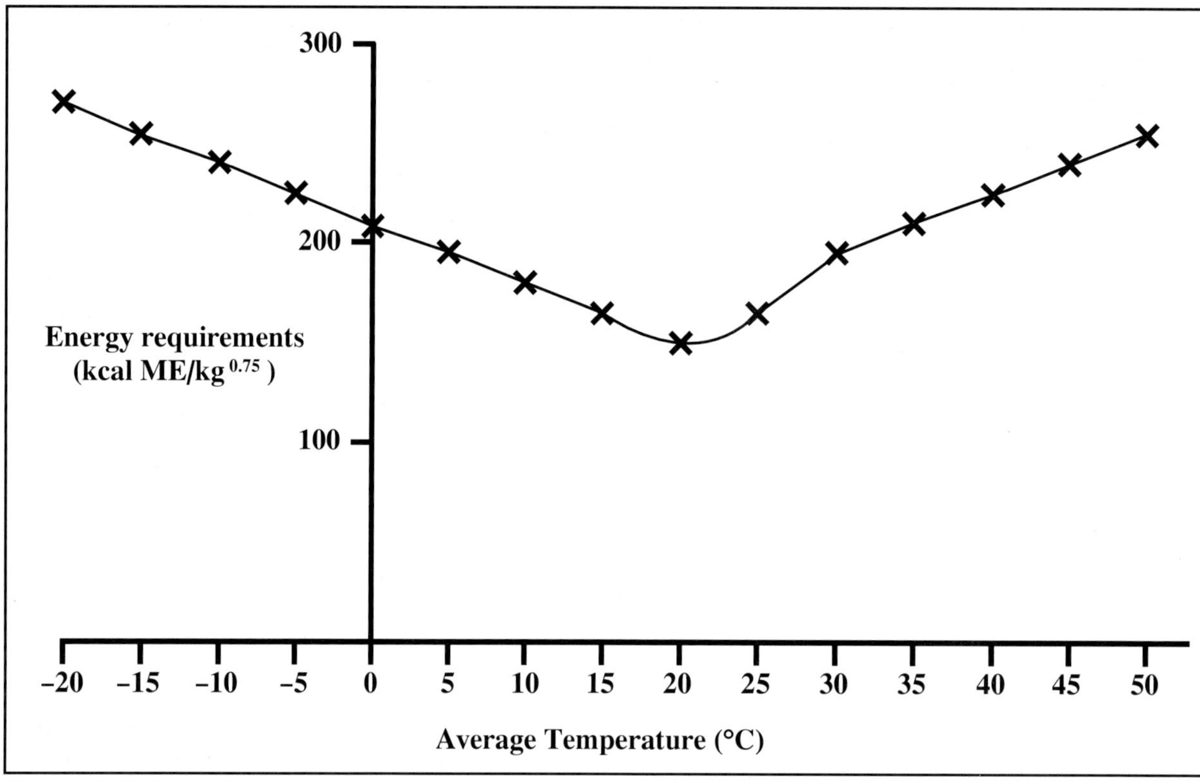

Figure 6.4: *Variations in energy requirements as a function of temperature (a dog working for one hour).*

Energy Availability

Primarily, energy must be digested and then metabolised if it is to arrive at its final site of utilisation. Given the alterations in gastrointestinal motility and physiological adaptations that are encountered in racing dogs, it is therefore important to consider the behaviour of various groups of nutrients which provide energy, i.e. fat (approximately 35.5kJ (8.5kcal) ME/g), nitrogen free extract (approximately 14.7kJ (3.5kcal) ME/g) and protein (approximately 14.7kJ (3.5kcal) ME/g).

Gastrointestinal Utilisation of Energy

The acceleration in **gastrointestinal transit time** brought about by exercise must be taken into account so that the food energy is usefully employed.

First of all, the **gastric transit time** must be optimised. There is a predisposition to diarrhoea caused by poor pre-digestion of proteins and accentuated by stress when this time is too short, while gastric stasis which may encourage vomiting and gastric torsion.

While no reliable scientific study has been made of the problem as yet, experience shows that the physical form of the food provided affects the results. The best results are obtained in racing dogs when dry, extruded foods are lightly rehydrated 10 minutes or so before meals. Kibbles which keep their initial shape after rehydration and do not become souplike are desirable.

The **digestibility** of food sources must also be considered. In fact, the time available for gastrointestinal enzyme attack is limited when the rate of transit is increased.

As far as starches are concerned (the predominant share of nitrogen free extract), digestion often levels off since amylase activity is sometimes mediocre in the dog, especially in working breeds such as German Shepherd and Nordic Dogs.

In the intestine, the rapidity with which amylase attacks starches depends essentially on the plant origin of the starches.

It is vital for the starch sources used in racing dogs to be highly digestible. In fact, compared to fats with a calorific value practically two and a half times higher, starches notably increase the volume of the food intake in animals requiring high energy levels for racing purposes. But even a low increase in the volume ingested results in lowered digestibility and wetter faeces (Paul and Issekutz, 1967).

In addition, carbohydrate digestion can alter the absorption of other ingredients in the food, such as proteins, certain electrolytes and water. Poor starch digestibility reduces precaecal and total digestibility of proteins in the dog, while at the same time a sharp drop in sodium and potassium absorption is observed (Metcalf, 1985; Kienzle *et al.*, 1990). Finally, a highly negative factor in racing dogs is that water turnover in the intestine is also altered by the ingestion of poorly digestible carbohydrates producing an increase in ileocaecal water flow (Mieir, 1987), and an increase in hydration of faeces.

The dog can digest large amounts of **proteins**, especially those of animal origin. Whilst gastrointestinal problems caused by protein intake are relatively rare in ordinary dogs, they can be more extensive in racing dogs.

The consumption of proteins which are resistant to pancreatic proteases but biodegradable (scleroproteins in feathers, collagen in tendons and udders, inadequately cooked eggs etc.) may lead to microbial abnormalities in the intestine which compromise the overall digestibility of the food intake, increase faecal volume and cause diarrhoea.

Lipids constitute, in most cases, the preferential source of energy in racing dogs. They are extremely palatable and highly digestible and well tolerated by the dog. At this point, it should be noted that two groups of fatty acids have a qualitative advantage in digestive terms in racing dogs:

- short or medium chain fatty acids (coconut, copra and palm fats etc.) whose digestion is facilitated since it occurs passively and without the participation of bile salts
- essential fatty acids of the *n*-3 series (basically purified fish oils) which play a part in maintaining the integrity of the intestinal mucosa, due to their local anti-inflammatory properties (Grandjean, 1991a).

Since energy must be made easily available and rapidly convertible by the body during exercise, it is essential to use low bulk **highly digestible foods** which produce little faeces and which have been prepared bearing the factors mentioned previously in mind. In simple terms, the optimum volume of faeces is 40–50g per 100g of ingested dry matter for a racing dog. This objective is difficult to obtain with home-prepared food and is still rarely achieved in the case of industrially prepared foods.

Metabolic Fate of the Energy

Hormonal factors play a major role in the mobilisation and utilisation of various energy substrates by muscle cells.

In brief, hormonal factors act either at membrane receptors by stimulating the production of a second hormonal messenger, or by crossing the membrane and binding to a cytosol receptor. The first mode of action is a modification of the activity of certain enzyme or other reactions (a short-term process), whereas the second increases the amount of enzyme and only has effects over the longer term.

All the hormonal messages are called into play during physical exercise, the degree of variation depending on two factors; intensity and duration of exercise (Figure 6.5). It should be noted that the drop in serum insulin and increase in glucagon and catecholamines during exercise are all factors capable of increasing the production and utilisation of carbohydrate reserves, with the mobilisation of adipocyte lipid reserves only controlled by an increase in plasma catecholamines and a drop in serum insulin levels (Gollnick *et al.*, 1970).

While the mobilisation of lipid reserves from adipose tissue is subject to control by several hormones, the utilisation of free plasma fatty acids (FFA) appears to be subject to the effect of relation-

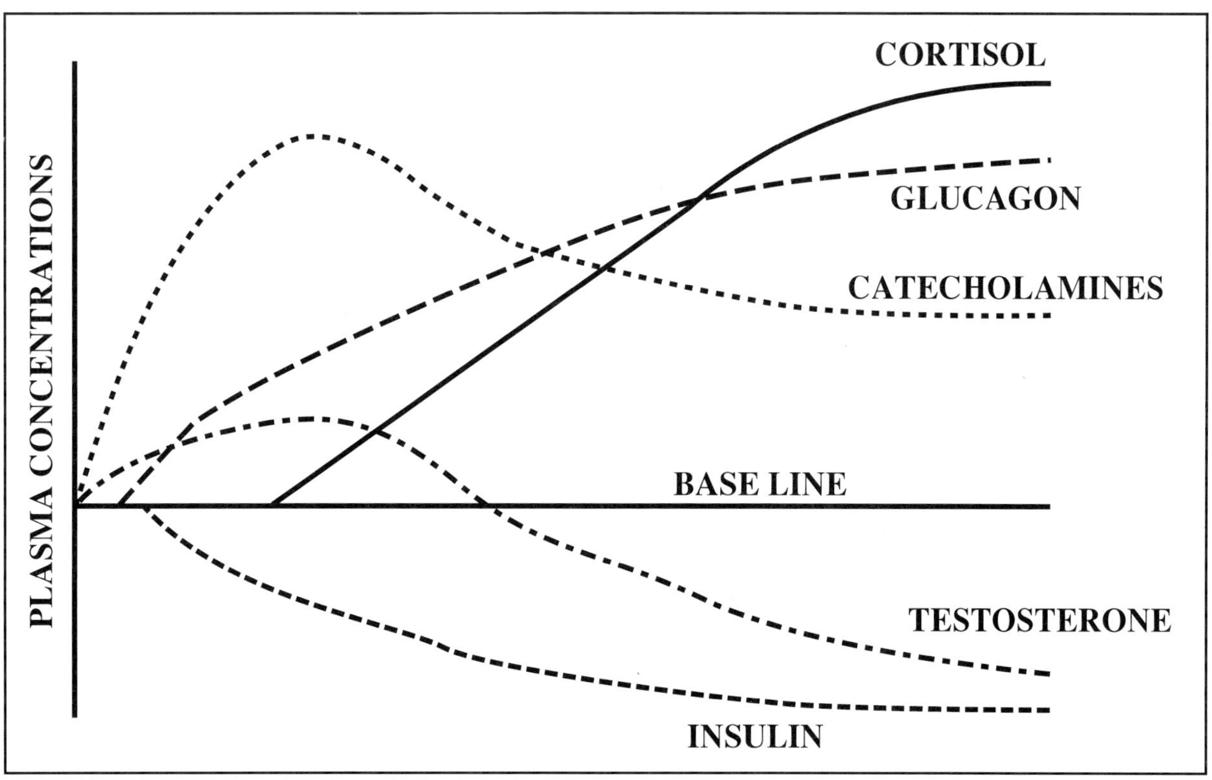

Figure 6.5: *Changes in plasma concentrations of various hormones involved in metabolic regulation as a function of muscle exercise time (Wolter, 1989).*

ships between metabolites which are relatively independent of hormones. FFA penetrate into muscle cells by diffusion and their oxidation in the cell is controlled by enzyme stages whose activity is regulated by the activity of other metabolic pathways, such as glycolysis.

Endocrine and enzyme adaptive data must be taken into account for **energy optimisation**. An excessive supply of starches and sugars to racing dogs can aggravate glycogen overstorage, promoting lactic anaerobiosis during exercise accompanied by excessive lactate production. In addition, the distribution of rapidly metabolised sugars before training or races will cause marked secondary hypoglycaemia at the start of the exercise due to a rebound hyperinsulin reaction.

During prolonged exercise, the food energy supply will be derived mainly from fats. But the fats must be incorporated progressively into the food intake for reasons of hormone and enzyme adaptation as previously mentioned. Under these conditions, high levels of fats can produce a considerable improvement in the performance of dogs during endurance exercise, whilst at the same time reducing the volume of the daily food intake and limiting the impact of stress-induced diarrhoea (Grandjean, 1983; Wolter *et al.*, 1983).

Factors Determining Variations in the Energy Yield

The energy supplied to dogs must be qualitatively adjusted to the required physiological objective and the type of energy metabolism involved. Subsequently, the muscle energy yield can be considerably reduced by an accumulation of metabolic waste or by metabolic blockade.

An excessive accumulation of lactates in blood can hamper tissue lipolysis and consequently reduce the efficacy of aerobic metabolism (Spitzer, 1974; Grandjean and Mateo, 1985), while the resulting release of protons causes a drop in intramuscular pH which hinders all energy reactions. An accumulation of extracellular potassium can further aggravate these phenomena (Haralambie, 1981).

Similarly, the nitrogenous hypercatabolism due to exercise may exaggerate the release of ammonia and increase muscle fatigue (Wolter, 1989). A collapse in blood glucose or deficiency in glucose-forming amino acids (insufficiency in protein intake) can, during severe endurance exercise, lead to actual metabolic blockade resulting from the accumulation of ketone bodies. However, this risk is minor in the dog, given its capacity for putting ketone bodies to good use in energy production.

Adaptation of the qualitative energy intakes should therefore offset these risks, especially since certain ergogenic nutrients improve the muscle energy yield:

- L-Carnitine, which transports long chain fatty acids across the mitochondrial membrane
- Fatty acids of the *n*-3 series, which improve erythrocyte deformability and the permeability of the membrane to oxygen (Guezennec, 1982)
- Arginine, an amino acid which prevents hyperammonaemia
- Vitamin B complex, which plays a recognised, vital role in the correct functioning of the cell energy mechanism.

Application to Greyhounds

Greyhounds are genetically selected for their sprinting performance and therefore have a much greater proportion of rapidly contracting muscle fibres than other breeds (Guy and Snow, 1981) (Table 6.4). Because of this, glycogen stores in muscle and the liver constitute an important determining factor in the performance of such dogs.

The glycogen concentration is easily affected by food and exercise or a combination of the two. When the glycogen concentration in muscle drops, the lactate levels in muscle and blood following exercise are lower than when the basal glycogen content is higher (Heigenhauser *et al.*, 1983; Serresse *et al.*, 1988). In the past, such a relationship led to the introduction of dissociated diets in man designed to produce a tran-

	GREYHOUNDS	CROSSBREEDS	FOXHOUNDS
Number of animals	6	5	4
M. deltoïdius	99.8 ± 0.3	74.4 ± 3.0	56.6 ± 6.8
M. triceps brachii caput longum	94.2 ± 5.4	77.2 ± 2.7	64.9 ± 4.4
M. vastus lateralis	96.6 ± 1.7	61.4 ± 10.2	80.7 ± 8.2
M. gluteus medius	97.4 ± 0.7	68.6 ± 5.6	65.3 ± 4.9
M. biceps femoris	88.6 ± 2.2	67.2 ± 1.3	63.0 ± 1.5
M. semitendinosus	98.9 ± 0.8	85.3 ± 2.6	69.6 ± 6.8

Table 6.4: *Percentage of muscle fibres with high myosin ATPase activity (rapid contraction fibres) in various groups of muscles in Greyhounds, cross-breeds and Foxhounds (Guy and Snow, 1981).*

sient glycogen overload (Hultman *et al.*, 1971; Philip, 1984; Evans and Hughes, 1985): an exclusive dietary carbohydrate overload follows glycogen depletion induced by a carbohydrate-deficient diet and intensive exercise, leading to re-synthesis of stores of glycogen at a higher concentration than initially (Topliff *et al.*, 1983; Topliff *et al.*, 1985). The massive ingestion of carbohydrates causes the release of insulin, thereby making more glucose available for the purposes of glycogenesis and increasing the intracellular concentration of glucose-6-phosphate (the allosteric activator of glycogen synthetase) (Ivy, 1983). Such excessive accumulation of glycogen followed by rapid destruction and subsequent accumulation of lactic acid as a result of exercise causes rhabdomyolysis and damage to cell membranes (Kronfeld, 1973; Lindholm *et al.*, 1974).

It is preferable to prevent such excessive lactic acidosis by avoiding glycogen overload in muscle: this is achieved by providing the animal with specific consistently balanced food, in amounts which are suited to its needs. The use of pure carbohydrates should thus be limited and the administration of sucrose and other rapidly metabolised sugars prohibited.

Warming-up before the race is important, in the same way that active recovery is vital in promoting the aerobic combustion of accumulated lactates. At this stage, optimum training should take place at the animal's anaerobic threshold, thus contributing to an improvement in aerobic capacity (which covers practically 30% of energy expenditure during racing).

Consequently, the **optimum distribution of dietary energy sources** in Greyhounds should be as follows:

- carbohydrates: 40–45%
- fats: 20–25%
- proteins: 35%.

The value of short or medium chain fatty acids might ideally represent 25% of the Greyhound's daily fat intake (Grandjean, 1991b); on the other hand it has been suggested that these medium chain fatty acids may cause vomiting and anorexia if given in large amounts (Hill, 1995).

Application to Huskies

The Husky is the prototype for endurance racing and its energy metabolism is geared to aerobiosis. However, given the changes occurring in this sport and the different types of competition encountered, there are different approaches in their nutrition:

- during **long distance races** (Iditarod, Yukon Quest, Beargrease, etc.), the dogs run at a rapid trot or even a limited gallop, probably between 30 to 40% of their VO_2 max. (maximal oxygen consumption), using a totally aerobic energy metabolism
- during **middle distance races**, or races in stages (Alpirod, etc.), the teams can momentarily increase their speed (in the zone of aerobic–anaerobic transition in energy terms) and exceed their anaerobic threshold for short periods
- during **speed racing**, (7–20km per leg), particularly in small categories or Scandinavian pulka, lactic anaerobiosis can play a significant role, estimated at 10–15% coverage of total energy expenditure.

As the length of the race increases, the fat content of the food intake assumes increasing importance at the expense of residual starches.

In overall terms, carbohydrate oxidation covers only 10–15% of the energy supply to muscles in huskies, whereas free plasma fatty acids account for 70–90% (Hultman *et al.*, 1971; Mutch and Bannister, 1983).

Kronfeld and Dunlap (1977) studied food intakes containing (on the basis of metabolisable energy) 0, 23 or 38% carbohydrate (CHO) and 61, 45 or 34% fats, respectively and demonstrated:

- that there were no pathological disturbances in harnessed Huskies fed on the first of these diets (high fat and CHO-deficient)
- that there was an improvement in endurance performance at the same time, combined with a better response by the body, both in haematological and metabolic terms.

Moreover, the same author had carried out unpublished trials in 1971 whose failure had led him to permanently abandon high CHO diets ('carbohydrate loading') in Huskies (Kronfeld *et al.*, 1981). In addition, work conducted by Hammel *et al.* (1977) using the same diets showed that that there was a greater capacity for mobilising body fatty acids in dogs receiving food containing 0% CHO and 61% fats. This obviously confers a certain advantage on such dogs during prolonged effort when there is a predominance of FFA oxidation.

Methodology which produced reproducible, programmable and quantifiable exercise in the dog (Wolter *et al.*, 1984), employing treadmill walking and a Latin square experimental protocol, showed that an increase in fat content (to 50% of the dry matter (DM)) in dog food intake led to a marked improvement in the dog's sporting performance and its biological repercussions during endurance exercise (Grandjean, 1983).

Philip (1984) studied a team of seven Siberian Huskies throughout one racing season and showed that the shift from 45% of fats (based on dry matter) to a diet with a 33% fat content, without any gradual transition, decreased the part played by fatty acids in energy metabolism during exercise, and decreased that of glucose by means of an increase in protein gluconeogenesis (Nicolas, 1978).

To summarise, the inclusion of too high a proportion of carbohydrates as energy source in the food intake of dogs undergoing endurance exercise leads to a drop in performance (Downey *et al.* 1980) which may even go so far as to cause clinical signs such as muscular stiffness, malaise, myositis and coprophagy (Wyatt, 1963; Kronfeld, 1973).

Although not ideal from the gastrointestinal point of view, working dogs can quite happily tolerate a food intake which is entirely deficient in CHO, without any lowering of blood glucose (by means of an increase in gluconeogenesis from glucose-forming amino acids) or pathological complications (Kronfeld *et al.*, 1976). This is in contrast to man who requires a minimum of 15% CHO in his diet .

In practice, the acceptable minimum content of CHO intake of Huskies is 30%: this ensures that a high energy concentration is maintained and any problems are avoided. This figure of 30% is used in suitably treated CHO sources (e.g. extruded dry food) under maintenance or racing conditions (such as speed racing in small categories). Any augmentation in CHO intake above this threshold may trigger an episode of acute diarrhoea, which regresses immediately once the food intake is corrected.

Between 25 and 40% of fats should be incorporated in the dry material, the optimum being 35% under normal racing conditions: this has been confirmed by all our field trials. Fats thus occupy a large share of the food intake with a corresponding decreased CHO intake.

Attention should also be paid to the **quality of the fats** used for Huskies. These can be organised into three categories:

- saturated long chain fatty acids
- short and medium chain fatty acids
- essential polyunsaturated fatty acids of the *n*-3 and *n*-6 series.

The supply of fats with a high concentration of **long chain saturated fatty acids** in the diet allows the dog to build or rebuild stores of adipose tissue from empty calories. Calling aerobic metabolism into play during exercise leads to tissue lipolysis: this increases free plasma fatty acids concentrations and the latter are finally oxidised in muscle cells so as to provide ATP.

Short or medium chain fatty acids can be defined (Bach *et al.*, 1977) as a mixture of fatty acids with 6 carbon atoms (1 to 2%), 8 carbon atoms (65 to 75%) and 12 carbon atoms (1 to 2%). These are of obvious nutritional value in Huskies. The digestive action of pancreatic lipase is facilitated by their low molecular weight, and they require no solubilisation by bile.

Triglycerides containing short or medium chain fatty acids are thus hydrolysed more rapidly and more completely than those with long chains. In metabolic terms, a second advantage derives from the low incorporation of these fatty acids into adipose tissue (Scheig, 1968). In addition, they do not require carnitine to penetrate mitochondrial membranes (Groot and Huismann, 1973); in this way, intramuscular oxidation is more rapid than in the case of long chain fatty acids.

Finally, they have a restraining effect on the synthesis of fatty acids from scratch in adipose tissue (Lavau and Hashim, 1978). The inclusion of short chain fatty acids into the food intake conserves carnitine and thus improves the global energy yield, whilst at the same time preventing certain forms of muscle diseases frequently found in Huskies. In practical terms, we recommend the introduction of short or medium chain triglycerides into the food intake, with an optimum of up to 25% of fats.

The intake of essential fatty acids should be doubled (in comparison with maintenance standards) for essential fatty acids (EFA) in the *n*-6 series because of their role in membrane structures. It is vital that provision be made for an adequate intake of fatty acids in the *n*-3 series, given their anti-inflammatory properties and the points already mentioned: a dose of 50mg/kg should be supplied, care being taken to maintain an *n*-6:*n*-3 ratio of around 5-6:1.

Figure 6.6 shows diagrammatically the various qualitative contributions made by energy sources in Huskies.

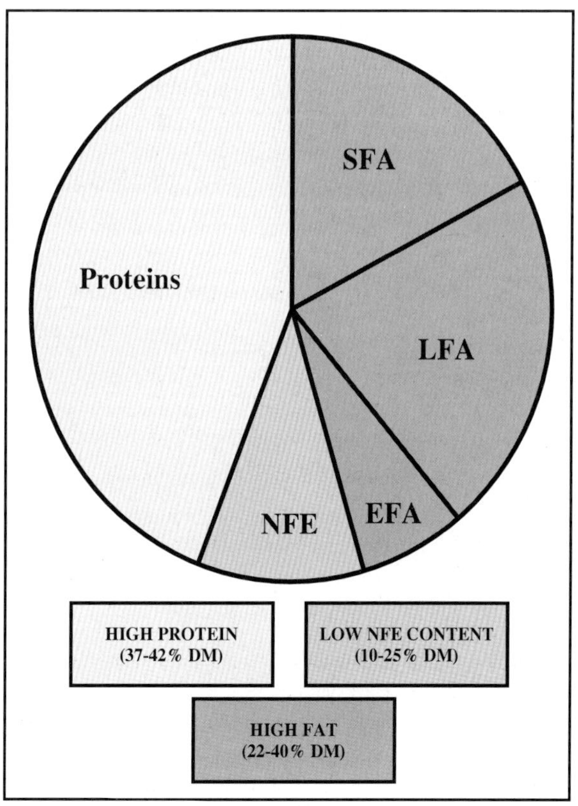

Figure 6.6: *Optimum distribution of dietary energy in Huskies.*

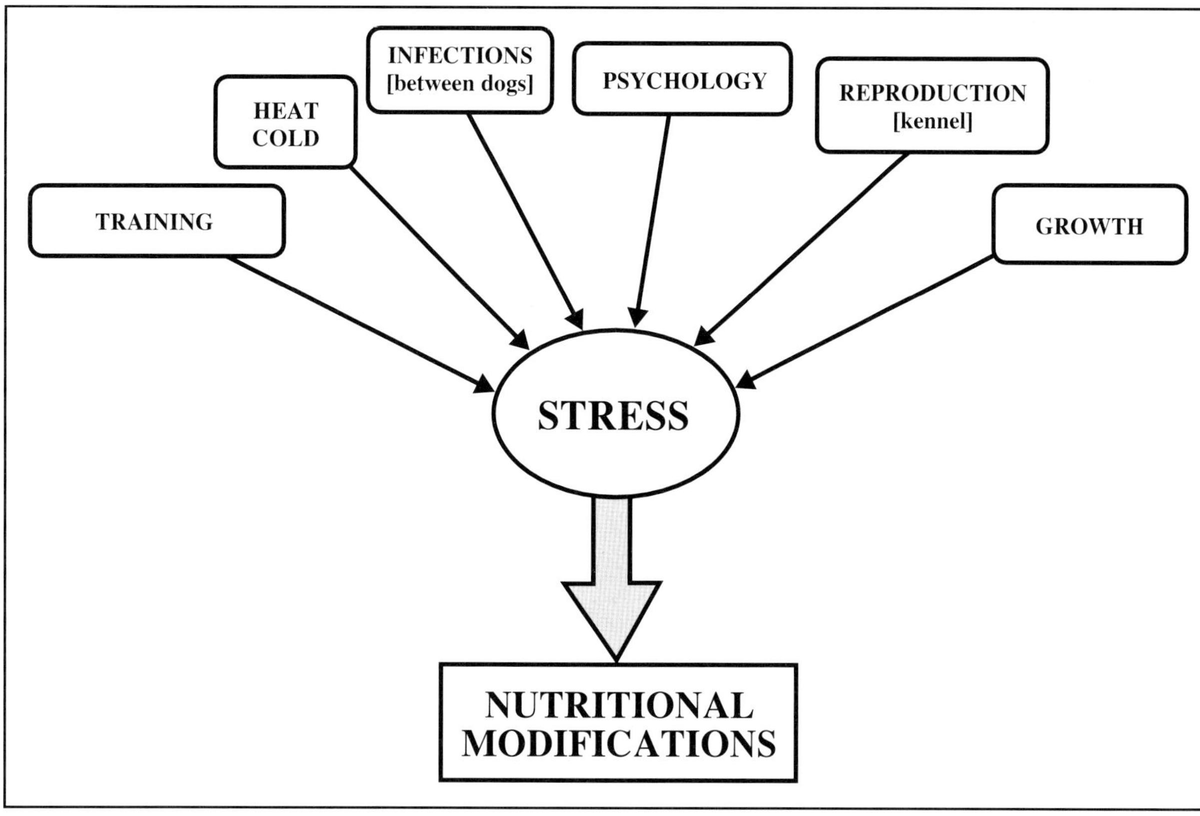

Figure 6.7: *Sources of stress in racing dogs (taken from Kronfeld and Downey, 1981).*

As far as **other racing dogs** are concerned, qualitative energy intakes must in fact be derived from the two extreme models represented by racing Greyhounds and Huskies. The fat concentration should take precedence over CHO intakes as the exercise becomes more prolonged and consequently less intense. The fat content should thus rise from 14% for relatively brief exercise to 22% for competitions or prolonged work, while the protein content should similarly progress, rising from 33-34 to 40% of the dry matter so as to preserve a high protein:energy ratio (more than 30% of energy being of protein origin).

Nutritional Impact of Stress

While the sources of stress as defined by Selye (1976) are vast, it is certain that racing dogs, like any other sporting animals, experience both organic stress (training, competition etc.) and psychological stress (transportation, psychological environment, spectators, temperature, noise etc.). Just as with the energy expenditure strictly due to exercise, such stress contributes to alterations in the animal's nutritional requirements (Figure 6.7).

Stress and Proteins

Stress due to exercise has a modifying effect on the regulation of cerebral serotonin (5-hydroxytryptamine or 5HT) synthesis and activity (Chaouloff *et al.*, 1985). This neurotransmitter participates in the regulation of numerous physiological functions (ingestion, sleep, blood pressure, energy metabolism etc.). The precursor of serotonin is tryptophan.

Exercise increases the transport of tryptophan to the brain, due to the effect of catecholamines released (Dominici *et al.*, 1969). Tryptophan penetrates the cephalic compartment thanks to a saturable stereospecific transporter (Panda *et al.*, 1991) which is itself controlled by the supply of neutral amino acids (valine, leucine, isoleucine, methionine, tyrosine, phenylalanine, threosine and histidine) (Fernstrom and Wurtan, 1972; Panda *et al.*, 1991). The overall cerebral metabolism of serotonin is increased by exercise, to an extent depending on the type of training (Chaouloff *et al.*, 1987).

In dogs, the first nutritional consequence of exercise stress is therefore an increased demand for neutral amino acids and tryptophan, i.e. for good quality protein with a high essential amino acid content (high biological value); at the present time, it is not possible to be more specific in quantitative terms.

Numerous studies have been conducted in dogs (Kronfeld *et al.*, 1976; Adkins and Kronfeld, 1982; Kronfeld, 1983; Grandjean and Mateo, 1985) and demonstrated that stress is linked to the appearance of anaemia, which can sometimes be serious. It can be prevented by a minimum dietary intake of protein corresponding to at least 30% of the metabolisable energy in the food intake, in the form of good quality proteins (Kronfeld e*t al.* 1976; Kronfeld and Downey, 1981; Kronfeld, 1983) (Figures 6.8 and 6.9). A recent study by Billerey (1989) involved the annual monitoring of laboratory parameters in Greyhounds and showed that there was a progressive drop in the haemoglobin concentration (less than 18g/dl), haematocrit level and number of red blood cells after 5 months of training and racing.

Regarding the energy concentration of the food intake, the protein content must therefore account for more than 35% dry matter. In dogs, the range of protein requirements - which is very broad under maintenance conditions - is narrowed (Figure 6.10).

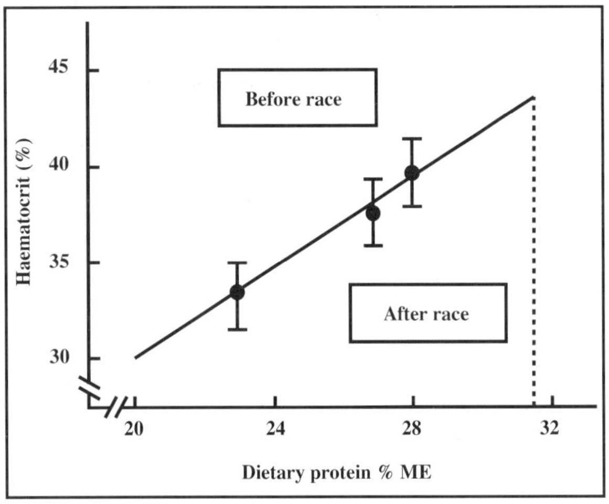

Figure 6.8: Changes in haematocrit level as a function of dietary protein content: in the case of Huskies in long distance races (Iditarod; Adkins and Kronfeld, 1982).

Stress and Acidosis

A large amount of stress can produce lactic acidosis in highly nervous subjects before any exercise whatsoever. This has many harmful effects:

- exacerbation of catecholamine secretion, with glycogenolysis and increased production of lactic acid
- bradycardia contributing to the development of cell anorexia
- reduced irrigation of the liver, slowing down gluconeogenesis from lactates
- inhibition of myocardial oxidation of free fatty acids.

Whatever the type of exercise involved, any lactic acidosis developed before a race only increases the effects of the acidosis which develops as a result of lactic anaerobic work.

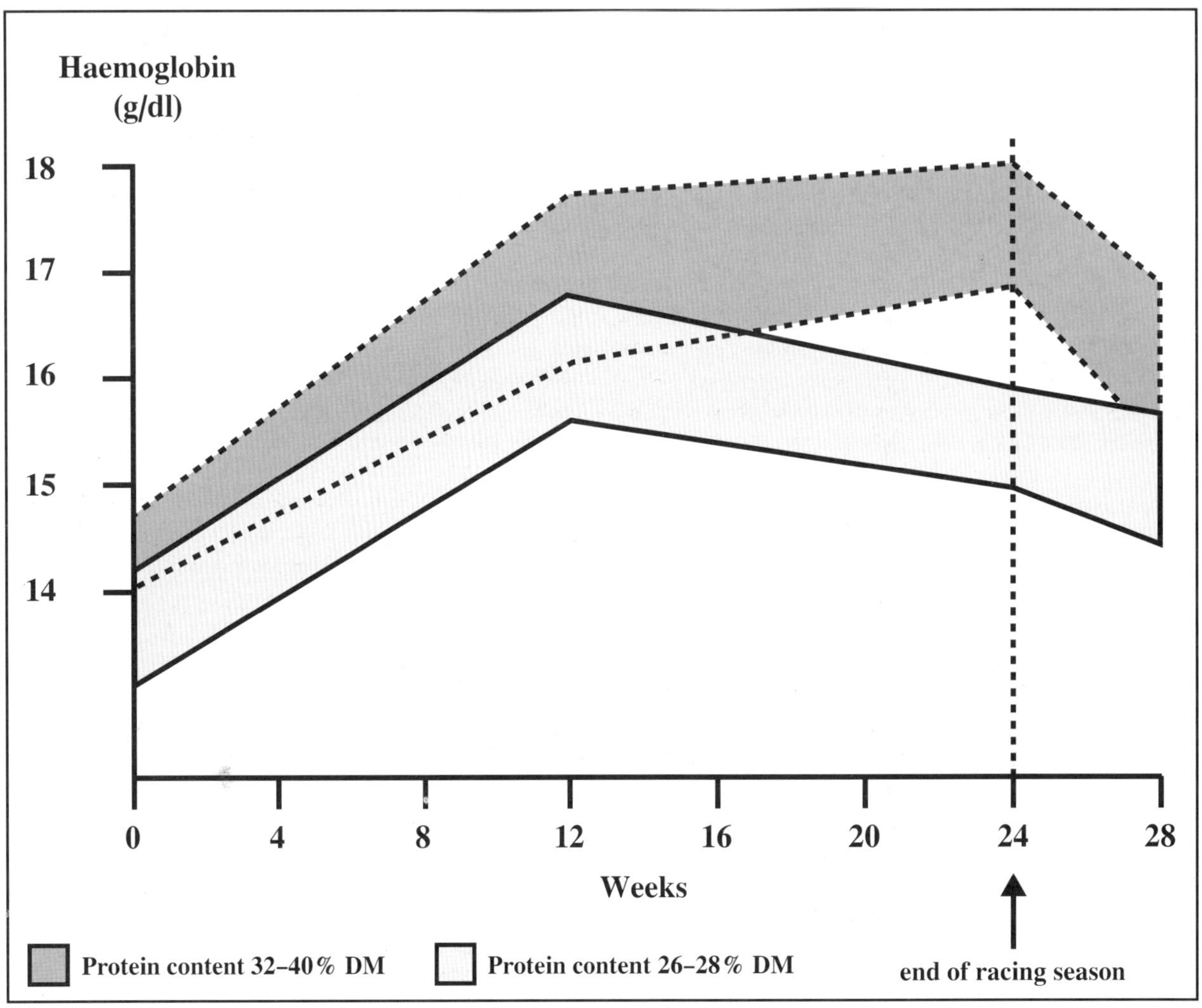

Figure 6.9: Changes in serum haemoglobin as a function of the percentage of proteins in the food intake during a racing season (Kohnke, 1983).

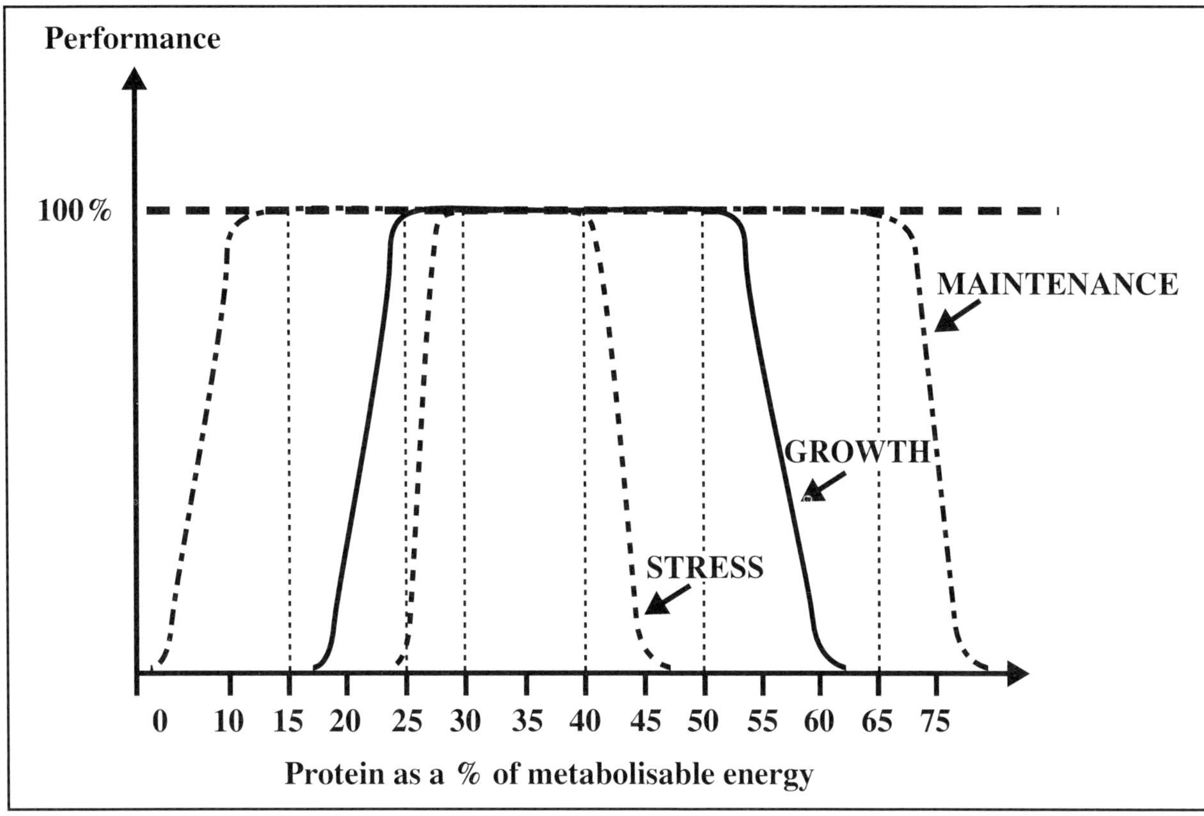

Figure 6.10: Concept of 'optimum' protein level: the range of variation in protein requirements narrows under conditions of stress (Kronfeld and Downey, 1981).

It is therefore important to prevent acidosis by reducing the stress felt by the animal, by means of training (repetition of supramaximal exercise enables the body to endure greater lactacidaemia) or the preventive provision of a nutritional buffer such as sodium carbonate in the drinking water supplied before exercise, at a dose of 300mg/kg.

Stress and Vitamins

Ascorbic acid (**vitamin C**), although synthesised physiologically by the dog, induces a marked improvement in the organic and metabolic response to exercise stress in dogs, at a dosage of 0.23mg/kJ (1mg/kcal) ME (Donoghue *et al.*, 1987). Ascorbic acid derivatives are co-factors for numerous hydrolases (Hornig *et al.*, 1984). One such derivative participates in the synthesis of carnitine which facilitates the transport of fatty acids across the mitochondrial membrane.

In a recent trial, performance was correlated with the plasma concentration of ascorbic acid (Kronfeld, 1983) and a concurrent decrease in serum levels of vitamins C and E was noted in Huskies with the cumulative stress of a racing season (Figure 6.11).

On the other hand, the dietary intake of pyridoxine (**vitamin B_6**) is usually boosted when the protein intake is increased (as in racing dogs), so as to bring about transamination (Kohnke, 1983). But because of the role assumed by vitamin B_6 in gluconeogenesis, the concentrations of energy substrates might be altered if this vitamin is too readily available during exercise.

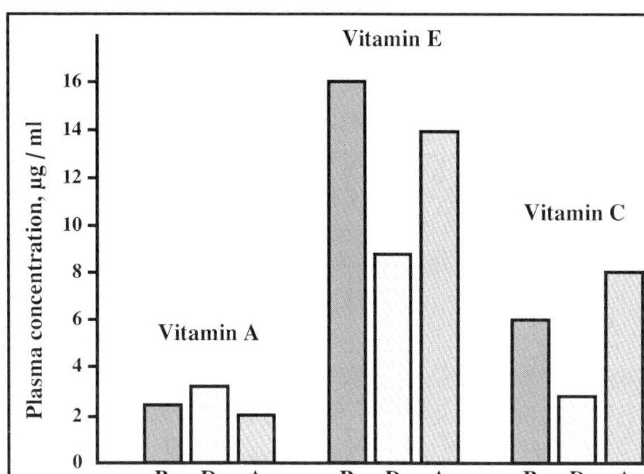

Figure 6.11: Serum vitamin levels: before (B), during (D), and after (A) a period of stress in the dog. Significant drops in serum (but not retinal) levels of α-tocopherol and ascorbic acid occur during season in a top class Husky team (Donoghue and Kronfeld, unpublished).

An exaggerated pyridoxine intake increases the concentration of glycogen phosphorylase in muscle and this may give rise to excessively rapid utilisation of muscle glycogen (Black *et al.*, 1977). Defective energy metabolism may result in unwanted overproduction of lactic acid, particularly during brief exercise (Manore and Leklem, 1988). On the basis of these data, it is recommended that pyridoxine supplements should not be exaggerated in racing dogs undertaking brief exercise and receiving a diet containing a high concentration of carbohydrates.

Stress and Cell Membranes

The stress of intensive exercise brings about the release of peroxides and free radicals which affect the integrity of cell membranes. The membranes contain polyunsaturated fatty acids and their oxidation is prevented by **selenium** in conjunction with **vitamin E**: these preserve the membranes intact, especially in the muscles.

This explains why vitamin E is the vitamin most frequently employed as a single nutritional supplement in racing dogs. Its reputation is based on its antioxidant effect in the tissues (skeletal muscles and myocardium), on the clinical improvement it produces in performance capability, as well as reduced muscle tiredness.

Vitamin E is also widely praised for its efficacy in preventing and treating acute rhabdomyolysis, mainly in combination with selenium. The recommended preventive dosage during brief, intense exercise is 100mg of vitamin E daily for a dog weighing 30kg, with the dose being raised to 400mg on the morning of the race. However, it should be pointed out that this practice is not supported by any scientific literature (Kronfeld and Ferrante, 1990).

Biological membranes contain numerous **essential fatty acids**; the permeability of the membranes is increased according to their degree of polyunsaturation, and the intensity of energy metabolism and sporting capability is consequently improved (Bourre *et al.*, 1988). These must therefore be incorporated into the diet of racing dogs, in the proportions mentioned previously.

It is evident that the nutritional impact of stress must always be taken into consideration and should make it possible to prevent many specific pathological disturbances - such as rhabdomyolysis, anaemia due to racing and stress diarrhoea - which lead to an inferior performance.

Dehydration and its Effects on Fluid Balance

Dehydration constitutes one of the major problems encountered in racing dogs. It affects electrolytic homoeostasis and acid-base balance in the animal, thus increasing the risk of rhabdomyolysis, collapse or exertional tetaniform symptoms (Heneghan, 1977; Hauler, 1983, 1989; Grandjean and Paragon, 1986; Grandjean *et al.* 1986; Lassen *et al.* 1986; Gannon, 1980).

Work by Blythe and Hansen (1986) in racing Greyhounds has shown some interesting results. Dogs are weighed prior to races in America, and any variation of more than 1kg in excess of the announced weight leads to disqualification of the animal from the race.

Dogs which are within weight are then kept in a common kennel without any water (to avoid the risk of doping) until the time of the race. This period lasts from 2 to 6 hours. The dogs are weighed again 20 minutes before the race and the race veterinarian is called in for any weight loss exceeding 1.5kg between the two weighings. The veterinarian decides whether or not to allow the dog to compete. The water losses in urine and saliva linked to the stress of such waiting are important causes of dehydration.

At this stage, 5% of dogs show more than 2.4% dehydration, though without any deleterious effects on their performance. Since it is well known that the conditions causing dehydration are repeated, and there is a clear relationship between the time spent waiting in the kennel before the race and the level of dehydration and systematic involvement of the dogs affected, the author has drawn the conclusion that such dogs should be identified and only participate in the first five races in any race meeting so that their waiting time in the kennel is shortened.

Such a regulation which prohibits watering the animals whilst waiting is spreading to European races and highlights the drastic side of anti-doping regulations. The objective of such rules is, after all, the well-being of the animals.

While the actual impact of extracellular dehydration during brief, intense exercise in dogs has not yet been clearly defined, it is still no less true that important changes are observed after exercise:

- increase in serum sodium, correlated with hyperlactacidaemia
- drop in serum potassium and bicarbonates
- constant lowering in serum magnesium
- return to normal after 2 hours of recovery.

The value of bicarbonate supplementation has already been discussed. However, it should be pointed out that according to Hauler (1989) such supplementation does not correct bicarbonate deficiency: on the contrary, it increases disturbances in fluid equilibrium by increasing the urinary output of potassium.

In Hauler (1983) optimum performance entails a serum sodium level of around 5.0mEq/litre. The serum potassium level becomes a primary limiting factor in performance in such an approach.

Actual potassium requirements depend on two essential factors: prior potassium status in the athlete's body, and potassium losses induced by exercise (Haralambie, 1979). Previous work has shown that there is an increase in potassium concentration in the muscle of trained animals (Mutch and Banister, 1983); it thus appears that the potassium concentration of non-fatty masses in the body is appreciably higher in suitably trained subjects than in sedentary subjects.

Consequently, short training programmes lead to an increase in total potassium in the body, but this appears to be due to an augmentation in relative body weight. Accordingly, athletes in training need a high potassium dietary intake so as to satisfy the increased demand related to increases in muscle mass and the intramuscular potassium concentration.

Experimental observations on dogs led Knochel and Carter (1979) to believe that hypokalaemia following exercise is not necessarily indicative of potassium deficiency, but that on the other hand there is a risk of hyperkalaemia as a result of exhausting exercise.

Whatever the case may be, hypokalaemia can also arise from digestive losses due to stress diarrhoea (as with Huskies), excessive sodium intake, and exercise performed under conditions of excessive heat. An increase in muscular and cardiac excitability, leakage of intracellular enzymes and even supraventricular ectopic beats may result, all leading to a considerable drop in performance (Mott *et al.*, 1972; van Dam and Haralambie, 1977; Dyckner and Wester, 1978).

It therefore seems clear that potassium supplementation is required in racing dogs and may be given in a complete diet.

Magnesium is the cation responsible for activating some 300 enzyme systems. In particular, in the membrane it activates Na-K-ATPase which operates the sodium pump and allows potassium to enter the cell.

An increase in magnesium has been demonstrated in the cells of trained animals (Yakovlev, 1977). Changes which affect serum magnesium levels during physical activity are basically dependent on the duration of exercise. Brief physical exercise (Greyhound race) causes a significant increase in serum magnesium (10 to 20%, connected to the increase in the haematocrit level) (van der Linde *et al.*, 1979; Grandjean and Paragon, 1986; Grandjean, 1991a), whereas prolonged exercise of whatever nature (hunting, sled etc.) is accompanied by a drop in serum magnesium of 2-5mg/litre (Haralambie, 1975; Berg, 1977; Haralambie and Berg, 1979; Grandjean, 1983; Grandjean and Mateo, 1985). The latter is all the more important physiologically since it affects the free fraction of plasma magnesium (Usher and Deegan, 1970) (approximately 65% of the total magnesium concentration in the blood).

Magnesium leaving the plasma is taken up by red blood cells (Straden, 1989), muscle cells (Costill *et al.*, 1981) and adipocytes (Wolter *et al.*, 1984). Given the lack of labile organic reserves of magnesium, this exertional hypomagnesaemia can sometimes lead to clinical muscle spasm (sometimes tetaniform) in poorly trained animals who have undergone intense tissue lipolysis (Grandjean *et al.*, 1986). Yet again, it seems necessary to raise the level of dietary magnesium intake in racing dogs, all the more so since an increase in the fat content of the food intake affects the digestibility of magnesium.

A rise in **serum calcium** is often the result of brief exercise (Rose and Bloomberg, 1988; Pibot, 1991) and appears to be associated with plasma extravasation phenomena. Nevertheless, Haralambie (1979) believes that the combined electrolyte disturbance involving mild hypokalaemia, hypomagnesaemia and hypercalcaemia is liable to increase muscle pain and rhabdomyolysis, all the more so because the drop in intracellular pH slows the inward calcium current in the cell (Sutton and Dirks, 1978).

During intense exercise, this mechanism may give rise to changes in membrane contractility and stability, with leakage of potassium and enzymes out of the muscle cell. Nevertheless, hormonal regulation ensures that calcium remains one of the most stable electrolytes, with usually minute variations in serum calcium occurring upon exercise. The largest drops in serum calcium in Huskies following exercise (3 to 9%) were observed by Hammel *et al.* (1977) and Philip (1984); they appear to be linked to an increase in the urinary excretion of calcium.

Most cases of dehydration and disturbances in fluid equilibrium observed in racing dogs result from inadequate watering (water requirements are multiplied by 2 or 3 during prolonged exercise), stress, or changes brought about in mineral metabolism (Bjotvedt *et al.*, 1984).

Required Vitamin and Mineral Adaptations

Mineral requirements during prolonged exercise are different from those of brief exercise periods.

The calcium intake must be slightly increased in dogs undertaking exercise of short or medium duration, so as to prevent joint pain and osteofibromatous

Type of exercise	Ca:P ratio		mg/kg Body weight	g/1000 kcalME	per cent DM
Brief exercise (Greyhounds, agility, ring)	1.3 to 1.6:1.0	Ca P	250-300 190-240	3.2-4.0 2.5-3.0	1.25-1.50 1.0-1.2
Prolonged effort or stress (sled dog sprint races)	1.4 to 1.6:1.0	Ca P	300-400 200-250	3.5-4.0 2.7-3.1	1.4-1.5 1.0-1.3
Prolonged endurance (sled dog distance races)	1.5 to 2.0:1.0	Ca P	400-500 200-300	4.0-5.0 2.7-3.1	1.8-3.0 1.0-1.5

Table 6.5: *Phosphorus and calcium requirements in racing dogs.*

processes which are frequent in racing dogs; however, in such cases strict standards must be adhered to so as not to increase the risk of osteochondrosis (Huxtable and Davis, 1976; Johnson and Davis, 1979; Hazewinkel *et al.*, 1985, 1990; Voorhout *et al.*, 1987). This work and our own observations lead us to make the recommendations shown in Table 6.5.

High fat diets given to dogs engaged in prolonged exercise can stimulate faecal losses of calcium and magnesium. It therefore appears necessary to establish a relationship between the fat content of the food intake and its calcium concentration (Table 6.5).

Unpublished trials conducted in French Husky teams showed us that serum calcium dropped considerably (from 120mg/litre to 80mg/litre) when the proportion of fats was increased from 30 to 40% of the dry matter whilst maintaining a constant calcium intake of 2.2% with respect to the dry matter. Such trials lead to the recommendation of a calcium concentration close to 2.5% when the fat content of food exceeds 30%.

We have discussed changes in plasma magnesium during exercise and believe that its concentration should be increased in food, especially when the food has a high fat content. Chronic magnesium deficiency in racing dogs results in the following:

- decreased endurance and resistance
- less habituation to heat and cold
- loss of motivation
- changes in neuromuscular excitability
- asthenia associated with cramps
- ligamentous laxity.

The **sodium chloride** intake must be restricted since the dog sweats very little through interdigital spaces. Overconsumption of salt, based on the use of quantities recommended for men or horses, readily leads to polyuria associated with polydipsia (Robinson and Robinson, 1954; Brossard 1975; de Mondenard 1980, 1981; Kjeldsen *et al.*, 1980). Extracellular dehydration and collapse can ensue in both hot and very cold climates. Diarrhoea can also occur when solutions of electrolytes intended for horses are used (as frequently happens in the world of dog racing).

The intake of all **trace elements** should be doubled compared to the intake under maintenance conditions. This allows a margin of safety, takes into account the higher energy concentration of foods and compensates for the antagonistic effects of calcium on their digestibility. Special attention should be paid to the following trace elements:

- **iron**, which helps to prevent anaemia. It is important to avoid excess of iron for strictly digestive reasons, since salts of iron are frequently responsible for the haemorrhagic appearance of stress diarrhoea and rectal bleeding;
- **copper**, which can also help in preventing certain types of anaemia (Griess, 1987), and improves the solidity of bone framework and cartilage;
- **zinc**, which takes part in muscle contraction (Richardson and Drake, 1979) and is the active metal in the enzyme lactate dehydrogenase (LDH) and the plasma protein which transports vitamin A;
- **iodine**, which activates thyroid function and can help in preventing myodystrophy;
- **selenium**, which – in combination with vitamin E – preserves muscle cell integrity.

As far as **vitamins** are concerned, two different aspects must be considered, i.e. long-term biological preparation, and a kind of 'doping' often carried out at the actual time of the race. While the former practice has a sound basis, vitamin overdosage in the days or hours before a race is of little or no value.

Vitamins C, B and E alone appear to be of some slight occasional value, although this has only been demonstrated empirically. Much work has been published concerning the effect (or lack of effect) of any given vitamin on exercise metabolism and physical performance. However, there are numerous obstacles to the objective interpretation of such work since:

- the subjects were nutritionally saturated with the vitamin under test
- vitamin action requires chronic and repeated administration (action latency period)
- a vitamin is often a co-factor in metabolic pathways, without value in the process itself, and generally has an influence on only one of the steps involved in an entire metabolic pathway
- vitamins may, depending on the dose employed, give rise to unwanted pharmacological effects.

In general, the intake of vitamins A, D and K can be doubled, while that of vitamin E may be tripled compared to maintenance standards. The same is true for vitamin B complex, and this is applied most of the time in practice.

An understanding of metabolism, physiological changes and nutritional requirements (shown in Tables 6.6 to 6.8) in the various categories of racing dogs should now enable us to arrive at a formula for food intakes in practice.

	Maintenance	Brief Exercise	Prolonged Exercise	Endurance
Energy (kcal ME/kg$^{0.75}$)	132	150-190	200-400	400-800
Proteins (g/1000 kcal ME)	50	70-80	80-90	80-90
Proteins (% ME)	20	30	35	35-40
Proteins (% DM)	20-27	30-35	35-40	35-40
Fats (% DM)	5-10	12-20	20-30	35-40
FA *n*-6 (% DM)	1	2	3	3
FA *n*-3 (% DM)	0.2	0.4	0.6	0.6
Short chain FA (% DM)	-	2.5-5	5-7	8-10
Fibres (% DM)	2-5	3	2.5	2
Calcium (mg/kg)	200	250-300	300-400	400-500
Calcium (% DM)	0.9-1.1	1.25-1.5	1.4-1.5	1.8-3.0
Phosphorus (mg/kg)	170	190-240	200-250	200-300
Phosphorus (% DM)	0.7-0.9	1.0-1.2	1.0-1.3	1.0-1.5
Potassium (mg/kg)	130	130-150	150	150
NaCl (mg/kg)	240	240	240	240
Magnesium (mg/kg)	8	20-25	25-30	25-30
Magnesium (% DM)	0.04	0.10	0.15	0.15

Table 6.6: *Nutritional recommendations for racing dogs.*

PRACTICAL FEEDING

Any practical diet formulation for racing dogs must be as follows:

- nutritionally balanced
- concentrated and very easy to digest
- suitably adapted to and eaten by the dogs concerned.

Diets for racing dogs involve a series of specific adaptations based on the following four themes:

- coverage of maintenance requirements
- increase in energy and nutrient concentration of the food, combined with a reduction in the amount of faecal material
- enrichment of the food solely for exercise purposes (provision of empty carbohydrate or fat joules)
- enrichment of the food to meet the demands of exercise and induced stress.

The choice or evaluation of any type of food will depend in the first place on its energy concentration, insofar as energy requirements are significantly affected by the amount and intensity of exercise required, making the volume of the food intake a limiting factor.

Under such circumstances, it is therefore clear that there is a place only for those manufactured dry, complete feeds to which supplements adapted to the specific requirements of each sporting discipline can be added (home-made feeds and wet foods being impractical).

Observations in the Field

It is surprising to note that the attitude of many owners towards the way that their racing dogs should be fed, is lacking in logic.

Whatever the canine sport considered, no secret magical powder will make an animal a winner. If races are to be won, a diet which encompasses all known nutritional data and is programmed over an entire season must be planned and adhered to.

The Relationship between Training and Diet

Training schedules should include the concept of customised basic training, followed by an increase in the importance of specific sequences (speed, resistance, power) in order to reach a plateau coinciding with the racing period.

VITAMIN		Limit	Optimum	Supplement
A	min	61	76	45
	max	*610*	*110*	–
D	min	550	700	375
	max	*5500*	*1050*	–
E	min	1200	1900	1500
	max	*24000*	*3600*	–
K	min	–	0	30
	max	–	*105*	–
Thiamin	min	54	100	24
	max	*1620*	*210*	–
Riboflavine	min	100	160	65
	max	*2000*	*290*	–
Niacin	min	450	850	340
	max	*13500*	*1800*	–
Pantothenic acid	min	400	750	68
	max	*12000*	*1600*	–
Pyridoxine	min	60	110	25
	max	*1800*	*230*	–
Folic acid	min	8	15	6
	max	*240*	*31*	–
B_{12}	min	1	1.9	0.7
	max	*30*	*3.9*	–
Biotin	min	–	0	–
	max	–	*14*	–
Ascorbic acid	min	–	0	–
	max	–	*150*	–
Choline	min	50	53	5
	max	*150*	*60*	–

Table 6.7: *Limits and optimum intake of vitamins in the dog (mg/kg) (Kronfeld and Downey, 1981).*

TRACE ELEMENTS		Limit	Optimum	Supplement
Iron	min	1.7	2.3	0.600
	max	*20.0*	*3.5*	–
Copper	min	0.16	0.5	0.005
	max	*12.5*	*1.4*	–
Zinc	min	1.9	3.3	0.150
	max	*50.0*	*6.7*	–
Iodine	min	0.03	0.05	0.005
	max	*0.64*	*0.09*	–
Manganese	min	0.28	1.00	0.006
	max	*25.00*	*2.8*	–
Selenium	min	0.006	0.013	–
	max	*0.250*	*0.025*	–

Table 6.8: *Limits and optimum daily intake of trace elements in the dog (mg/kg) (Kronfeld and Downey, 1981).*

When the racing season is over, the dog should not be allowed to rest immediately but should, on the contrary, be put through a progressive running-down of training. Consequently, the diet should be finely attuned to changes in training:

- **rest period**: good quality maintenance diet;
- **training period**: progressive transition to a working food intake (allowing one week for each change), or progressive addition of a working diet supplement to the maintenance diet intake;
- **racing period**: stress is added to work and may require additional nutritional adjustments. Quantitatively, food intake is adjusted to changes in the animal's weight;
- **detraining period**: progressive return to the maintenance diet.

In qualitative terms, it is possible to define the adjustments required, by specifically adapting the amount of fats to the length of the aerobic training sessions. Thus, except in the case of Huskies, the fat content can be close to 20% at the start of training and return to 14-16% during the racing period in dogs whose exercise performance does not last more than 20 to 30 minutes during competition.

Choice of Foods

In racing dogs, the quality of starting materials or complete foods used to satisfy nutritional requirements is of prime importance - the food intake must be very easy to digest, provide an optimum energy yield, and optimise detoxification processes.

Sources of Proteins

Any source of protein with low amino acid bioavailability and poor biological value (essential amino acid equilibrium) should be avoided; the same is true of poorly digestible, collagen-rich proteins (the collagen:total protein ratio must not exceed 15%). Accordingly, the following are recommended:

- meats (red or white)
- fish meal and meat flour with a protein content of at least 55-60% on dry matter
- powdered whole eggs
- lactose-free casein (to which approximately 2% of methionine should be added for perfect balance).

Sources of Carbohydrates

Foods or starting materials with a high starch content should be selected on the basis of quality and undergo optimum heat treatment so as not to give rise to microbial abnormalities in the intestine. Rapid sugars should be banned. Fibres should be introduced in reduced amounts (2 to 3% of cellulose in the food) since they are bulky, lower the total digestibility of the food intake, and lead to water retention in the faeces, adversely affecting hydration in the dog.

FORMULA (g/120g)		**ANALYSIS**	
Magnesium sulphate	3		
Iron sulphate	1.08	Minerals	42%
Copper sulphate	0.025	Calcium	10%
Manganese sulphate	0.5	Phosphorus	6%
Zinc sulphate	0.003	NaCl	6%
Potassium iodide	0.0002	Magnesium	350 ppm
Sodium chloride	2	Iron	1800 ppm
Vit. A (500)	0.004	Copper	75 ppm
Vit. D_3 (500)	0.001	Manganese	60 ppm
Vit. E (acetate)	0.1	Zinc	1500 ppm
Calcium phosphate	30		
Calcium carbonate	13	Vit. A	200.000IU/kg
Brewer's yeast	42	Vit. D_3	5.000IU/kg
Vit. B_1	0.02	Vit. E	500IU/kg
Vit. B_2	0.04		
Vit. B_6	0.02		
Vit. B_{12} (1000 μg/g)	0.2		
Fish hydrolysate	0.6		

Table 6.9: *Example of a formulation for a vitamin and mineral supplement for home-made feed, suitable for racing dogs.*

Fat Sources

These should be considered as the vehicles of particular fatty acids, and great care must be taken to avoid oxidation and rancidity:

- pork fat, suet, poultry fat (saturated long chain fatty acids)
- coconut, copra, and palm oils (short or medium chain fatty acids)
- sunflower, soya bean and corn oils (essential fatty acids in the *n*-6 series)
- purified fish oils (essential fatty acids in the *n*-3 series).

Mineral and Vitamin Sources

Mineral sources which are perfectly assimilated - such as calcium phosphates and carbonates - should be sought. Yeasts can be used systematically as an excellent source of vitamin B complex. Liposoluble vitamins should be provided in commercially available forms. Table 6.9 gives an example of a formulation for a vitamin and mineral supplement suitable for racing dogs eating home-made feed.

Lean meat	750g
Cooked rice	450g
Bone meal	2 teaspoons
Corn oil	1 teaspoon
Liver	30–60g
Supplement of vitamins and trace elements	

Table 6.10: *Example of home-made feed for a racing Greyhound weighing 30kg (Kronfeld and Downey, 1981).*

Manufactured Complete Feeds

For numerous reasons already mentioned, only complete feeds in a dry or even semi-moist form should be employed in racing dogs.

Maintenance Diet

Some owners adopt the simplest approach of increasing the daily food intake in proportion to increasing energy requirements, without changing the feed. In this case, no special approach to diet is envisaged, and the resulting performance is inferior.

The following alternatives might conceivably be more effective:

1) **The same maintenance diet is used throughout the year;** it is simply progressively supplemented during training and the racing period. In this case, the best basis is provided by a '25/10' type feed (25% protein and 10% fat in the raw product, corresponding to approximately 27% of protein and 11% of fat with respect to the dry material), with high digestibility (optimum of 50g of faeces passed per 100g of dry matter ingested). By retaining this feed as an unchanging basis throughout the year, training supplements and then racing supplements can consist of lean meat or fish for brief exercise, and fat meat or fish for prolonged exercise. In this way, a food intake containing one quarter to one third of dry feed and three quarters to two thirds of meat or fish can progressively be attained at the peak of training. A suitable vitamin and mineral supplement is then mandatory at this point.

→ **Complete dry maintenance diet**		500g/day for a 30kg dog	
Proteins	Approx. 25–27%		
Fats	Approx. 10%		
Fibres	Approx. 3%		
NFE	Approx. 55%		
Calcium	Approx. 1.2%		
Phosphorus	Approx. 1.0%		
Energy	Approx. 3600 kcal ME		
+ other minerals, trace elements, vitamins			
→ **Maintenance home-made feed**		1370g/day for a 30kg dog	
Red meat	Approx. 450g	3	Parts
Cooked rice	Approx. 750g	5	
Vegetables or fruits	Approx. 120g	1	
Vegetable oils	Approx. 10g		
Minerals/Vitamins	Approx. 40g	1	
Energy	Approx. 1340 kcal ME/kg		

Table 6.11: *Maintenance food intakes in racing dogs.*

→ **Semi-manufactured feed**	
Meat flour (60% proteins)	Approx. 50%-60% ↖ anaerobic training
Powdered egg	Approx. 15%
Fats	Approx. 10%-20% ↙
Yeast	Approx. 5%
Calcium carbonate	Approx. 2%
Calcium phosphate	Approx. 1%
Minerals, trace elements, vitamins	Sufficient quantities
Energy	Approx. 3500 kcal ME/kg

$$\text{Average quantity} = \frac{\text{Energy requirements linked to training} - 1700 \text{ [maintenance energy requirements]}}{3500} \text{ kg}$$

***Table 6.12:** Composition of a work supplement for brief exercises in racing dogs (e.g.: Greyhound).*

→ **Complete dry specialised diet**	650g/day for a 30kg dog
Proteins	Approx. 30%
Fats	Approx. 15%
Fibres	Approx. 2%
NFE	Approx. 43%
Calcium	Approx. 1.4%
Phosphorus	Approx. 1.0%
Energy	Approx. 3900 kcal ME
+ other minerals, trace elements, vitamins	

→ **Specialised home-made feed**	1200g/day for a 30kg dog	
Red meat	Approx. 60%	→ Proteins → 33%
Cereal flakes	Approx. 30%	Fats → 14%
Soya bean oil	Approx. 2%	NFA → 45%
Copra oil	Approx. 2%	Energy → 2250 kcal ME/kg
Fish oil	Approx. 2%	
Specific vitamin/mineral supplement	Approx. 4%	

***Table 6.13:** Composition of a specialised diet for brief exercise in dogs.*

Proportion Dry feed[1]/supplementary[2]	kcal ME/kg	Protein (% DM)	Fats (% DM)	Original Cal. Protein (%)[3]
80/20	Approx. 4550	37	24	32.5
70/30	Approx. 4650	38	26	32.6
60/40	Approx. 4750	39	28	32.6
50/50	Approx. 4850	40	30	32.7
40/60	Approx. 5000	41	32	32.8

***Table 6.14:** Practical rationing for Huskies on the basis of distribution of a complete dry feed and a suitable work complement.*

1 Complete dry feed, type '35/20' 2 Work supplement, type '45/45' 3 Basic adherence to protein:calorie ratio.

2) **The maintenance diet is only used during the rest period**; it should satisfy the qualitative conditions mentioned and give way progressively to a specific complete feed once training becomes intensive. Transitions in diet should be made over a period of 1–2 weeks.

Specific Diets

Ideally, a '30/15' type food should be aimed at for short to medium exercise, and '35/20' type food for prolonged exercise. Once again, high digestibility and low intestinal and faecal volume are required, while quantities must be adapted to weight changes in the dog.

Since there are wide variations in the exercise demanded of Greyhounds and Huskies, Tables 6.10 to 6.14 pick out individual requirements. For Huskies, '35/20' type food is perfectly suitable for most of the training period, as well as for team races in the 'small' categories (three or six dogs).

Otherwise, specific protein, fat, mineral and vitamin supplements appear to be necessary, either in home-made or manufactured form (Figures 6.12 to 6.14, Tables 6.10 to 6.14). For long-distance purposes, the progressive transition to a semi-moist complete feed of the '35/36' type appears to be an excellent solution (Figure 6.15).

In any case, a rationing schedule in which the proportion of specific supplement included in the daily food intake is progressively increased is feasible.

Useful Supplements

Without going into details of possible nutritional supplements (ergogenic aids) for racing dogs, those which are of real value, especially in terms of improving the energy yield and combating stress as mentioned later, are as follows (See Figures 6.16 and 6.17.). Pangamic acid (vitamin B_{15}) appears to be effective during brief exercise at a dose of 1.5mg/kg, while supplements of L-carnitine (50mg/kg), ascorbic acid (vitamin C, 1mg/kg, i.e. 24mg/kJ (100mg/kcal) on average) and vitamin B_{12} seem to be effective whatever the exercise required (Grandjean *et al.*, 1993).

CONCLUSION

A certain number of scientific data now appear to be clearly established where the specific nutritional needs of racing dogs are concerned. They may seem disproportionate but constitute the keys to racing success in an area which is undergoing constant development.

Scientific data relating to Greyhounds and Huskies are accumulating, which is reasonable, given the extremes which these two sports represent. How-

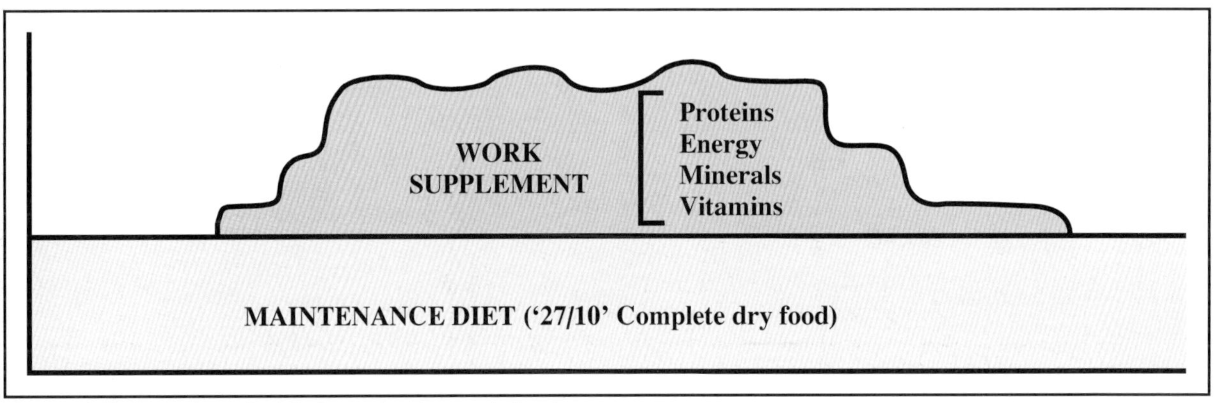

Figure 6.12: *Rationing schedule for racing dogs; solution 1.*

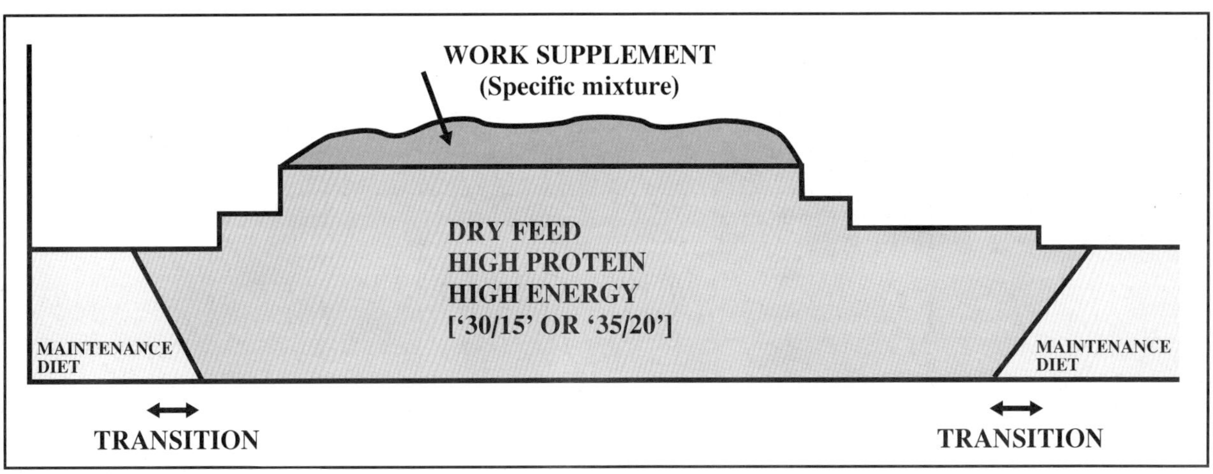

Figure 6.13: *Rationing schedule for racing dogs; solution 2.*

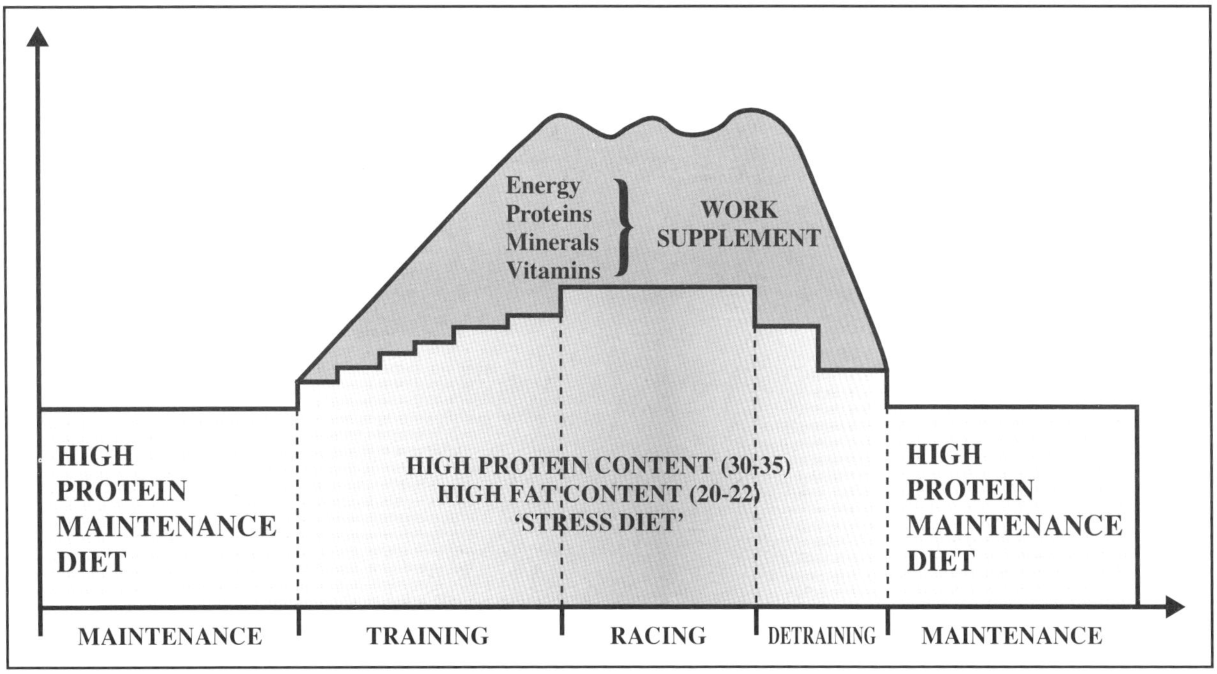

Figure 6.14: *Theorical approach to rationing schedule for Huskies.*

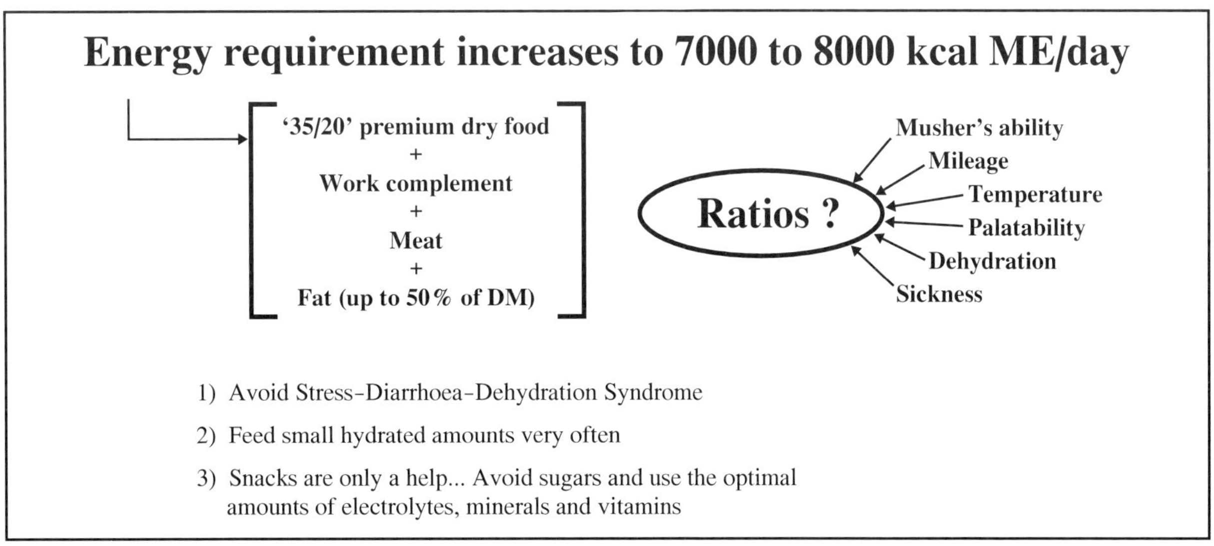

Figure 6.15: *Practical rationing for Huskies (example of Iditarod type race).*

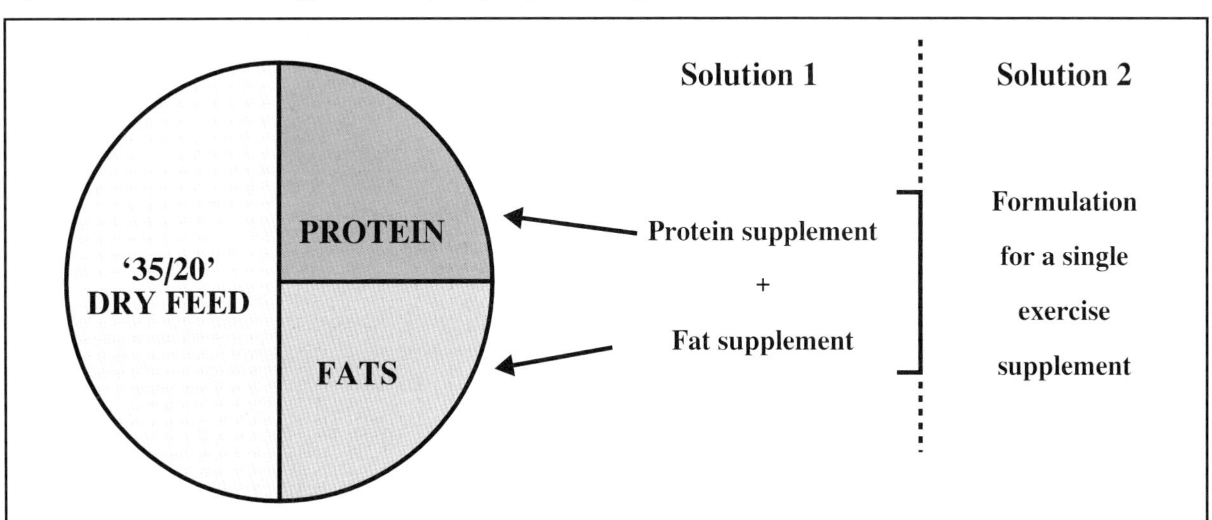

Figure 6.16: *Exercise supplementation for Huskies. Theoretical features.*

SOLUTION 1

PROTEIN SUPPLEMENT (2/3)

- Meat flour (60%)
- Fish meal (10%)
- Powdered egg (15%)
- Yeast (5%)
- Calcium phosphate (1%)
- Calcium carbonate (2%)
- Trace elements and vitamins

FAT SUPPLEMENT (1/3)

- Poultry fat

• Fatty acids (*n*-3) (purified salmon oil)
• Short chain fatty acids (coconut oil)
• Fatty acids (*n*-6) (vegetable oil)

SOLUTION 2

or

Specific manufactured supplements

(45 to 50% of proteins and
40 to 45% of fats in the dry matter)

- Meat flour (40%)
- Fish meal (10%)
- Powdered egg (10%)
- Poultry or dehydrated pork fat (25%)
- Sunflower, corn or soy bean oil (5%)
- Coconut oil (5%)
- Purified salmon oil (2%)
- Minerals and vitamins

Figure 6.17: *Exercise supplementation for Huskies. Practical application.*

ever, numerous gaps still remain regarding other canine activities. Nutrition in racing dogs should be logical and not capitulate in the face of numerous witches' brews whose only value is to flatter the owner's psyche.

REFERENCES

Adkins TO and Kronfeld DS (1982). Diet of racing sled dogs affect erythrocyte depression by stress. *Canadian Veterinary Journal* **23,** 260-263.

Bach A, Schirardin H, Weryha A and Bauer M (1977). Ketogenic response to medium chain triglyceride load in the rat. *Journal of Nutrition* **107,** 1863-1870.

Berg A (1977). Skilanghauf und Elektrolytveranderunger. *Schweizerische Zeitschrift für Sportmedizin* **25,** 185-189.

Billerey E (1989). Contribution à l'étude des paramètres biologiques chez le lévrier de course: variations chez le greyhound et le whippet au cours d'une saison de course. *Thèse Doc. Vet., Alfort 7.7.89* 118pp.

Bjotvedt G, Weems CW and Foley K (1984). Strenuous exercise may cause health hazards for racing greyhounds. *Vet. Small Anim. Clin.* **79,** 1481-1487.

Black AL, Guirard BM and Snell EE (1977). Increased muscle phosphorylase in rats fed high levels of vitamin B6. *Journal of Nutrition* **107,** 1962-1968.

Blaza SE (1982). Energy requirements of dogs in cool conditions. *Canine Practice,* **9,** 10-15.

Blom P (1982). Régime alimentaire et processus de récupération. *2ème cours international de physiologie et de biochimie de l'exercie et de l'entralnement physique Nice, 29 oct.-ler nov. 1982.*

Blythe LL and Hansen DE (1986). Factors affecting prerace dehydration and performance of racing greyhounds. *Journal of the American Veterinary Medical Association* **189,** 1572-1574.

Bourre JM, Dumont O, Piciotri M, Pascal G and Durand G (1988). Controle par les acides gras polyinsaturés de la composisiton des membranes. Minimum alimentaire necessaire en acide linoleique et linolénique. *Bullétin de la Société de Sci. Hyg. Alim.* **73 (4),** 43-50.

Brossard JJ (1975). Influence de l'apport liquide sur la capacité physique. Plan de réhydratatlon a l'effort. *Colloque médicosportif FFC-FFHB, Paris 22.02.75.*

Brzezinska Z, Kaciuba-Uscilko H and Nazar K (1980) Physiological responses to prolonged physical exercise in dogs. *Archives of International Physiology and Biochemistry* **88,** 285-291.

Cerretelli P (1980). Oxygen debt : its role and significance. In: *Lactate, physiologic, methologic and pathologic approach.* Eds PR Morel, J Weber, JC Haissly. Springer, Berlin.

Cerretelli P, Di Prampero PE and Piiper J (1969). Energy balance of anaerobic work in dog gastrocnemius. *American Journal of Physiology* **217,** 581-585.

Chaouloff F, Elghozi JL, Guezennec Y and Laude D (1985). Effects of conditioned running on plasma, liver and brain tryptophan and on brain 5-hydroxytryptamine metabolism of the rat. *British Journal of Pharmacology* **86**, 33-41.

Chaouloff F, Laude D, Serrurier B, Merino D, Guezennec Y and Elgozi JL (1987). Brain serotonin response to exercise in the rat; the influence of training duration. *Biogenic Amines* **4,** 99-106.

Costill DL (1981). Fats and carbohydrates as determinants of athletic performance. In: *Nutrition and athletic performance. Proc. Nutr. Determinants Athlet. Perf.* Ed. Haskell pp16-28.

Costill D, Cote R and Fink W (1976). Muscle water and electrolytes following varied levels of dehydration in man. *Journal of Animal Physiology* **40,** 6-11.

de Mondenard JP (1980). L'alimentation de l'effort bases physiologiques. *Can. Nutr. Diet.* **15,** 285-294.

de Mondenard JP (1981). La diététique du sportif. *Ann. Kines.* **8,** 103-111.

Dominici G, Rottini E, Milia U and Cozzolino G (1969). Protéinurie de fatigue: détermination quantitative de certaines fractions protéiniques. In: *Biochemistry of exercise. Medicine and Sport.* Karger, Basel. pp 365-370.

Donoghue S, Kronfeld DS and Banta CA (1987). A possible vitamin C requirement in racing sledge dogs trained on a high fat diet. In: *Nutrition, malnutrition and dietetics in the dog and cat.* Ed. H Meyer Hanover, Pub: British Veterinary Association. pp 57-59

Downey RL, Konfeld DS and Banta CA (1980). Diet of beagles affect stamina. *Journal of the American Animal Hospital Association* **16,** 273-277.

Dyckner T and Wester PO (1978). Ventricular extrasystoles and intracellular electrolytes in hypokalaemic patients before and after correction of the hypokalaemia. *Acta Medica Scandinavica* **204,** 375-379.

Evans WJ and Hughes VA (1985). Dietary carbohydrates and endurance exercise. *American Journal of Clinical Nutrition* **41,** 1146-1154.

Fernstrom J.D and Wurtan RJ (1972). Brain serotonin content: physiological regulation by plasma neutral aminoacids. *Science* **178,** 414-416.

Freminet A (1986). Origine et destinée du lactate dans l'organisme in: La zone de transition aérobie-anaérobie. *INSEP, Paris Mars 1986.*

Freund H and Zouloumian P (1981a). Lactate after exercise in man: I. Evolution kinetics in arterial blood. *European Journal of Applied Physiology* **46,** 121-133.

Freund H and Zouloumian P (1981b). Lactate after exercise in man: IV. Physiological observations and model predictions. *European Journal of Applied Physiology* **46,** 161-176.

Gannon JR (1980). Exertional rhabdomyolysis (myoglobinuria) in the racing greyhound. In: *Current Veterinary Therapy, Edition VII.* Ed RW Kirk. WB Saunders, Philadelphia pp 783-787.

Gazzola A, Valeite JP, Grandjean D and Wolter R (1984). Les acides gras libres plasmatiques chez le poney et le chien en effort prolongé. *Receuil de Médecine Vétérinaire* **160,** 69-77.

Gollnick PD, Soule RG, Taylor AW, Willlams C and Ianuzzo D (1970). Exercise induced glycogenolysis and lipolysis in the rat: hormonal influence. *American Journal of Physiology* **219,** 729-733.

Grandjean D (1983). Nutrition hyperlipidique et aptitudes sportives à l'effort d'endurance chez le chien étude des paramètres physiologiques, plasmatiques et hématologiques *Thèse Doct. Nutrition Unlv. Paris VI 1983* 376pp.

Grandjean D (1987). Préparation du lévrier de course à la compétition: approche globalisée du plan d'entramement. *Congrès National CNVSPA* Paris France 27.11.87.

Grandjean D (1991a). Diététique clinique et diarrhées chroniques chez le chien. *Forum Européen de Nutrition Annecy 23-24 février 1991.*

Grandjean D (1991b). Nutritional particularities of racing greyhound. *Eastern Veterinary Conference Annual Congress Orlando, Florida 6-9 Jan.1991.*

Grandjean D, Cadore JL and Paragon BM (1986). Les tétanies hypomagnésémiques du chien de sport. In: *Compte-rendu de la joumée pathologie musculaire et tendineuse du chien de sport. CNVSPA ed. IXème World Congress WSAVA Paris 4-7/12/86* pp 35-52.

Grandjean D and Mateo R (1985). Aspects métaboliques de l'exercice musculalre chez le chien. In: *Première Journée de Médecine Sportive Canine.* Point Veterinaire, Alfort pp 1-67.

Grandjean D and Paragon BM (1986). Alimentation du chien de traineau 1. Bases physiologiques et métaboliques. *Receuil de Médecine Vétérinaire* **162,** 1167-1180.

Grandjean D and Paragon BM (1987). Alimentation du chien de trameau 3. Rationnement pratique. *Receuil de Médecine Vétérinaire* **163,** 213-240.

Grandjean D and Paragon BM (1992). Nutrition of racing and working dogs. Part I. *Compendium of Continuing Education* **14,** 1608-1615.

Grandjean D and Paragon BM (1993a). Nutrition of racing and working dogs. Part II. *Compendium of Continuing Education* **15,** 45-76.

Grandjean D and Paragon BM (1993b). Nutrition of racing and working dogs. Part III. *Compendium of Continuing Education* **15,** 203-211.

Grandjean D, Paragon BM and Grandjean R (1987). Sled dog nutrition and feeding. In: *Die Ernährung, Fehlernährung und Diätetik bei Hund und Katze Int. Symp., Meyer H ed., Hannover 3-4/09/87* 86-87.

Grandjean D, Valette JP, Jouglin M, Gabillard C, Bacque H, Bene M and Guillaud JP (1993). Intérêt d'une supplémentation en L Carnitine, Vitamine C et Vitamine B12 chez le chien de sport; Etude experimentale conduite chez le chien de traineau en situation. *Receuil de Médecine Vétérinaire* **169,** 543-551.

Griess D (1987). L'alimentation particulière à l'effort bref. In: *Société Française de Cynotechnie Séminaire sur le chien au travail.* Queinnec G. ed., Toulouse, France 1.03.87 138-158.

Groot PHE and Huismann WC (1973). The activation and oxidation of octanoate and palmitate by rat skeletal muscle mitochondria. *Biochimica Biophysica Acta* **316,** 124-135.

Guezennec CY (1982) Influence d'un régime riche en acides gras polyinsaturés sur la réponse hémorragique à l'exercie physique en hypoxie. *Medicine d'Armées* **16,** 583-588.

Guy PS and Snow DH (1981). Skeletal muscle fibre composition in the dog and its relationship to athletic ability. *Research in Veterinary Science* **31,** 244-248.

Hammel EP, Kronfeld DS, Ganjan YK and Dunlap HL (1977). Metabolic responses to exhaustive exercise in racing sled dogs fed diets containing medium, low or zero carbohydrate. *American Journal of Clinical Nutrition* **30,** 409-418.

Haralambie G (1975). Changes in electrolytes and trace elements during long-lasting exercise. In: *Metabolic adaptations to prolonged physical exercise.* Eds J Howald and J Poortmans. Bickhauser, Basel pp 340-351.

Haralambie G (1979). Magnesiumstoffwechsel bei korperlicher Belostung. *Krankenhausartz* **52,** 293-299.

Haralambie G (1981). Electrolytes, trace elements and vitamins in exercise. In: *Physiological chemistry of exercise and training. Medicine and sport.* Karger, Basel **13,** pp 134-152.

Haralambie G and Berg A (1979). Veranderungen physiologischer und biochemischer Grosser nach Ausdauerbelostung bei frauen mit und ohne Kalziumsubstitution. *Med. Welt* **30,** 1233-1238.

Hauler AD (1983). Dehydration and electrolytes in the racing greyhound. In: *Proceedings of the University of Sydney Referral Course for Veterinarians.* **64,** 472-489.

Hauler AD (1989). Electrolyte metabolism in Greyhound. In: *Greyhound medicine and surgery. Proceedings of the University of Sydney Referral Course for Veterinarians.* **122,** 393-404.

Hazewinkel HA, Goedegebuure SA, Poulos PW and Wolvekamp WT (1985). Influences of chronic calcium excess on the skeletal development of growing great danes. *Journal of the American Animal Hospital Association* **21,** 377-391.

Hazewinkel HA, van den Brom WE, van't Klooster AT, Voorhout G and van Wees A (1990). Calcium metabolism in great dane dogs fed rations with varying calcium and phosphorus levels. *Journal of Nutrition* **11S**, S99-S106.

Heigenhauser GJF, Sutton JR and Jones NL (1983). Effects of glycogen depletion on the ventilatory response to exercise. *Journal of Applied Physiology* **54,** 470-474.

Heneghan T (1977). Haematological and biochemical variables in the greyhound. *Veterinary Science Communications* 277-284.

Hill RC (1995). Clinical nutrition in the athletic dog. In: *Proceedings 11th Annual Int. Canine Sports Medicine Symposium, Orlando Florida, 14-15/01/95.* Ed. M. Bloomberg. pp 10-11.

Hornig D, Glatthaar B and Moser U (1984). General aspects of ascorbic acid function and metabolism. In: *Ascorbic acid in domestic animals.* Royal Danish Agricultural Society, Copenhagen pp 3-23.

Hultman E, Bergstrom I and Roch-Norlund AE (1971). Glycogen storage in human skeletal muscle. In: *Muscle metabolism during exercise.* Plenum Press, New York pp 273-313.

Huxtable CR and Davis PE (1976). The pathology of polyarthritis in young greyhounds. *Journal of Comparative Pathology* **86,** 323-333.

Issekutz B (1979). Energy mobilization in exercising dogs. *Diabetes* **28,** Suppl.1 39-44.

Issekutz B, Miller H, Paul P and Rodahl K. (1965). Aerobic work capacity and the plama free fatty acids turn-over *Journal of Applied Physiology* **20,** 293-296.

Ivy JL, Sherman WM, Miller W, Farrell S and Fishberg B. (1983). Glycogen synthesis: effect of diet and training. In: *Biochemistry of exercise.* Eds HG Knuttgen, JA Vogel and J Poorimans. Human Kinetics Publications pp 29-269.

Johnson KA and Davis PE (1979). Osteochondritis dissecans in the greyhound stifle. *Australian Veterinary Practice* **12,** 339-341.

Kienzle E, Schneider R and Meyer H (1990). Investigations on palatability, digestibility and tolerance of low digestible food components in cats. *International Symposium on Nutrition of Small Companion Animals, UC Davis, CA 1990.*

Kjeldsen B, Komme J and Aasmundrud O (1980). Sport et dietétique. In: *Etude sur l'alimentation du sportif.* Documents consulat de Norvège, Lyon.

Knochel JP and Carter W (1979). Electrical hyperpolarization of muscle cells and potassium tolerance induced by exercise and training. *Commun. 4th International Symposium on the Biochemistry of Exercise, Brumels 1979.*

Kohnke JR (1983). Nutrition of the racing greyhounds; vitamins, amino acids, additives. *Proceedings of the Greyhound Course, University of Sydney* **64,** 681-718.

Kronfeld DS (1973). Diet and the performance of racing sled dogs. *Journal of the American Veterinary Medical Association* **162,** 470-473.

Kronfeld DS (1983). Stress supplements: protein and vitamin C. *Pure Bred Dogs Kennel Gazette* **100**(10), 8-9.

Kronfeld DS and Downey RL (1981). Nutritional strategies for stamina in dogs and horses. *Proceedings of the Nutrition Society of Australia* **6,** 21-29.

Kronfeld DS and Dunlap HL (1977). Common clinical and nutritional problems in racing sled dogs. *Team and Trail* **14**(7), 16-17.

Kronfeld DS, Dunlap HL and Adkins T (1981). The red blood cells connection. *Team and Trail* **18**(9), 4-6.

Kronfeld DS and Ferrante PL (1990) Evaluation of ergonomic diets and nutrients for stressed dogs. In: *Colloque International Medecine Sportive Canine,* Royal Canin, Blagnac.

Kronfeld DS, Hammel EP, Ramberg CF and Dunlap HL (1976). Haematological and metabolic responses to training in racing sled dogs fed diets containing medium, low and zero carbohydrates. *American Journal of Clinical Nutrition* **30,** 419-430.

Lacour JR (1983). Facteurs limitants de l'exercice de longue durée. *3ème Congès National Scientifique de la Société Française de Médecine du Sport. Toulouse 12-14 mai 1983.*

Lassen ED, Craig AM and Blythe LL (1986). Effects of racing on haematologic and serum biochemical values in greyhound. *Journal of the American Veterinary Medical Association* **188,** 1299-1303.

Lavau MM and Hashim SA (1978). Effects of medium chain triglyceride on lipogenesis and body fat in the rat. *Journal of Nutrition* **108,** 613-620.

Lindholm A, Johanson HA and Kjaersgaard P (1974). Acute rhabdomyolysis in standard bred horses. A morphological and biochemical study. *Acta Veterinaria Scandinavica* **15,** 325-329.

Manore MM and Leklem JE (1988). Effect of carbohydrate and vitamin B6 on fuel substrates during exercise. *Med. Sci. Sport Exerc.* **20,** 233-241.

Margaria R, Cerretelli P, di Prampero PE, Massari C and Torelli G (1963). Kinetics and mechanism of oxygen debt contraction in man. *Journal of Applied Physiol*ogy **18,** 371-377.

Metcalf J (1985). MSM, a dietary derivative of DMSO. *Journal of Equine Veterinary Science* **3,** 148-151.

Meyer RA, Dudley GA and Terjung AL (1980). Ammonia and IMP in different skeletal muscle fibre after exercise in rats. *Journal of Applied Physiology* **49,** 1037-1041.

Mieir PJ (1987). In: *Carnitine in medecine.* Ed H Gitzelman. Schattauer, Stuttgart pp 101-104.

Mott CB, Sarles H. and Tiscornia O (1972). Action différente des triglycérides à chaînes courtes, moyennes ou longues sur la sécrétion pancréatique exocrine de l'homme. *Biol. Gastro. Enterol.* **5,** 79-84.

Mutch BJC and Banister EW (1983). Ammonia metabolism in exercise and fatigue: a review. *Med. Sc. Sport and Exercise* **15,** 9-84.

Nicolas F (1978). Pathologie hydro-électrique et rénale aigüe due aux activités sportives. *Medicine and Sport* **52,** 176-185.

Panda P, Reiser S, Scholfield D, Behall K, Ahrens R and Canary J (1991). Carbohydrate tolerance in humans as influenced by sex, age, and eruthrocyte superoxide dismutase activity. *Journal of Nutritional Biochemistry* **2,** 222-228.

Paul P and Issekutz B (1967). Role of extramuscular energy sources in the metabolism of exercising dogs. *American Journal of Physiology* **22,** 615-622.

Philip J (1984). Comparaison de deux régimes alimentaires chez le chien de traîneau en situation. Applications en nutrition comparée. *Thèse Doct. Méd. Université Paris XI 1984* 173 pp.

Pibot P (1991). La digestibilité des aliments pour chiens. *Forum Euripéen de Nutrition, Annecy 23-24 février 1991.*

Richardson JH and Drake PD (1979). The effects of zinc on fatigue of striated muscle. *Journal of Sports Medicine and Physical Fitness* **19,** 133-134.

Rieu M (1988). *Bioenergetique de l'exercice musculaire et de l'entrainement physique.* Presses Universitaires de France 462 pp.

Robinson S and Robinson A (1954). Chemical composition of the sweat. *Physiological Reviews* **54,** 202-220.

Rodahl K (1964). Plasma free fatty acids in exercise. *Journal of Applied Physiology* **19,** 489-492.

Rose RJ and Bloomberg MS (1988). Responses to sprint exercise in the greyhound: effects on haematology, plasma biochemistry and muscle metabolites. In: *International Racing Greyhound Symposium, Florida Veterinary Medical Association 1988.*

Sahlin K (1983). Effect of acidosis on energy metabolism and force generation in skeletal muscle. In: *Biochemistry of exercise.* Eds HG Knuttgen, JA Vogel and J Poortmans. Human Kinetics Publications pp 151-160.

Scheig R (1968). Hepatic and extrahepatic metabolism of medium chain fatty acids. In: *Medium chain triglycerides.* Ed. JR Senior. University of Pennsylvania Press, Philadelphia PA pp 39-49.

Segers A (1969). Reprecussions des activités physiques modérées sur le taux de la protéinurie intermittente des adolescents. In: *Biochemistry of exercise. Medicine and Sport.* Karger, Basel **3,** pp 361-364.

Selye H (1976) *The Stress of Life.* MacGraw Hill, New York.

Serresse O, Lortie G, Bouchard C and Boulay MR (1988). Estimation of the contribution of the various energy systems during maximal work of short duration. *International Journal of Sports Medicine* **9**, 456-460.

Spitzer JJ (1974). Effects of lactate infusion on canine myocardial free fatty acid metabolism in vivo. *American Journal of Physiology* **226,** 213-217.

Straden R (1989). The exercise physiology of the racing greyhound. *International Symposium Racing Greyhound, Sydney 1989* pp 1-8.

Sutton J and Dirks J (1978). Renal handling of calcium. *Federation Proceedings* **37,** 2112-2119.

Topliff DR, Potter GD and Dutson RR (1983). Diet manipulation and muscle glycogen in the equine. *Proc. 8th Equine Nutrition and Physiology Symposium* pp 119-124.

Topliff DR, Potter GD and Dutson RR (1985). Diet manipulation, muscle glycogen metabolism and anaerobic work performance in the equine. *Proc. 4th Equine Nutrition and Physiology Symposium* pp 119-124.

Usher D and Deegan T (1970). An assesment of the use of Sephadex G25 in the estimation of serum protein-bound magnesium and calcium. *Clinica Chemica Acta* **29,** 361-367.

van Dam B and Haralambie G (1977). Die Anderungen einiger biochemischer Parameter durch sportartzspezifische Belastungen in Fechtsport. *Laitungssport* **7,** 285-292.

van der Linde A, Jooste P, Wolfswinkel J and Strydom N (1979). Magnesium changes during and after exercise. *Commun. 4th International Symposium on Biochemistry of Exercise, Brussels 1979.*

Vincent Falquet JC, Pernod A, Forichon J and Minaire Y (1972). Les acides gras libres comme source majeure d'énergie pour la thermogenèse chez les chiens *Life Science* **14,** 725-732.

Voorhout G, Herman A and Hazewinkel HA (1987). A radiographic study on the development of the antebrachium in great dane pups on different calcium intakes. *Veterinary Radiology* **28,** 152-157.

Wolter R (1986). L'alimentation du chien de sport. *Prat. Med. Chir. An. Comp.* **21,**129-146.

Wolter R (1989). L'alimentation du chien de sport *Receuil de Médécine Vétérinaire* **165,** 585-604.

Wolter R, Grandjean D and Valette JP (1983). Nutrition lipidique et aptitudes sportives en effort d'endurance. *Science Veterinaire et Medicale Comparative* **85,** 183-193.

Wolter R, Grandjean D and Valette JP (1984). Relations Nutrition-Aptitudes sportives. Méthodologie de l'étude expérimentale chez l'animal en effort d'endurance. *Receuil de Médécine Vétérinaire* **160,** 657-668.

Wolter R, Grandjean D, Valette JP and Mateo R (1984). Nutrition magnesique et effort applications à l'animal de sport. Interet en nutrition comparée- in: Le point sur le magnésium et le soufre en alimentation animale. *CMA INA, Paris 14/06/1984.*

Wyatt HT (1963). Further experiment on the nutrition of sledge dogs. *British Journal of Nutrition* **17** 273-280.

Yakovlev NN (1977). *Sportbiochemie.* Barth, Leipzig.

CHAPTER SEVEN

Feeding Older Pets

Ronald S. Anderson

INTRODUCTION

What do you say to the client who asks for advice on how to feed her old dog or cat? Since there are no published nutritional recommendations specifically for old pets, it would be technically correct to tell her to go on feeding as before. This advice would not, however, meet her expectation that there is something which she should and could do to take account of her pet's old age and prolong its quality of life. So, even though the nutrient requirements of geriatric dogs and cats are not well documented, there is considerable room for advice based on first principles and common sense.

OLD DOGS AND CATS

What characterises an old animal? Extreme old age is as readily recognised as extreme youth, most obviously by behavioural change such as slowing of movement and decreased responsiveness to stimulus, and also by change in appearance such as greying of pigmented hair, loss of skin elasticity and of coat condition. However, the onset and development of old age is less well defined than the period of puppyhood.

There is a long period after puppyhood when the behaviour, appearance and needs of the mature adult animal stabilise and a pattern of life is established in which feeding and management is much the same from year to year. The onset of old age towards the end of this period is usually a gradual process and many owners will not appreciate that their pet is old until there are quite obvious indications of ageing such as appearance, exercise intolerance or age-related disease.

Species, Breed and Size Variation in the Onset of Old Age

A US survey indicated that there were breed and size differences in the age at which dogs were considered to be geriatric (Table 7.1). The age at which cats were considered geriatric was greater than all categories of dogs. Individual cats have reportedly lived for 35 to 36 years but there is no apparent relationship between breed or size on longevity in cats (Morris, 1994) although females are more long lived than males (Griffiths, 1968).

Ageing

Veterinary care of ageing animals is dependent on a working knowledge of the underlying biological events associated with the ageing process. This process does not appear to differ between animals of different species, though it may occur at different ages in different breeds.

It is beyond the scope of this chapter to examine the biology of ageing on which there is extensive literature. For further details, see Morris (1994) and Simpson *et al.* (1993).

FEEDING OBJECTIVES AND REQUIREMENTS

Ageing has been described as the progressive accumulation with time of changes associated with or responsible for increasing susceptibility to disease and death. These changes occur in tissue structure and composition, rate of metabolism, cardiovascular and pulmonary function, renal and alimentary excretion, special senses, skin, reproductive system... indeed, virtually all functional and structural systems of the body. They compromise homoeostasis, immune competence and behaviour. Feeding objectives should, if possible take account of these changes and be adapted to minimise, reduce or at least not accelerate the rate of this ageing process. Objectives of the nutritional management of old dogs and cats are:

- enhancing the quality of life
- delaying the onset of ageing
- extending life expectancy
- slowing or preventing progression of disease
- eliminating or relieving clinical signs of disease
- maintaining optimal body weight.

Category	Body weight (kg)	Age of onset
Dogs		
Small	<9.1	11.48 $\pm$ 1.86
Medium	9.1–22.7	10.19 $\pm$ 1.56
Large	22.8–40.1	8.85 $\pm$ 1.38
Giant	>40.1	7.46 $\pm$ 1.27
Cats		11.88 $\pm$ 1.94

Table 7.1: *Age at which dogs in various weight groups, and cats, were considered to be 'geriatric' (from Goldston, 1989).*

Digestion

There is little or no evidence that healthy old dogs are less able to digest their food than younger dogs (Simpson *et al.*, 1993). Several experimental studies have shown that old dogs make as efficient or more efficient use of dietary nutrients than younger dogs. Likewise, there is no evidence of decreased digestive efficiency associated with age in cats (Morris, 1994). Young (1 year old) cats may have marginally lower digestive efficiency than mature and older animals.

Digestion and digestibility do not, therefore, appear to be important factors in considering the dietary requirements of most normal old dogs and cats. Individual animals may, however, show deterioration in digestive efficiency with age and it remains to be shown whether longitudinal studies, i.e. measuring the digestive efficiency of one group of animals over a 10 year period, will uncover some consistent effects of ageing.

Nutrient Requirement

Since there is no apparent effect of ageing on digestion, any general nutrient recommendations and intake specifically designed for old animals must take account of factors other than digestive efficiency and digestibility.

Energy

One of the most apparent characteristics of ageing is reduced physical activity; even the active old dog probably expends less energy than it did when it was younger.

If, therefore, old dogs or cats retain their appetites and are fed as much as in the past, it is almost inevitable that they will become obese. If, on the other hand, their appetite is very substantially reduced, they may in fact lose weight unless the appropriate dietary measures are taken.

Energy intake. Although energy requirement is the primary drive for energy intake, other factors, such as the palatability, energy density and digestibility of the food also affect intake.

Energy density. Proprietary dog and cat foods vary in metabolisable energy density by a factor of 4 or more. In general, dry foods contain 3 or 4 times the energy density of moist (canned) foods, largely due to the diluting effect of the water - (70–80%) in the latter. This necessitates the consumption of three or four times more of the moist than the dry foods (on a weight basis) to obtain an equivalent energy intake.

Digestibility. Dry foods are, in general, less digestible than wet foods primarily due to their higher vegetable fibre content. The metabolisable energy content *of the dry matter* in dry foods is, therefore, less than in wet foods - but this difference is of minor importance in offsetting the effect of water content on the energy density of dry and moist foods.

Palatability (and cost). Moist or canned foods, being largely of meat and meat by-products, are generally more palatable than dry foods which are largely cereal-based. Because of the higher costs of their ingredients, processing and packaging, moist foods cost more per unit of energy than dry foods. These interrelated factors, energy density, digestibility and palatability, have an important bearing on the energy intake of all dogs and cats, but particularly older animals.

Old dogs have a reduced energy requirement, lowered appetite and increased taste thresholds. It is, therefore, logical to offer at least part of their diet as low energy, high palatability moist foods. Because of the reduced overall food requirement to maintain energy balance, the increased unit cost of moist *versus* dry foods is at least partially offset by the reduced intake. If the food has previously been mainly dry, the increased bulk afforded by low energy moist foods may help to offset the effect of decreasing energy intake on the manifestation of hunger.

Requirement. There are no published recommendations for the energy requirement of old dogs and cats. If there were, they would be on a sliding downward scale from the requirements of mature animals. It is likely that decreased energy requirement is due to both a reduction in resting metabolic rate and in elective energy expenditure (as it is in the ageing human). The only useful criterion is the body condition of the animal; if too fat, decrease total food offered and change to food of lower metabolisable energy density. If too thin, offer higher palatability foods at increased frequency and at body temperature. For animals that are already obese, it is reasonable to pursue a reduced calorie dietary regimen (see Chapter 9 - obesity). The choice of diet and the assessment of energy requirement in old dogs and cats must be on an individual basis. There is clearly a greater need for an effective weight reducing regimen if obesity is contributing directly to impaired body function such as locomotion and thermoregulation. In old animals the successful implementation of a weight reducing regimen may be more difficult and at the same time more important than for younger animals for the following reasons:

1) Both the animal and its owner may be more resistant to fundamental dietary change because of long habituation to the existing diet.

2) The underlying deterioration in other regulatory systems will be more advanced and thus more vulnerable to imposed metabolic change than younger animals.

3) The option of hospitalisation and radical reduction in food intake is inappropriate, since such treatment may be less tolerable for an old animal, both physiologically and psychologically, than for a younger one.

4) The owner may, not unreasonably, argue that, with a relatively short life expectancy anyway, they would prefer their pet to die fat and happy rather than lean and miserable!

Protein

Ageing is associated with a reduction in muscle and bone mass and a loss of tissue protein reserves. Although total body weight may be unaltered the decrease in muscle mass and protein reserves is marked by a proportional increase in fatty tissues. A brief period of anorexia in old dogs and (particularly) cats results in a much more rapid depletion of this reduced muscle mass and protein reserves than in younger animals.

Cats are particularly susceptible to protein depletion since (unlike dogs) liver enzymes (aminotransferases) continue to degrade dispensable amino acids regardless of the level of protein intake. There is, therefore, a continuous loss of nitrogen through gluconeogenesis in normal healthy cats; in aged cats with reduced muscle mass and protein reserves, the effects of such losses are likely to be accentuated.

Requirement: Because of the reduced protein reserves in old animals the avoidance of negative nitrogen balance is important. On the other hand, the relatively high incidence of renal insufficiency in older dogs reduces their capacity to excrete the end products of protein catabolism. While protein requirement is, therefore, more finely balanced in old dogs and cats, it would be unrealistic to lay down arbitrary rules. Nevertheless, some general principles should be followed.

Biological value (BV): The BV is the proportion of a food protein which can be utilised for synthesising body tissues and compounds. The higher the BV the greater the efficiency of the protein in replenishing or maintaining tissue protein and the less, in proportion to intake, is excreted. In healthy animals with fully functional kidneys, protein of relatively low biological value can maintain nitrogen balance without overloading the urinary system, provided sufficient is present in the diet. In renal insufficiency an equivalent quantity and quality of protein is likely to overload the kidneys and cause uraemia. Dietary control of renal failure is discussed in detail elsewhere (Chapter 11), but for the old dog, particularly if renal insufficiency is present, it is clearly more important to provide high, rather than low quality protein. Good quality animal protein (meat, fish, eggs, milk, cheese) has substantially higher BV than cereal protein. High quality canned proprietary foods have protein of higher BV than cheaper canned foods or cereal-based dry foods. An additional benefit for the old dog is the generally higher palatability of high quality protein. It is, however, important to monitor renal function by the appropriate methods and, if necessary, reduce the amount of protein fed. The use of specially formulated low protein diets may be useful in such circumstances as a component of the diet. It is, however, essential that energy intake be maintained and it is preferable to achieve this by fat supplementation rather than carbohydrate.

Where protein intake is decreased due to poor appetite, appetite can be stimulated by warming the food, feeding smaller meals more frequently and vitamin supplementation (particularly the vitamin B complex).

Carbohydrate

Most of the dietary carbohydrate in canine and feline diets is provided by cereal or legumes. It is a useful and cheap source of energy but not a dietary essential. Although expanded cereal-based foods are palatable they are less so than meat-based foods. Mixed meat and biscuit mixer is the traditional dietary regimen for dogs - but not cats - in Britain, the meat providing palatability and high quality protein, minerals and vitamins, the biscuit providing primarily a source of energy as carbohydrate. Complete dry (cereal-based) foods are, however, providing an increasing proportion of the total food intake of dogs and cats. Where the regular diet is a mixture of meat and cereal, any reduction in energy intake is more effectively accomplished by reduction in the cereal proportion of the diet. This will increase palatability and the BV of the protein.

Some semi-moist dog foods have a high sucrose content to act as a preservative. Because of the age-related incidence of obesity and of diabetes mellitus, such foods should provide only a small proportion of the daily ration.

The popularity of dry cat foods has resulted in a relatively higher proportion of carbohydrate in cats' diets than in the past. Despite their essentially carnivorous nature, cats appear to have adapted well to this significant change in their nutrient intake and there is no reason to propose that dry cat foods should not form part of the senior cat's diet.

Fat

Fat provides energy, essential fatty acids, a vehicle for fat-soluble vitamins and palatability. It is essential for the health of both old dogs and cats. However, because of its high energy density, the most effective way to reduce energy intake is by reduction of the dietary fat content. Several reducing diets are on the market for both dogs and cats, all of which have low, but sufficient fat levels. The simplest and safest way of reducing fat (and energy) intake is to use such products.

Fibre

Because of the bulking effect of dietary fibre on gut contents and the consequent beneficial effects on constipation to which some older animals are predisposed, dietary fibre has a potentially useful role in the old pet diet. Furthermore, because of its low digestibility, it can play a part in low energy diets. The addition of the various forms of fibre available has, however, the effect of lowering palatability. Many dogs are, nevertheless, happy to consume added fibre in the form of wheat bran and this has a useful regulatory effect on faeces frequency and consistency. The inclusion of cooked vegetables two or three times a week has a similar effect.

Minerals

Calcium

Most proprietary complete foods contain sufficient calcium to meet the requirements for growth and thus much more than is required for maintenance. The reduction in phosphorus intake which is indicated for old animals with renal insufficiency (see below) requires that calcium intake should also be reduced to maintain an acceptable calcium:phosphorus ratio. It is, therefore, inappropriate to use calcium supplementation in the diet of old animals unless there is clear evidence of calcium depletion. In such cases vitamin D supplementation should also be given to ameliorate the increased Ca:P ratio.

Phosphorus

Dietary phosphorus restriction is recommended for dogs with renal insufficiency – to offset the hyperphosphataemia consequent upon impaired phosphate excretion. The amounts of phosphorus in most diets is generous and therefore some reduction could be beneficial for old dogs. Again, the simplest way to achieve this is to include a proprietary low phosphorus product as part of the diet. Antacids, such as aluminium hydroxide or carbonate, which bind phosphorus may also be used in conjunction with low phosphorus diets. Reduction in the phosphorus content of home-made diets can be achieved by substituting calcium carbonate for bone flour or fish meal and using white bread or cooked rice as a carbohydrate source instead of cereal.

Sodium

Most dogs and cats, whether fed prepared foods or receiving a proportion of table scraps, receive substantially more than their minimum requirements. The role of sodium in hypertension and cardiac or renal dysfunction is unclear. There is no good evidence that healthy dogs or cats of any age are predisposed to any disease as a result of an increased salt intake. However, on the grounds that ageing is associated with a progressive impairment in homoeostatic mechanisms, it is prudent to ensure that old pet's diets do not contain excessive salt. The total avoidance of table scraps (high in salt) is essential if a low salt intake is to be achieved.

Zinc

There is some evidence that zinc absorption and plasma zinc concentration is decreased in old dogs. Zinc absorption is impaired in the presence of high calcium or phytate levels in the food. Although primary or secondary zinc deficiency occurs in a wide range of breeds and ages, the zinc status of old dogs is more likely to be vulnerable, particularly if fed on a cereal-based diet with a liberal calcium level. The inclusion of zinc (zinc sulphate) in a dietary supplement should be considered if there is any clinical evidence (see Chapters 2 and 14) of zinc deficiency.

Vitamins

The use of vitamin supplements is controversial. The argument against supplementation is that a food or diet which is 'complete' (see Chapters 2, 3, 4 and 5) already contains all the required nutrients in the correct balance and the nutrient status can at best be unimproved by supplementary vitamins and at worst become unbalanced.

In the case of old dogs and cats, however, there is a counter argument. Commercial diets are formulated to contain adequate levels of nutrient per unit of energy in the diet, the assumption being, the bigger the animal, the greater the food and, therefore, vitamin intake. In old dogs and cats, however, food intake may be voluntarily reduced or restricted as part of a weight control programme. Thus the intake of vitamins and other nutrients is also decreased.

Although there is no quantitative evidence of a need for vitamin supplementation in old dogs or cats, there is a qualitative and anecdotal rationale for vitamin supplementation particularly after a period of illness accompanied by reduced food intake and antibiotic therapy.

While there are specific justifications for supplementation with individual vitamins (for instance the antioxidant properties of vitamin E help to maintain cell membrane integrity by scavenging away free radicals which cause peroxidation of unsaturated fatty acids – thus defending against the membrane damage associated with old age), it is unlikely that the potentially reduced vitamin status of a convalescent and elderly dog or cat will be confined to one vitamin. There is, therefore, sound nutritional rationale for prescribing in moderation one of the many multivitamin preparations which are available. It is a fundamental characteristic of old age that tissue reserves of many essential nutrients are depleted and this will apply particularly to the vitamin B complex.

Food Types

The main food types – dry, semi-moist and wet or canned – are described in detail elsewhere (see Chapter 2).

For old dogs and cats the most appropriate type of food depends on the circumstances.

For all types, it may well be that, because of habituation to a particular diet by the owner or the pet, change to a new type may not be popular. If, however, there is a good reason for change, the importance of the change should be made clear to the owner. A new type should, of course be introduced gradually over 3 or 4 days, particularly when the old type has been fed consistently over a long period. There are various reasons why change from one food type to another may be advisable.

Reduced food intake and weight loss: Decreased appetite and weight loss is not uncommon in old dogs and cats. This may be due to a multiplicity of clinical causes - renal, cardiac, hepatic insufficiency, periodontitis, neoplasia etc. If, however, there is no apparent clinical cause, it may well be that the appetite can be restored by changing from one type of food to another - or introducing variety into the dietary regimen. An old animal that displays less interest in a food that it has been fed for many years may well show a revived interest in a new type of food, particularly if it has higher quality and palatability. The inclusion of some cat food (dry or wet) as part of the regimen for an old dog is an effective stimulus to appetite. Generally speaking, dry foods are less palatable than canned and their palatability and ease of consumption can be increased by moistening with warmed water, soup or gravy. Substitution or mixing with canned food is also effective.

Obesity: If food intake and appetite is maintained and energy expenditure reduced, obesity results. For the old dog or cat obesity is even more undesirable than in the younger animal because of the added strain on arthritic joints and other degenerating body systems. Weight reduction by the use of low calorie diets is described elsewhere (Chapter 9) but in the old dog or cat this regimen requires greater persistence due to the underlying decrease in energy expenditure and reduced exercise tolerance associated with old age. It may also be more difficult to achieve owner compliance since the owner has become used to the animal in its obese state and so may lack the motivation and discipline to change it. The maintenance of lean body mass while shedding fat is more important in the old animal because of its reduced protein reserves. Dry foods have a much higher energy density than wet foods and reduced energy intake can be achieved without reducing bulk intake by replacing part or all of a dry food with a canned food. The generally higher biological value of the protein and its higher protein-calorie percentage is also beneficial in maintaining protein reserves and appetite.

Dry Food

Its convenience and cost have considerable advantages in feeding dogs and cats. Other factors to be taken into account are:

Palatability. Fed dry it is less palatable than good quality canned foods. This can be largely offset by mixing with gravy, warm water or meat.

Energy. Higher energy density than canned food may contribute to obesity.

Nutritional value. Cheaper foods have lower digestibility and protein biological value. Higher phytate levels may reduce zinc absorption. Faecal consistency may, however, be improved by fibre content.

Fluid balance. Relatively higher fluid intake is required with dry than with wet foods. Not a disadvantage so long as water is constantly available. In older dogs and cats, impaired renal concentrating capacity may mean water balance is particularly vulnerable.

Feeding frequency. Older animals benefit from increased feeding frequency. Dry food availability may encourage voluntary increase in frequency.

Dental and oral health. Dry foods have the reputation of being less associated with dental calculus and periodontal disease. Kittens reared on dry foods have been shown to have less dental plaque than controls. However, there is little evidence that dry foods can reduce dental calculus in adult dogs.

Semi-Moist Food

Convenient, like dry foods - more palatable (and costly). Other factors are:

Palatability. Intermediate between dry and canned. Use of sugars, syrups or polyhydric alcohols as preservatives contribute to palatability for dogs.

Energy. Energy density similar to dry, some energy from simple sugars. Inappropriate for obese or diabetic animals.

Nutritional value. May have less cereal and higher protein biological value than dry.

Fluid balance. As for dry food, a plentiful supply of drinking water is essential.

Additives. Tend to have higher levels of preservatives and colouring agents. May have added acid to prevent bacterial spoilage.

Canned Foods

More palatable (and expensive) than other types. Often

fed with dry mixers. Should make up reasonable proportion of the diets of old dogs and cats.

Palatability. There is a wide range, proportional to quality of ingredients and, therefore, cost. Canned cat foods are often highly palatable to dogs and can be used to stimulate failing appetites in old dogs.

Energy. Energy density about 25 to 30% of dry but increased by the addition of mixer (see Chapter 2).

Nutritional value. Higher digestibility and protein quality than most dry foods, therefore, have a useful role in replacing lean body mass. High protein-calorie ratio may be contraindicated where old age is associated with renal failure.

Storage. Opened cans stored in fridges have low palatability especially for old animals. Increase palatability by warming to blood heat. Remove leftovers to prevent spoilage.

Specialist Foods

It is not surprising that there are few products designed specifically for old dogs and cats since there are few or no consistent data on their nutrient requirements. The old dog or cat may be characteristically obese or thin, it may have renal, hepatic or cardiac dysfunction. It may be losing lean tissue mass and/or it may be retaining fluid, salt, phosphorus or nitrogen. The dietary indications for many of these conditions are conflicting. More 'Senior pet' dietary products are, nevertheless, likely to appear in future and will undoubtedly have a useful role in the feeding options for ageing dogs and cats.

Regimen

Dogs

Many mature dogs of medium and large size are satisfactorily maintained on one meal per day. Small dogs usually require to be fed twice daily.

Although old dogs may continue on a single meal per day, experience suggests that their reduced appetite may be insufficient to stimulate the consumption of their daily needs in a single meal. Feeding twice a day is recommended for dogs of medium size and above, and three times a day for small dogs.

Cats

Domestic cats are frequent feeders if given the opportunity. The advent of dry cat foods allows them access to fresh food throughout the 24 hours. Dry food should not, however, be put down in large quantities and should be replenished daily.

Wet food should be fed once or twice per day and any leftovers discarded. Cats in particular find cold food from the refrigerator unpalatable and should if possible receive their food at room temperature or slightly warmed.

Assessment of Suitability of Feeding Over Time

Old dogs and cats have a short life expectancy and during the last year or so of their lives will probably show progressive deterioration in health and organ function.

Experience shows that significant alleviation of this deterioration can be achieved by recognition of their changing metabolism and needs during this period.

Deterioration in health should not be shrugged off as 'just old age'. Loss of appetite may be due to the toxaemia and pain of periodontitis which can often be significantly improved. Other organ dysfunctions such as chronic renal failure may respond to protein and phosphorus restricted diets. Obesity may aggravate the locomotor disabilities and should be tackled determinedly. Progressive reduction in exercise tolerance must be accompanied by progressive reduction in energy intake. The reduction in total food intake may create a need for multivitamin supplementation.

Although the effects of dietary alleviation of age-related problems in dogs and cats are inevitably relatively short term, they can be extremely rewarding if introduced thoughtfully and with the quality of life of the patient as the main criterion.

REFERENCES

Goldston RT (1989). Geriatrics and gerontology (Preface). *Veterinary Clinics of North America : Small Animal Practice* **19,** ix-x.

Griffiths BCR (1968). The geriatric cat. *Journal of Small Animal Practice* **9,** 343.

Morris JG (1994). Feeding the senior cat. *Veterinary International* **6,** 28.

Simpson JW, Anderson RS and Markwell PJ (1993). *Clinical Nutrition of the Dog and Cat.* (Chapter 6.) Blackwell Scientific Publications, Oxford.

FURTHER READING

Bush BM (1989). Geriatric nursing. In: *Jones's Animal Nursing,* 5th edn. Ed DR Lane. Pergamon Press, Oxford. pp. 392-397

Goldston RT (ed.) (1989) Geriatrics and gerontology. *Veterinary Clinics of North America: Small Animal Practice* **19,** 1-202.

Lewis LD, Morris ML and Hand MS (1987). Feeding the aged dog or cat. In: *Small Animal Clinical Nutrition III.* Mark Morris Associates, Kansas. pp. 3.22-3.25.

Mosier JE (1989). Effect of ageing on body systems of the dog. *Veterinary Clinics of North America: Small Animal Practice* **19,** 1-12.

Mosier JE (1990). Caring for the ageing dog in today's practice. *Veterinary Medicine* **85,** 460-471.

PART III

Clinical Nutrition – Dog and Cat

CHAPTER EIGHT

The Underweight Patient

Susan Donoghue

INTRODUCTION

Underweight dogs and cats present to veterinarians with less than optimal levels of body fat and lean tissue, and often it is the practitioner who must solve the mystery of the pet's undesirable condition. In the first instance, what is considered underweight and what is considered optimal? The body condition considered to be optimal varies with age and breed. For example, a young Saluki or Siamese in optimal condition looks and feels much leaner than middle-aged individuals representative of other breeds, such as the Bulldog or Maine Coon Cat.

Underweight body condition may serve as a signal of disease or mismanagement. Not every underweight pet has been starved; chronic organ failure, for example, produces thin dogs and cats despite exemplary care. In addition, not every underweight dog or cat is ill. Racing sled dogs, for example, carry substantially less fat when in peak condition than when sedentary in the off-season. Veterinarians unfamiliar with the dogs or the sport may consider racers to be underweight, yet these athletes race most successfully (as do human marathoners) when in lean condition. Usually, though, underweight conditions in pets prompt veterinary investigation. This chapter considers underweight body condition as an undesirable finding in dogs and cats presenting to veterinary clinics.

PREVALENCE

Few data exist on the prevalence and distribution of underweight body conditions in pet dogs and cats. Mostly, data have been collected for animals (healthy and sick) presenting to veterinary hospitals. While these data are not necessarily representative of the entire pet population, the information is valid and useful for establishing guidelines on the assessment of underweight veterinary patients and their subsequent care.

Dogs

In a study of 3729 dogs presenting to a referral teaching veterinary hospital in the USA, 0.5% of dogs were considered cachectic and 10% were underweight, compared to 66% which were considered to be in optimal condition for the patient's age and breed (Kronfeld *et al.*, 1991). In this and another study of body condition, many of the underweight dogs were less than one year of age or over 12 years (Donoghue *et al.*, 1991; Kronfeld *et al.*, 1991). In earlier surveys of dogs presenting to veterinary clinics in the UK, 3.5% and 15% were considered underweight (Edney and Smith, 1986; Mason, 1970).

Cats

Of 1620 cats presenting to a referral teaching veterinary hospital, 2% were considered cachectic and 17% considered underweight, compared to 64% considered to be in optimal condition (Kronfeld *et al.*, 1994). In a study of 2050 cats presenting to private veterinary hospitals in the USA, about 3% of cats were considered cachectic and about 15% were underweight (Scarlett *et al.*, 1994).

These data from dogs and cats suggest that, in a veterinary clinic, up to about 20% of patients will present with less than optimal body condition. The underlying cause(s) for the underweight dog or cat determines treatment strategies.

CAUSES OF UNDERWEIGHT CONDITIONS

Loss of body weight may represent loss of water (dehydration), fat (condition), protein (muscle wasting), or mineral (osteoporosis). Many of the causes of underweight conditions in animals are summarised in Table 8.1. Any condition, however, which may suppress appetite, impair voluntary food consumption, increase energy demands, or lead to neglect by the patient's caretaker should be considered when assessing underweight dogs and cats.

Energy

Animals lose weight when energy intake fails to meet energy needs. Energy intake may be poor because of partial or complete anorexia due to disease and stress, or such factors as appetite-suppressing medication, jaw fractures, and old age. In addition, energy intake will be compromised with poor diets, including rations containing low energy density, low protein content, or

Physiological Changes
Pregnancy
Lactation
Old age; senescence, senility
Exercise
Feeding Mismanagement
Deprivation of food
Low dietary energy or protein
Malnutrition
Abrupt changes in diet
Trauma
Pain-induced anorexia
Head injuries
Maxillary fracture, mandibular fracture, dislocation
Inability to access food
Diseases
Tooth loss
Oral disease
Pain- or nausea-induced anorexia
Parasitism
Malabsorption; chronic diarrhoea
Diabetes mellitus; endocrine disorders
Chronic failure of liver, pancreas, heart
Chronic infection
Cancer
Theriatrogenic Causes
Medication and supplements (such as mineral oil)
Drug use; ephedrine, amphetamines
Hospitalisation
Neglect or abuse by owner; abandonment
Physical or mental incompetence/ignorance of owner
Ambient Conditions
Exposure to cold, wind

Table 8.1: *Causes of underweight body conditions in dogs and cats.*

unbalanced nutrient content. Abandoned and stray dogs and cats often suffer from starvation; many will be underweight and some will be cachectic. In these patients, underfeeding and parasitism often combine to create large energy deficits, cachexia, and life-threatening debilitation.

Energy needs increase with above-maintenance physiological conditions, such as exercise and lactation, and with certain disease states, such as infection and wound healing. If food intake fails to keep up with increased energy demands, weight is lost.

Feeding Management

Poor feeding management may lead to weight loss. In these cases, the animal's diet may be balanced, but the amount offered may be inadequate, poorly timed, or placed in a competitive or distracting setting.

Another type of feeding management leading to poor body condition arises from intentional withholding of food by owners of large and giant breed puppies, in futile attempts to prevent or mitigate musculoskeletal problems such as osteochondrosis dissecans (OCD) or wobbler syndrome. While gross overfeeding is not recommended nor considered to be a healthy practice for animals, feeding for optimal growth, with diets of optimal energy and protein, is not associated with the development of OCD or other disorders that have been studied (Nap *et al.*, 1991; Slater *et al.*, 1992). Dietary factors other than energy, such as high and low calcium intakes and anion-cation balance, may impact on these disorders (Hazewinkel *et al.*, 1985; Hazewinkel *et al.*, 1991; Kealy *et al.*, 1993; Nap *et al.*, 1991; Slater *et al.*, 1992). In the author's opinion, restricting dietary energy for puppies to the degree that body condition is poor or growth is impaired, is medically unsound and ethically unjustifiable.

Diet

Dietary inadequacies may also lead to weight loss or failure to grow. In practice, this may be seen with vegetarian diets, because plant-source ingredients such as rice, potato, tofu, and oatmeal, contain fewer calories than animal-source ingredients, such as meat, cheese, and eggs. Although vegetarian diets can be formulated by professionals to meet nutritional needs of some adult dogs at maintenance, these rations rarely meet nutritional needs of dogs for growth, reproduction, or activity, and invariably fail to meet the needs of any cat.

Another nutritional cause for weight loss is the feeding of inappropriate commercial diets. For example, maintenance-type diets fed to puppies may result in growth failure, and when fed to lactating bitches may lead to poor milk production. Diets that pass tests for weight control under optimal ambient conditions, such as the feeding trial protocols of the Association of American Feed Control Officials (AAFCO) fail to maintain animals outdoors in cold temperatures. These problems of mismatched diets may become evident in a carefully taken history.

Specific nutrient deficiencies also lead to weight loss. Protein deficient diets are seen in pets fed homemade diets comprised mainly of carbohydrate-rich ingredients such as breads, potatoes, rice, or diets with too much fat added for palatability. Empty calories induce subclinical multiple nutrient deficiencies and insidious loss of performance. The condition has been seen in sled dogs worked hard in cold temperatures and fed diets with added vegetable oils or tallow for energy.

Vitamin and mineral deficiencies may lead to weight loss but, as distinct entities, are less common in practice. Oversupplementation with vitamin/mineral products is occasionally associated with underfeeding of diets. Some supplements claim (erroneously) to improve digestibility, thereby implying that less food can be offered, thus exacerbating the problem of underfeeding.

Home-made diets that are imbalanced with regard to energy and several nutrients may result in an underweight dog or cat. Recipes of balanced and complete home-made diets for dogs and cats are easy to prepare (Donoghue and Kronfeld, 1994).

Because so many different causes of weight loss are possible, investigation of the thin patient is painstaking and time consuming. Throughout the course of patient workup, many diseases must be considered, and the reader is referred to the appropriate sections of this text for diagnostic aids concerning specific disease processes. Emphasis here focuses on nutrition-related aspects of patient evaluation.

PATIENT ASSESSMENT

History

The patient's history may provide valuable clues regarding the cause of its underweight condition. A history of anorexia and vomiting in an old thin dog, for example, may signal chronic renal failure. One of the first aspects of a dietary history is to estimate if the thin dog or cat is taking in too few calories, or if calorie intake appears adequate. The latter finding prompts careful investigation of energy expenditure.

Care is necessary when taking a dietary history, in order for the information to be valid. For example, clients may be distraught and unable to recollect accurately, the current diet may not reflect the patient's usual intake, the client may not be the one who feeds the pet, and information may be withheld if clients suspect the feeding regimen will be judged to be inappropriate. Collection of valid dietary information usually involves a standardised approach. It is often most productive to begin gently, with minimal prompting that may bias responses, and to eventually ask the crucial questions — what is fed, how much, how often — more than once to test the reliability of the reporting.

When taking a dietary history, owners may be asked about the pet's current, usual, and prior diets, including brands and varieties (flavours) of pet foods, home-made diets, free choice foods and meals, commercial and home-made snacks, treats and table foods, and unsupervised activities such as hunting and scavenging. Also ascertained are the individuals responsible for the purchase of pet foods and the actual feeding. Information is obtained on pet food purchases (number of packages per week) and compared with meal offerings (volume per day). These should match.

To assess energy intake, general approximations may be used to assess energy contents of foods. Canned (wet) premium dog and cat foods often contain about 1-1.3kcal/g (4.2-5.4kJ/g) as fed (AF) (wet weight); maintenance-type canned pet foods, about 0.8-1kcal/g (3.3-4.2kJ/g) AF. Dry premium dog and cat foods contain about 4-4.5kcal/g (16.7-18.8kJ/g) AF; maintenance-type dry pet foods, about 3.5-4kcal/g (14.6-16.7kJ/g) AF. Diets intended for weight loss contain about 70 to 85% of the calories found in premium and maintenance pet foods. Biscuit-like treats for dogs are similar to maintenance-type dry pet foods. Medium-sized (about 5g) dog treats contain about

Food	Energy (kcal/g as fed)[1]	Protein	Fat	Carbohydrate
		← (% calories)		→
Chicken,				
w/ skin	2.3	42	58	0
w/o skin	2.0	56	44	0
Lamb	2.8	36	64	0
Beef, lean	2.7	37	63	0
Liver, beef	1.6	63	28	9
Salami	3.8	23	76	1
Gravy	0.5	27	39	34
Egg	1.5	33	64	3
Cottage cheese,				
creamed	1.0	48	40	12
low fat	0.7	86	5	9
Cheddar cheese	4.0	25	74	1
Yogurt,				
low fat	0.6	31	26	43
Ice cream	2.0	7	48	45
Rice	1.3	8	2	90
Potato	1.1	8	1	91
Green beans	0.4	18	7	75

Table 8.2: *Energy content of table foods commonly fed to dogs and cats.*

1 To convert results from kcal to kJ, multiply by 4.184

Body Weight		Multiples of Maintenance (kcal ME/day)[1]							
lb	kg	0.75	1.0	1.5	2.0	2.5	3.0	3.5	4.0
2.5	1.1	91	121	181	242	303	363	424	484
5	2.3	153	203	305	407	509	611	713	815
7.5	3.4	207	276	414	558	690	828	966	1104
10	4.5	257	342	514	685	856	1027	1199	1369
15	6.8	349	464	696	928	1161	1392	1624	1857
20	9.1	432	576	864	1152	1439	1727	2017	2304
25	11.4	510	681	1020	1361	1702	2042	2383	2724
30	13.6	585	781	1170	1561	1952	2344	2731	3122
40	18.2	726	969	1453	1937	3301	2905	3389	3873
50	22.7	859	1145	1718	2589	2862	3434	4007	4580
60	27.3	985	1313	1969	2625	3281	3938	4594	5250
70	31.8	1105	1474	2210	2947	3683	4421	5157	5894
80	36.4	1221	1628	2445	3257	4071	4886	5700	6515
90	40.9	1334	1779	2669	3558	4448	5338	6227	7117
100	45.4	1444	1925	2888	3850	4813	5775	6739	7705
120	54.5	1656	2207	3311	4415	5519	6623	7727	8830
140	63.6	1858	2478	3717	4957	6196	7435	8674	9913
160	72.7	2054	2739	4109	5478	6848	8218	9588	10957

Table 8.3: *Average daily energy required by dogs. Calories were calculated as multiples of maintenance (M) energy, where M, kcal/day =* $110W_{kg}^{0.75}$.[2]

1 *To convert results from kcal to kJ, multiply by 4.184.*
2 *This is an average value; the coefficient of variation is about 20%, so that, for example, about one dog in seven needs 20% more, and another from the same seven needs 20% less (Kendall* et al.*, 1983).*

Body Weight		Multiples of Maintenance (kcal ME/day)[1]							
lb	kg	0.75	1.0	1.5	2.0	2.5	3.0	3.5	4.0
4.0	1.8	95	127	191	254	318	382	445	509
4.5	2.0	107	143	215	286	358	430	501	573
5.0	2.3	119	159	239	318	398	477	557	636
5.5	2.5	131	175	262	350	438	525	612	700
6.0	2.7	143	191	286	382	477	573	668	764
6.5	3.0	155	207	310	414	517	620	724	827
7.0	3.2	167	223	334	445	557	668	780	891
7.5	3.4	179	239	358	477	596	716	835	954
8.0	3.6	190	254	382	509	636	764	891	1018
8.5	3.9	202	270	406	541	676	811	946	1082
9.0	4.1	214	286	430	573	716	859	1002	1145
10.0	4.5	238	318	477	636	795	954	1114	1273
10.5	4.8	250	334	501	668	835	1002	1169	1336
11.0	5.0	262	350	525	700	875	1050	1225	1400
11.5	5.2	274	366	549	732	915	1098	1281	1464
12.0	5.4	286	382	573	764	954	1145	1336	1527
13.0	5.9	310	414	620	827	1034	1241	1448	1654
14.0	6.4	334	445	668	891	1114	1336	1559	1782
15.0	6.8	358	477	716	954	1193	1432	1670	1909
16.0	7.3	382	509	764	1018	1273	1527	1782	2036

Table 8.4: *Average daily energy required by cats. Calories were calculated as multiples of maintenance (M) energy, where M, kcal/day =* $70W_{kg}$.[2]

1 *To convert results from kcal to kJ, multiply by 4.184.*
2 *This is an average value; the coefficient of variation is about 20%, so that, for example, about one cat in seven needs 20% more, and another from the same seven needs 20% less (Kendall* et al.*, 1983).*

15kcal (63kJ); small soft cat treats (about 1.5g) contain about 5kcal (21kJ). Calorie contents of some table foods often fed to dogs and cats are summarised in Table 8.2.

Estimates of energy expenditure are based on the dog or cat's weight, age, and physiological state, such as growth, lactation, activity, and health. Calculated energy needs based on body weights are presented for dogs (Table 8.3) and cats (Table 8.4). Maintenance levels are those energy intakes sufficient to maintain weight in adult healthy dogs and cats, that are at rest or mildly active, living in comfortable surroundings. Estimates drop below maintenance for inactive dogs and cats, such as those that are very old, or kept in a confined space or cage at home or in the hospital. Severely underweight animals decrease voluntary activity in order to spare energy and protein mobilisation.

Energy needs increase above maintenance for many reasons, including physical activity, physiology, health, and ambient conditions (Table 8.5). For animals considered to be below or above maintenance, the calculated maintenance energy intake is multipled by an appropriate number to account for altered caloric needs (Table 8.5).

Estimates can be made of calories taken in and expended, based on a thorough dietary history, the patient's energy needs relative to maintenance, and reference to Tables 8.2–8.5. In this way, one ascertains appropriate strategies for patient management. Further workup is needed for many cases, however, to diagnose underlying disease or other potential causes of weight loss.

		Adjustment
Growth:	Preweaning	3.0
	Postweaning	2.0
	Half mature size	1.5
Gestation:	First trimester	1.0-1.1
	Second trimester	1.1-1.4
	Third trimester	1.2-1.5
Lactation:	Early	2.0-3.0
	Late	1.5-2.0
Hot environment		1.0-1.1
Cold environment		1.0-2.0
Physical activity		1.0-6.0
Physical inactivity		0.7-0.9
Starvation		0.5-0.7
Trauma:	Mild	1.0-1.1
	Moderate	1.1-1.4
	Severe	1.2-2.0
Cancer		1.0-1.8
Sepsis		1.2-1.5
Burns:	Moderate	1.1-1.5
	Severe	1.2-1.8

Table 8.5: *Individual adjustments recommended for adjustment of maintenance energy (M), where M = maintenance energy/day in dogs and cats. Additional adjustments are made upward for hyperactivity and steroid therapy, or downward for paralysis and coma (Donoghue, 1989).*[1]

1 *This list is intended only as an approximate guide for groups of animals. Prediction of a specific energy goal for an individual must accumulate all relevant factors: breed, age, weight, body condition, physiological states, physical activity, environment, and pathological conditions.*

Physical Examination

Underweight conditions are usually diagnosed by observation and palpation of the patient. Fat cover over ribs and lumbar region is noted, as well as muscling over the skull, lumbar regions and limbs. From observation and palpation, a score describing body condition is assigned (Table 8.6) (Donoghue, 1989). Body condition scoring utilises numerical or pictorial systems (Table 8.6) (Donoghue *et al.*, 1991; Donoghue and Kronfeld, 1993; Kronfeld *et al.*, 1991; Scarlett *et al.*, 1994).

In a study of 250 dogs, body condition scoring was highly correlated (r=0.90) to a measure of total body fat utilising dual energy x-ray absorptiometry (DEXA) (Laflamme *et al.*, 1994). Body condition scoring adds a few seconds to a physical examination and costs little, in contrast to DEXA estimates of body fat which require 20 minutes and a large financial investment. The information return on investment in body condition scoring is exceptional.

Most scoring systems consider amounts of fat over ribs. For many cats, ventral abdominal and inguinal fat needs to be considered as well as rib cover (Donoghue and Kronfeld, 1993; Scarlett *et al.*, 1994). Recent work suggests that body condition scoring accurately assesses these extra fat stores. Body condition scores derived from pictorial silhouettes discriminated cats of different weights and girth measurements with a relatively high degree of accuracy, with correlation coefficients of 0.77 and 0.75, respectively (Scarlett and Donoghue, unpublished data). Body weights and abdominal girth measurements for cats considered thin and cachectic are provided (Table 8.7).

Score	Condition
1	Cachectic; no obvious body fat.
2	Thin; limited body fat evident.
3	Optimal; ribs and lumbar musculature palpated easily but not observed readily.
4	Overweight; ribs difficult to palpate.
5	Obese; large amounts of subcutaneous fat, obvious impairment.

Table 8.6: *Example of one five-point body condition scoring system (Donoghue and Kronfeld, 1993). Specific conditions will vary according to age and breed. For example, a Labrador Retriever puppy in optimal condition carries more fat than an adult Greyhound in optimal condition.*

Condition	BCS	Weight (kg)	Girth (cm)	Percent of Study Population
Cachectic	1	3.1	32.3	3
Lean	2	3.7	36.3	15
Optimal-lean	3	4.3	39.5	26
Optimal	4	5.2	44.1	30

Table 8.7: *Body weights and abdominal girth measures from underweight cats presenting to US veterinary hospitals (Scarlett* et al.*, 1994; Scarlett and Donoghue, unpublished data). A six-point body condition scoring (BCS) system was used (Scarlett* et al.*, 1994).*

Laboratory Aids

Dogs and cats that are underweight because of chronic underfeeding but are not suffering severe starvation may have normal blood profiles. Other non-starved underweight patients that are sick from disease may provide test results reflective of the underlying disease process, such as elevated globulin concentration with chronic infection or elevated creatinine concentration with renal failure. There are no practical, readily available blood tests that are specifically diagnostic for weight loss due to underfeeding in dogs and cats. Anaemia is used in AAFCO feeding trials as a non-specific indication of an inadequate diet.

Blood tests from severely starved dogs may show:

- moderate hypoglycaemia or normoglycaemia
- decreased insulin:glucagon ratios
- decreased plasma T3 concentration
- increased free fatty acids
- decreased concentrations of gluconeogenic amino acids
- increased concentrations of branched chain amino acids

(Donoghue, 1989; Hendrick *et al.*, 1990).

Starved cats may show similar changes, but little has been published on the subject. Although ketogenesis and ketolysis increase in starved dogs, and presumably starved cats, plasma ketone concentrations appear to stay within normal ranges (Donoghue, 1989).

Several techniques, in addition to body condition scoring, have been investigated for applicability in assessment of body condition in dogs and cats. These include ultrasound, DEXA, and bioelectrical impedance (Booles *et al.*, 1994; Munday *et al.*, 1994; Toll *et al.*, 1994; Wilkinson and McEwan, 1991). Also, techniques for assessing energy needs, in addition to observation and calculation, have been tested, such as doubly labelled water and calorimetry (Ballevre *et al.*, 1994; Burger, 1994). To date, none of these techniques is suited for clinical practice and none has been shown to impact patient outcome better than accurate history-taking, observation and calculation, and clinical judgement.

Necropsy

Patients only mildly underweight may show few specific lesions at necropsy, except for those dogs and cats with specific diseases. Underweight dogs and cats mobilise fat before protein, so serous atrophy may be observed at necropsy of those patients with moderate or severe weight loss. For most species, fat depletion begins with the coronary and perirenal adipose sites, then proceeds to subcutaneous fat, and, lastly, omental fat. With longstanding energy deprivation, serous atrophy disappears and there are little or no traces of fat visible.

Muscle wasting, indicative of protein mobilisation, is also visible with severe or longstanding energy deprivation. Tissue loss may be observed in the muscles of the skull, loins, forearms, and rear quarters. The size of the latter muscles also changes with activity.

Animals mobilise relatively more protein with catabolic stress than with simple fasting. Thus dogs and cats suffering from trauma or infection, for example, will exhibit relatively more muscle wasting relative to weight loss than patients that are underfed only.

DIETARY STRATEGIES

Dietary management of underweight dogs and cats depends on the underlying cause of the animal's poor condition. For example, special commercial diets are available for dogs with advanced renal disease or intestinal malabsorption. The former are low in protein, the latter may be low in fat, so both may be unpalatable. How to feed an unpalatable diet to an anorexic dog or cat so as to overcome the cause of its anorexia is a challenge for clinicians.

Regardless of underlying cause, an understanding of the metabolic state precipitated by weight loss aids formulation of general dietary strategies. Thin dogs and cats may be categorised as exhibiting effects of simple or complicated starvation. Simple starvation describes those patients that have been underfed while growing or housed in the cold, for example. Complicated starvation describes thin patients that are also catabolic. These animals may have serious infection, multiple injuries, advanced cancers, or thermal burns.

Simple Starvation

Underfed dogs and cats utilise hepatic glycogen stores to supply necessary glucose for cells in the brain, blood, and kidneys. After about 36h of fasting, amino acids are mobilised for glucose synthesis. Fat is mobilised from adipose tissue to supply energy needs for remaining cells. Thus dogs and cats that are totally or partially starved are utilising fat and protein as energy sources.

For starved dogs and presumably cats, fatty acid utilisation accounts for 70–85% of energy expenditure, ketones up to 15%, protein up to 25%, and carbohydrate less than 10% (Donoghue, 1989). Provision of limited (<30% of calories) carbohydrate to fasted dogs is not harmful, but excessive (>50%) carbohydrate upsets the metabolic balance of a fat-adapted dog. Carbohydrate is unnecessary for cats at any time.

Complicated Starvation

In addition to the above changes, patients suffering from complicated starvation may exhibit a 'diabetes of injury' characterised by peripheral insulin resistance and glucose intolerance (Donoghue, 1989). In addition, dogs and cats with trauma and wounds mobilise amino acids not just for energy but also for anabolic activities such as antibody production and tissue growth.

Patients with complicated starvation may be termed hypermetabolic (because of increased energy needs) and catabolic (because of protein mobilisation and subsequent nitrogen loss). Degrees of hypermetabolism and catabolism are graded according to the degree of injury or illness (Table 8.5).

Diet Selection

The metabolic changes outlined above suggest that diets containing relatively more protein and fat than carbohydrate are better suited for underweight patients. The one exception is those thin patients with a disease such as lymphangiectasia, that is managed specifically by fat restriction (minimal amounts of safflower or sunflower oils).

Other diet characteristics include palatability, and high protein quality, digestibility, and nutrient bioavailability. These characteristics, along with optimal levels of fat and protein, are more likely to be found in commercial or home-made (freshly made) diets that are comprised of mainly animal-source rather than plant-source ingredients, or in commercial liquid enterals. Since nutrient balance is critical for optimal utilisation of food in starved patients, home-made diets are recommended only if balanced and complete (Donoghue and Kronfeld, 1994).

Amounts to Feed

When feeding underweight patients, the goal is to achieve a suitable energy intake, which has usually been calculated or estimated from tables (Tables 8.3–8.5). For cases of simple underfeeding, the patient can be brought up to the desired food level usually within 2 to 4 days. Occasionally, sudden increases in dietary fat causes soft stools but such faecal changes are transient.

For patients with severe or complicated starvation, transitions must be more gradual, usually in more than 4 days. The animal is started at a level as low as 50% of maintenance. The level is increased to maintenance over about 2 weeks. Although starved enterocytes begin renewal almost immediately upon feeding, some malabsorption and diarrhoea may be evident during the first week in cachectic patients. For these animals,

Product	Energy (kcal/ml)[1]	Protein	Fat (% kcal)	Carbohydrate	Comments
Pedigree® Canine Instant Concentration[2]	1.5	3.8	35	27	Dry form, hydrolysed protein
Whiskas® Feline Instant Concentration[2]	1.24	37	41	22	Dry form
CliniCare®[3]					
Canine	0.99	20	55	25	Liquid and dry forms
Feline	0.92	30	45	25	Liquid and dry forms
RenalCare®[3]					
Canine	0.88	11	63	26	Phosphorus = 0.10%
Feline	0.84	22	57	21	Phosphorus = 0.10%
Ensure®[4]	1.06	14	31	55	Available in groceries
Enrich®[4]	1.08	14	31	55	Contains 10mg fibre/ml
Criticare HN®[5]	1.06	14	3	83	Low fat; hydrolysed protein
Traumacal®[5]	1.5	22	40	38	Higher energy density
Pulmocare®[5]	1.5	17	55	28	Higher energy density

Table 8.8: *Nutritional characteristics of commercial liquid enteral products. All of these products contain essential nutrients in relatively balanced amounts.*

1 To convert results from kcal to kJ, multiply by 4.184
2 WALTHAM Veterinary Diets, Masterfoods Austria
3 Pet-Ag, Elgin, IL, 60120, USA.
4 Ross Laboratories, Columbus, OH, 43216, USA.
5 Mead Johnson, Evansville, IN 47721, USA.

feeding strategies should be checked to ensure that the patients are not overfed and the patient may be treated symptomatically. The problem resolves within days.

Patients failing to consume at least 85% of goals for energy intake are candidates for involuntary feeding (see Chapter 17). Generally, feeding via indwelling tube creates less stress and physical damage than repeated intubations. Meal feeding via tube is better tolerated metabolically than continuous feeding. Enterals or enterals blended with premium pet foods are superior nutritionally to pet foods blended with water. Enterals are sterile, highly digestible, and well balanced nutritionally, thus providing superior nutrition (Table 8.8).

Complications

Most of the weight gained during the early refeeding period is water and fat, not protein which is vital for recovery. Factors other than weight, such as the patient's attitude and activity may be better than body weight as determinants of successful refeeding in the early stages.

Overfeeding patients with severe debilitation is associated with life-threatening hypokalaemia and hypophosphataemia, termed the refeeding syndrome. The problem is more common in patients fed intravenously or with continuous enteral feedings than in patients meal-fed by enteral means (Solomon and Kirby 1990). With starvation, whole body levels of potassium and phosphorus decrease; blood levels remain normal at the expense of intracellular concentrations. With refeeding, potassium and phosphorus enter cells rapidly with insulin and glucose, causing precipitous drops in circulating levels. This phenomenon has been shown in dogs and presumably occurs in cats (Silvis *et al.*, 1980). Dietary supplements fail to prevent refeeding syndrome (Maier-Dobersberger and Lochs, 1994); prevention is best achieved through cautious refeeding and monitoring.

REFERENCES

Ballevre O, Anantharaman-Barr G, Gicquello P, Piguet-Welsh C, Thielin A-L and Fern E (1994). Use of the doubly-labeled water method to assess energy expenditure in free living cats and dogs. *Journal of Nutrition,* **124,** 2594S-2600S.

Booles D, Poore DW, Legrand-Defretin V and Burger IH (1994). Body composition of male and female Labrador retriever puppies at 20 wks of age. *Journal of Nutrition* **124,** 2624S-2625S.

Burger IH (1994). Energy needs of companion animals: matching food intakes to requirements throughout the life cycle *Journal of Nutrition* **124,** 2584S-2593S.

Donoghue S (1989). Nutritional support of hospitalized patients. *Veterinary Clinics of North America: Small Animal Practice*, **19,** 475.

Donoghue S, Khoo L, Glickmann LT and Kronfeld DS (1991). Body condition and diet of relatively healthy older dogs, *Journal of Nutrition* **121**, S58.

Donoghue S and Kronfeld DS (1993). Feeding the Hospitalised Cat. In: *Handbook of Feline Medicine*. Eds J Wills and A Wolf. Pergamon Press. Oxford. pp 35-47.

Donoghue S and Kronfeld DS (1994). Homemade diets for dogs and cats. In: *The Waltham Book of Clinical Nutrition of the Dog and Cat.* Eds J Wills and K Simpson. Pergamon Press, Oxford. pp 445-449.

Edney ATB and Smith PM (1986). Study of obesity in dogs visiting veterinary practices in the United Kingdom, *Veterinary Record* **118**, 391.

Hazewinkel HAW, Goedegebuure SA, Poulos PW and Wolvekamp WTC (1985). Influence of chronic calcium excess on the skeletal development of growing Great Danes. *Journal of American Animal Hospital Association* **21**, 377.

Hazewinkel HAW, Van den Brom WE, Van 'T Klooster ATh, Voorhout G and Van Wees A (1991). Calcium metabolism in Great Dane dogs fed diets with various calcium and phosphorus levels. *Journal of Nutrition* **121**, S99.

Hendrick GK, Frizzell RT, Williams PE and Cherrington AD (1990). Effect of hyperglucagonemia on hepatic glycogenolysis and gluconeogenesis after a prolonged fast, *American Journal of Physiology* **258**, E841.

Kealy RD, Lawler DF, Monti KL, Biery D, Helms RW, Lust G, Olsson S-E, and Smith GK (1993). Effects of dietary electrolyte balance on subluxation of the femoral head in growing dogs, *American Journal of Veterinary Research* **54**, 555.

Kendall PT, Blaza SE and Smith PE (1983). Comparative digestible energy requirements of adult beagles and domestic cats for body weight maintenance, *Journal of Nutrition* **113**, 1946.

Kronfeld DS, Donoghue S and Glickman LT (1991). Body condition and energy intakes of dogs in a referral teaching hospital, *Journal of Nutrition* **121**, S157.

Kronfeld DS, Donoghue S and Glickman LT (1994). Body condition of cats, *Journal of Nutrition* **124:** 2683S-2684S.

Laflamme DP, Kealy RD and Schmidt DA (1994). Estimation of body fat by body condition score. *Proc Twelfth Annual Veterinary Medicine Forum* p 985.

Maier-Dobersberger T and Lochs H (1994). Enteral supplementation of phosphate does not prevent hypophosphatemia during refeeding of cachectic patients, *Journal of Parenteral and Enteral Nutrition* **18**, 182.

Mason E (1970). Obesity in pet dogs, *Veterinary Record* **86**, 612.

Munday HS, Earle KE and Anderson PA (1994). Changes in the body composition of the domestic shorthaired cat during growth and development. *Journal of Nutrition* **124,** 2622S-2623S.

Nap RC, Hazewinkel HAW, Voorhout G, Van den Brom WE, Goedegebuure SA and Van 'T Klooster ATh (1991). Growth and skeletal development in Great Dane pups fed different levels of protein intake, *Journal of Nutrition* **121**, S107.

Scarlett JM, Donoghue S, Saidla J and Wills JM (1994). Overweight cats - prevalence and risk factors. *International Journal of Obesity* **18**, S22.

Silvis SE, DiBartolomeo AG and Aaker HM (1980). Hypophosphatemia and neurological changes secondary to oral caloric intake, *American Journal of Gastroenterology* **73**, 215.

Slater MR, Scarlett JM, Donoghue S, Kaderly RE, Bonnett BN, Cockshutt J and Erb HN (1992). Diet and exercise as potential risk factors for osteochondritis dissecans in dogs, *American Journal of Veterinary Research* **53,** 2119.

Solomon SM and Kirby DF (1990). The refeeding syndrome: a review, *Journal of Parenteral and Enteral Nutrition* **14**, 90.

Toll PW, Gross KL, Berryhill SA and Jewell DE (1994). Usefulness of dual energy x-ray absorptiometry for body composition measurement in adult dogs. *Journal of Nutrition* **124,** 2601S-2603S.

Wilkinson MJA and McEwan NA (1991). Use of ultrasound in the measurement of subcutaneous fat and prediction of total body fat in dogs, *Journal of Nutrition* **121**, S47.

CHAPTER NINE

The Obese Animal

Peter J. Markwell and Andrew T.B. Edney

INTRODUCTION

Obesity is something of a paradox. Owners rarely present their animals for the treatment of accumulated body fat, whereas some 25% of dogs (Edney and Smith, 1986) and cats (Scarlett *et al.*, 1994) seen by veterinarians are fatter than the optimum. There is good evidence that the state of obesity is often associated with pathological changes and may eventually be life threatening (Markwell and Butterwick, 1994).

The condition of obesity is usually identified as having been reached when the accumulation of adipose tissue reaches a stage where there are pathological changes as a direct result. These changes are mainly associated with the additional load on various body systems. This is notable with the musculoskeletal system. As in humans, osteoarthritis is a common sequel of obesity (Edney, 1974). Similarly the demands on the cardiovascular system are likely to be excessive when an animal is too fat. Added to this, there are increased anaesthetic and surgical risks with obese animals (Clutton, 1988). The physical complications of operating through excessive fatty tissue are immediately evident. Adiposity also tends to insulate animals from heat loss. Although this can be advantageous in some circumstances, it results in discomfort and distress in high ambient temperatures. The first very hot day of the year can be a real trial for overweight dogs especially. The very close association between obesity and diabetes mellitus in man has been known for many years (Hundley, 1956), and a similar link has been established in the dog (Krook *et al.*, 1960) and cat (Panciera *et al.*, 1990). Liver disease may also be an important consequence of obesity. Fatty infiltration of the liver has been noted in obese dogs (Joshua, 1970; Lewis, 1978), but of particular importance is the relationship between liver disease and obesity in cats. Obesity is considered an important predisposing factor to idiopathic hepatic lipidosis (IHL) in this species, a condition carrying a poor prognosis (see Chapter 12). Typically cats presented with this condition will have a history of obesity followed by recent weight loss, and will have been partially or completely anorectic for a period of time (median two to three weeks). The anorexia may have been caused by some stress such as moving house or by attempts to change the cat's diet (Center, 1986; Hardy, 1989). There are no figures available for the effects obesity has on life span in companion animals, but it is reasonable to assume that excessive amounts of body fat will reduce the life span of all mammals.

ASSESSMENT OF PATHOLOGICAL STATUS - RECOGNISING OBESITY

The obese condition is one which is usually readily recognisable from a distance. However, there are other reasons for being overweight. Among these are oedema, ascites, tumours and even pregnancy. As with all conditions, a proper examination is necessary to establish a diagnosis. Not only do the differential diagnoses have to be considered, but any complications associated with obesity need to be identified.

By its very nature, obesity is an insidious condition. It may take many months to develop but there are certain characteristics which can be identified. Fat which is deposited subcutaneously is usually easily palpable. That which is found in the chest area eventually prevents the rib cage from being easily felt. Fatty deposits begin to alter the outline of dogs and cats as described by Joshua (1970). The effects of neutering lead to a modification of body outline in both dogs and more so in cats. Entire male cats tend to be very lean at the rear end and have strong muscular thick skinned heads. After castration, the head is seen to be more like the female in appearance. Folds of fat appear on the flank and especially in the inguinal region. Owners sometimes become concerned that these folds may be tumours or similar abnormalities.

As body composition determinations are not very practical in every day practice, a subjective assessment has to be made. Criteria for the assessment of body fat status in dogs were outlined by Edney and Smith (1986) (Table 9.1). It was found that most of the ill effects of obesity were associated with the gross category only, 3% of all dogs seen. Being a little overweight due to fat was not particularly harmful but it has to be remembered that the condition is likely to be progressive. The gross state is almost certain to result from a continuation of conditions which brought about the obese situation.

Classification	Observations
Thin	Pronounced underweight, no obvious body fat
Lean	Little body fat evident, skeletal structure obvious
Optimum	Moderate amount of body fat, rib cage easily palpable, but not showing too obviously
Obese	Rib cage not visible when dog moves, bones of the chest barely palpable, body weight noticeably more than normal for type
Gross	Unable to feel ribs, large amounts of subcutaneous fat can be grasped by hand, obvious incapacity due to excess fat

Table 9.1: *Criteria for the assessment of body fat status in dogs (from Edney and Smith, 1986).*

DEVELOPMENT OF OBESITY

As dogs are mainly opportunist feeders they are more likely to become obese, compared with cats. Feeding behaviour in any individual is a result in part of the innate characteristics and of the behaviour gained during development. Some breeds are prone to overeating. These include the hounds and certain gundogs, particularly the Labrador.

There is an indication that as far as dogs are concerned, neutering increases the probability of obesity in later life. This suggests that there are endocrine factors which influence the utilisation of food by individuals which have been castrated or spayed. However, very few cases of canine obesity appear to be a direct result of thyroid disturbances (A. Rijnberk, personal communication).

Once a dog has achieved a state of positive energy balance, that is it is taking on more energy than it is using, the effect is cumulative. Even small amounts of energy rich food in excess of requirements, if allowed to continue on a daily basis, will be steadily deposited as adipose tissue. Owners who feed a dog every time it will eat food and allow it to dictate the amounts of food provided, are moving towards having an obese animal in the household. Feeding from the table, giving special treats frequently if they are not included as part of the total daily ration, leaving food lying around, and constant scavenging will all add to the obese state. With cats the situation is complicated by hunting and when more than one household feeds the animal. Some owners do not realise that what they see as 'their' cat may be viewed in the same way at more than one other home.

DIETARY STRATEGY - REVERSING THE OBESE STATE

As a positive energy balance *at some time* is always the reason for the obese condition, a negative energy balance is required to reverse this state. That is the animal has to have an energy intake which is less than the energy it is using. When this situation prevails, the animal draws on its own adipose tissue as a source of energy. This principle is the basis for all slimming regimens. However, too drastic energy restriction leads to losses of lean body mass and can be harmful. Because of this, starvation regimens are not advised. Although dogs can withstand food deprivation for several days without apparent ill effect, there is no reason why risks should be taken when simple calorie controlled diets are both effective and have good owner compliance. Starvation is contraindicated in cats because of the risks of IHL.

Requirements

Energy

The quantity of diet to be fed initially should be calculated as a proportion of the animal's maintenance requirement at its **target weight** (see below).

For **dogs** it is recommended that maintenance (kcal/day) is calculated from the equation:

$$110 \text{ x body weight (kg)}^{0.75} \text{ (equation 1)}$$

The proportion of this maintenance requirement that is fed should be between 45 and 60% (Markwell and Butterwick, 1994). Weight losses averaging approximately 1% per week have been achieved by feeding 45% of maintenance energy requirements (Markwell *et al.*, 1994). Table 9.2 provides a summary of recommended energy allowances at various target weights, calculated as 45% of maintenance requirements. These can be converted readily into a food allowance by dividing by the energy content of the diet used. For example:

Target body weight = 10 kg
Maintenance at target weight (from equation 1) =
$110 \text{ x } 10^{0.75} = 619$ kcal/day
Recommended energy intake for weight loss =
$0.45 \text{ x } 619 = 279$ kcal/day
Food allowance (assuming 57 kcal/100 g) =
$279/0.57 = 489$ g/day.

Commercially prepared foods offer clear advantages over home-prepared diets when trying to assess amounts to feed, as the energy content will be both known and consistent.

Care should be taken with energy restriction in **cats**, because of the risks of IHL (as discussed above). The National Research Council (1986) suggested a

Current Body weight (kg)	Target Body weight (kg)	Energy Requirement at Target Weight (kcal[1]/day)	Recommended Energy Allowance for Weight Reduction (kcal[1]/day)
2	1.7	164	74
4	3.4	275	124
6	5.1	373	168
8	6.8	463	208
10	8.5	548	247
15	12.75	742	334
20	17	921	414
25	21.25	1089	490
30	25.5	1248	562
35	29.75	1401	630
40	34	1549	697
45	38.25	1692	761
50	42.5	1831	824
55	46.75	1967	885
60	51	2099	946

Table 9.2: *Recommendations for weight reduction in dogs.*

1 To convert kcal into kJ multiply by 4.184

Current Body weight (kg)	Target Body weight (kg)	Energy Requirement at Target Weight (kcal[1]/day)	Recommended Energy Allowance for Weight Reduction (kcal[1]/day)
4	3.4	204	122
4.5	3.83	230	138
5	4.25	255	153
5.5	4.68	281	168
6	5.1	306	184
6.5	5.53	332	199
7	5.95	357	214
7.5	6.38	383	230
8	6.8	408	245

Table 9.3: *Recommendations for weight reduction in cats.*

1 To convert kcal into kJ multiply by 4.184

range for maintenance energy allowance for cats of 70-80kcal/kg/day (293-335kJ/kg/day). However, recent studies suggested that the maintenance energy requirements of very inactive cats (which presumably apply to most obese individuals) may be much lower (Earle and Smith, 1991). Taking these data in conjunction with a recent report of a weight reduction study in which reductions averaging 13.5 ± 6.3% were safely achieved over a period of 18 weeks in client owned cats (Butterwick *et al.*, 1994), it is recommended that maintenance (kcal/day) at the target weight is calculated from the following equation:

60 x body weight (kg) (equation 2)

The animal should then be fed approximately 60% of the requirement calculated from equation 2 (Markwell *et al.*, 1994). Table 9.3 shows recommended energy allowances for various target weights calculated on this basis. These can be converted to food allowances as described above.

For both dogs and cats it may be necessary to reduce these allowances depending on an individual animal's response (monitored as described below). If weight loss is not occurring, a reduction of 10% in food allowance may be made. If reductions are made it is important, especially for cats, that the health of the animal is particularly closely monitored.

Nutrients

A number of adverse health problems during weight loss in man have been attributed to possible deficiencies in minerals or vitamins (Fisler, 1992; Weinsier *et al.*, 1984). There is no evidence to suggest that the mineral, vitamin or essential fatty acid requirement of the dieting individual is reduced. Thus, vitamin and mineral intake should be maintained at normal levels.

Some lean body mass in obese individuals is lost with effective dieting (Forbes and Drenick, 1979). However, excessive protein loss during weight reduction is not desirable, because functional tissue losses will need replacing. Some of the adverse effects of very low calorie diets in man may be related to inadequate protein intake and the subsequent loss of lean body mass (Weinsier *et al.*, 1984). For cats, in particular, excessive tissue protein loss should be avoided since protein or specific amino acid deficiencies may be causative factors in the pathogenesis of idiopathic hepatic lipidosis (Bauer and Schenck, 1989; Cornelius and Jacobs, 1989).

A dose response curve between preservation of lean tissue mass and increasing protein content of very low calorie diet formulations has been demonstrated in man during weight loss (Phinney, 1992). However, the protein requirement to maintain optimum well-being and minimise tissue protein loss during weight reduction has not been determined. It would appear prudent, therefore, to provide at least as much protein to the individual on a weight reduction programme as would normally be expected to maintain a non-dieting individual of comparable weight.

For these reasons, diets designed for feeding during weight reduction should have increased levels of essential nutrients relative to their energy content, when compared with normal foods, to take account of the lower energy intake of the dieting animal. This is because (as explained in Chapter 2) standard foods are formulated with their nutrients balanced to their energy content. One advantage of some commercial diets designed for weight reduction is that this point is addressed during their formulation.

In human and small animal medicine one attempt to overcome hunger during weight reduction programmes has been to include additional **dietary fibre**. A recent review indicated a variable response of different dietary fibres on satiety in man (Leeds, 1990). Although a number of studies in man have shown a short-term effect of fibre on intake (Bolton *et al.*, 1981) and on the perception of hunger (Levine *et al.*, 1989), there is no evidence to suggest that these effects are maintained, or whether compensation in energy intake occurs in the long term. There is some evidence to suggest that the type of fibre ingested may be important with regard to satiety. There is, however, little evidence to support the feeding of high levels of insoluble fibre for the treatment of obesity in the companion animal. Observations in the dog suggest that inclusion of raw materials containing high levels of insoluble fibre to a commercial low calorie diet has no apparent beneficial effect on satiety (Butterwick and Markwell, 1994). In contrast, a number of studies have suggested that soluble fibres may be more effective than insoluble fibres in inducing satiety (Delargy *et al.*, 1993; Stevens *et al.*, 1987). However, long-term studies need to be conducted in order to evaluate the potential benefits of soluble fibre in the obese companion animal. In addition, a high intake of soluble fibre is associated with gastrointestinal signs (bloating and flatulence) and loose stools (Krotkiewski, 1984; Stevens *et al.*, 1987) which may limit the levels of soluble fibre used in products for the treatment of obesity.

Method

A careful, methodical approach is crucial in the successful treatment of obesity in companion animals. Just advising on a diet, or worse simply telling an owner to feed the animal less, is usually not good enough. The case has to be *managed.* It has been recommended that three components are prescribed together for obesity therapy in man:

- diet
- behavioural/psychological support
- and exercise (Weinsier *et al.*, 1984).

These can be applied to a variable extent in the companion animal. Undoubtedly, the key to success is compliance from the owner and all who are involved in feeding the animal, as ultimately they will control its food intake. Thus, it may be argued that this is the area where behavioural/psychological support is provided, rather than directly to the patient. Exercise programmes may be beneficial as they can promote increased energy expenditure and fat loss, and help maintain lean body mass (Weinsier *et al.*, 1984). They are relatively easy to implement in dogs, but clearly difficult to apply to cats. Any exercise programme should be well within the capabilities of both patient and owner, and should be introduced with caution. Increased activity should be self-generating rather than forced. Practical experience has indicated that a step-wise approach to the management of companion animal obesity, working with the client, provides a good level of compliance

Dietary objectives	Reduce body weight Maintain health
Dietary characteristics	Nutrient levels increased to account for restricted intake Low energy density
Energy requirement	Dog - 50 x target weight[1] $(kg)^{0.75}$ kcal/day Cat - 36 x target weight[1] (kg) kcal/day
Specific nutrient requirements	Maintain intake of essential nutrients at normal levels
Food type	Commercial canned or dry Home-prepared
Regimen	Client counselling / patient evaluation Set target weight / calculate food allowance Re-assess and weigh fortnightly / adjust food allowance if necessary Calculate maintenance allowance Follow up regularly

Table 9.4: *Dietary management of obesity.*

1 Target weight based on 15% reduction from current weight.

(Butterwick *et al.*, 1994; Edney, 1974; Markwell *et al.*, 1990). Based on these experiences the following programme is recommended (Figure 9.1), and the overall approach to management is summarised in Table 9.4.

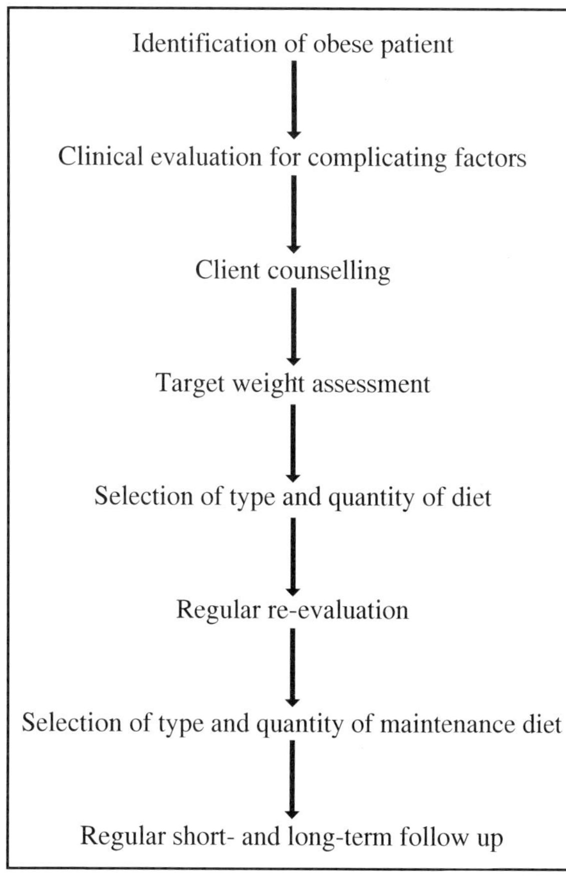

Figure 9.1: *Stages in controlled calorie reduction.*

1) **Identification of obese patient** (see above).

2) **Clinical evaluation for complicating factors**. The terms complicated and uncomplicated obesity differentiate between adiposity arising from overeating / underexercising, and that arising from other causes (Clutton, 1988). The most important causes of complicated obesity are endocrine disorders and drug induced polyphagia, although very rare cases may arise from hypothalamic lesions (de Bruijne and Lubberink, 1977). Even though these underlying conditions are relatively uncommon, it is necessary to determine their presence or absence to allow for appropriate therapy. Thus taking a history and performing a physical examination, and if necessary, thyroid and adrenal function testing, should be a part of initial case assessment.

3) **Client counselling.** This is probably the most important aspect. Once a diagnosis has been arrived at, the owner needs to be counselled on the necessity of taking the subject seriously enough to bring about the desired result. The client should be convinced of the clinical importance of the problem, the benefits that will be derived from weight reduction, and the need to follow the feeding regimen precisely. This means making sure everyone who comes into regular contact with the patient keeps to the regimen prescribed. One person feeding even small amounts 'illicitly' can mean the difference between success and failure. It may be necessary to have the whole family present when the plan is laid down, and at this point owner/animal interactions that may lie at the root of an individual obesity problem can be investigated and discussed.

One strategy worth considering to help with compliance is to set the charges for the whole course of treatment at the outset. This gives the owner some incentive to keep to the instructions and to ensure that the rest of their family does as well. Another device which can be used is to fit a conspicuous badge on the dog's collar indicating that it is not to be given extra food as it is on a strict dietary programme.

4) **Target weight assessment.** Two approaches may be considered, either targeting immediately for an ideal body weight, or a standard initial reduction followed by reassessment. The latter approach, although potentially taking longer to achieve an ideal weight for an individual, is recommended for several reasons. Firstly, it can be very difficult on initial presentation to judge the ideal weight for many individuals, particularly cross-bred dogs, although reference to breed standards and the type under treatment may allow an estimate to be made. With a gradual reduction through one or more targets a more accurate assessment is possible. Secondly, by using a standard and moderate reduction, the time likely to be required to achieve weight loss will be known to the veterinarian and can be indicated to the owner. This will facilitate monitoring of compliance and provide encouragement to the owner. If very large initial targets are set, the owner may despair of ever achieving them, and compliance may suffer. For these reasons an initial target of a 15% reduction from current body weight is recommended; it is likely that most dogs or cats assessed as obese will require at least this degree of weight loss. This result should be achieved in 10–15 weeks in dogs and 16–20 weeks in cats at the feeding levels recommended, although individual variation must be expected.

5) **Selection of type and quantity of diet.** Several aspects of this have been considered above, and some of the advantages of commercial diets designed for weight reduction described. Additional factors worthy of consideration are the palatability of the diet and the volume of food offered to the animal. The suggestion that provision of a bland or tasteless food to companion animals on weight reduction programmes will be beneficial since it will limit intake (Lewis, 1978) is clearly unhelpful. It could be argued that any mechanism by which palatability is reduced could be used as a method in designing a low calorie diet. However, it is important that any diet which is used as a part of a weight reduction programme is palatable, since long-term acceptance will influence compliance and ultimately the success of the programme. This is particularly important in cats which are recognised as 'finicky' eaters (Castonguay, 1981), since poor acceptance of an unpalatable diet can lead to withdrawal from weight reduction studies, or worse still, prolonged anorexia and the risk of hepatic lipidosis (Burrows *et al.*, 1981). Use of calorie-dilute, relatively bulky foods may assist in compliance; the owner sees their pet as receiving a reasonable volume of food despite the reduction in energy intake, which may help to assuage any feelings of guilt they have in restricting their animal's food intake.

   Once the diet has been prescribed, it is vital that no other food is allowed at all. Drinking water is the only supplement allowed. Owners who like to give the odd treat, say at bedtime, may still do so **but it must come out of the total dietary allowance**. This is more effective than trying to prohibit such practices. The whole allowance may be divided into several small frequent meals. The temptation to feed the whole allowance several times a day has to be resisted!

6) **Regular re-evaluation.** This is another key factor in achieving success. It provides an opportunity to monitor progress and the health of the animal, make any needed adjustments to the feeding regimen, and for practice staff to discuss progress with the owner. This provides encouragement and reinforcement of the need for compliance to the programme. It is recommended that animals are reassessed every two weeks, ideally weighed on the same set of scales and at the same time of day. Although it is useful for the clinician to keep a careful watch on progress, weighings and adjustments in food allowance can be made by a practice nurse. Any medical changes must be reported and a physical examination carried out by the clinician without delay. If there is serious impairment of the animal's health a clinical examination is needed at every weighing. If weight loss is not occurring, possible reasons can be explored with the owner, and if necessary reductions in food allowance made (see above). Simple graphs of weight loss can be plotted at these re-evaluations to demonstrate progress to the owner, as initially changes may not be apparent in the animal.

   If it proves impossible to enforce the necessary compliance by normal levels of supervision, it will probably mean that the animal has to be hospitalised. Even then it will be necessary to make sure the practice staff are aware of the need to be strict. Some animals are very skilled at looking very appealing when there is the prospect of additional food being given. Hospitalisation to achieve weight reduction is not really desirable, as it does not address the issues associated with the owner's feeding practices which led to development of the problem in the first place.

7) **Selection of type and quantity of maintenance diet and regular follow up.** These are important to try to prevent recurrence of the problem. Although understanding and helping the owner to bring about a change in the husbandry practices that contributed to, and maintained, the obese state are also very important. It is essential that the owner is advised very strongly that the case is not resolved until the animal is eating a diet which maintains it at the optimum body weight. All too often the discipline is lost and the animal and the owner are soon back where they started. There are currently few data on which to base feeding recommendations for animals following weight reduction programmes, therefore, it is recommended that initial maintenance levels are calculated using equations 1 and 2. However, it is essential that cases are followed up to make adjustments to food intake to maintain the animal at its ideal weight. It is recommended that commercially produced diets are used in preference to home-prepared foods, as their energy content will be both consistent and known, and thus they can be fed in a more controlled manner. To begin with, follow up examinations should be as frequent as the weighings which were carried out for the treatment. If all goes well these can be reduced to monthly and then three monthly intervals. Owners can be encouraged to weigh their own animals if this can be achieved reliably. After six months of success, the case can be reviewed annually, preferably at each appointment for booster vaccinations.
   Many practices provide ongoing feeding advice for their clientele. When this is available, the nurse or counsellor can keep a close eye on the body weight and general health of the practice patients.

Obesity Clinics

Some practices find that they like to treat their obese animals at particular clinics. One afternoon a week may be set aside to deal with all the obese animals. It is possible to make use of the supportive and competitive aspects of the shared problems of owners. This can be carried out in the style of 'Weight Watchers' or even 'Alcoholics Anonymous', providing a 'competitive' environment which may increase motivation amongst some owners. Owners can compare notes, provide mutual support and other social benefits.

REFERENCES

Bauer JE and Schenck PA (1989). Nutritional management of hepatic disease. *Veterinary Clinics of North America: Small Animal Practice* **19,** 513.

Bolton RP, Heaton KW, Burroughs LF (1981). The role of dietary fibre in satiety, glucose, and insulin: studies with fruit and fruit juice. *American Journal of Clinical Nutrition* **34,** 211.

Burrows CF, Chaipella AM and Jezyk P (1981). Idiopathic hepatic lipidosis: the syndrome and speculations of it's pathogenesis. *Florida Veterinary Journal* **10,** 18.

Butterwick RF and Markwell PJ (1994). Effect of level and source of dietary fibre on food intake in the dog. *Proceedings of BSAVA Congress*, p 157 (abstract).

Butterwick RF, Wills JM, Sloth C and Markwell PJ (1994). A study of obese cats on a calorie controlled weight reduction programme. *Veterinary Record* **134,** 372.

Castonguay TW, (1981). Dietary dilution and intake in the cat. *Physiology and Behaviour* **27,** 547.

Center SA (1986). Feline liver disorders and their management. *Compendium on Continuing Education* **8,** 889.

Clutton RE (1988). The medical implications of canine obesity and their relevance to anaesthesia. *British Veterinary Journal* **144,** 21.

Cornelius LM and Jacobs G (1989). Feline Hepatic Lipidosis. In: *Current Veterinary Therapy X, Small Animal Practice*. Ed. RW Kirk, WB Saunders, Philadelphia p 869.

De Bruijne JJ and Lubberink AAME (1977) Obesity. In: *Current Veterinary Therapy X, Small Animal Practice*. Ed. RW Kirk, Saunders, Philadelphia p 1068.

Delargy HJ, Burley VJ, Blundell JE, O'Sullivan KR and Fletcher RV (1993). The effects of fibre in the breakfast upon short-term appetite control: a comparison of soluble and insoluble fibre. *Proceedings of the Nutrition Society, Summer Meeting*. PC 52.

Earle KE and Smith PM (1991). Digestible energy requirements of adult cats at maintenance. *Journal of Nutrition* **121,** S45.

Edney ATB (1974). Management of obesity in the dog. *Veterinary Medicine/Small Animal Clinician* **49,** 46.

Edney ATB and Smith PM (1986). Study of obesity in dogs visiting veterinary practices in the United Kingdom. *Veterinary Record* **118,** 391.

Fisler JS (1992). Cardiac effects of starvation and semi-starvation diets: safety and mechanisms of action. *American Journal of Clinical Nutrition* **56**(Suppl), 230S.

Forbes GB and Drenick EJ (1979). Loss of body nitrogen on fasting. *American Journal of Clinical Nutrition* **32,** 1570.

Hardy RM (1989). Diseases of the liver and their treatment. In: *Textbook of Veterinary Internal Medicine*, Ed. SJ Ettinger, WB Saunders, Philadelphia p 1479

Hundley JM (1956). Diabetes - overweight: U.S. problems. *Journal of the American Dietetic Association* **32,** 417.

Joshua JO (1970). The obese dog and some clinical repercussions. *Journal of Small Animal Practice* **11,** 601.

Krook L, Larsson S and Rooney JR (1960). The interrelationship of diabetes mellitus, obesity and pyometra in the dog. *American Journal of Veterinary Research* **21,** 120.

Krotkiewski M (1984). Effect of guar gum on bodyweight, hunger ratings and metabolism in obese subjects. *British Journal of Nutrition* **52,** 97-105.

Leeds AR (1990). Mechanisms of action of dietary fibre in weight loss. In: *Progress in Obesity Research*. Eds. Y Oomura, S Tarui, S Inoue and T Shimazu. John Libbey and Company, London p 519.

Levine AS, Tallman JR, Grace MK, Parker SA, Billington CJ and Levitt MD (1989). Effect of breakfast cereals on short-term food intake. *American Journal of Clinical Nutrition* **50,** 1303.

Lewis LD (1978). Obesity in the dog. *Journal of the American Animal Hospital Association* **14,** 402.

Markwell PJ and Butterwick RF (1994). Obesity. In: *The Waltham Book of Clinical Nutrition of the Dog and Cat*. Eds. JM Wills and K Simpson. Pergamon Press, Oxford p 131-148.

Markwell PJ, Butterwick RF, Raiha M and Wills JM (1994). Clinical studies in the management of obesity in dogs and cats. *International Journal of Obesity* **18,** S39-S43.

Markwell PJ, Van Erk W, Parkin GD, Sloth CJ and Shantz-Christienson T (1990). Obesity in the Dog. *Journal of Small Animal Practice* **31,** 533.

National Research Council (1986). *Nutrient Requirements of Cats*. National Academy Press, Washington D.C.

Panciera DL, Thomas CB, Eiker SW and Atkins CE (1990). Epizootiologic patterns of diabetes mellitus in cats: 333 cases. *Journal of the American Veterinary Medical Association* **197,** 1504.

Phinney SD (1992). Exercise during and after very-low-calorie dieting. *American Journal of Clinical Nutrition* **56**(Suppl), 190S.

Scarlett JM, Donoghue S, Saidla J and Wills JM (1994). Overweight cats: prevalence and risk factors. *International Journal of Obesity* **18,** S22-S28.

Stevens J, Levitsky DA, Vansoest PJ, Robertson JB, Kalkwarf HJ and Roe DA (1987). Effect of psyllium gum and wheat bran on spontaneous energy intake. *American Journal of Clinical Nutrition* **46,** 812-817.

Weinsier RL, Wadden TA, Ritenbaugh C, Harrison GG, Johnson FS and Wilmore JH (1984). Recommended therapeutic guidelines for professional weight control programmes. *American Journal of Clinical Nutrition* **40,** 865.

CHAPTER TEN

Feeding the Cardiac Patient

Mike Davies

INTRODUCTION

All animals have basic nutritional requirements including the need for energy-producing nutrients and other essential nutrients. In the cat and dog these include essential amino acids, fatty acids, vitamins and minerals though there are significant differences between the two species. Cats and dogs do not have an absolute requirement for carbohydrates to be present in their ration providing other sources of glucose (gluconeogenic amino acids and glycerol) are present. In fact, most prepared pet foods do contain carbohydrate and both species can utilise them well. Dietary recommendations have been published based on the nutritional requirements of **normal** cats and dogs (National Research Council, 1985, 1986).

Although several veterinary publications contain chapters on nutrition in relation to cardiac disease (Ettinger and Suter, 1970; Ralston and Fox, 1988; Ross, 1987; Stepien and Miller,1994) very little work has been done to determine the precise nutritional requirements of animals with subclinical or clinical cardiac disease. However, it is possible to make value judgements about appropriate nutrition for individual cases by applying basic nutritional principles to our knowledge of the aetiopathogenesis and complications of cardiac disorders.

Consideration of nutrition is important in **all** cardiac patients because of its role:

1) As a causative factor in the onset of the disease
2) As a complicating factor in the presence of a cardiac disorder
3) In maintaining energy and essential nutrient status in the animal.

Nutritional management is a prerequisite to successful clinical management of all animals with cardiac disease.

NUTRITIONAL ASSESSMENT OF THE CARDIAC PATIENT

When decision-making in cardiac disease it is important to assess the nutritional status of the patient at the outset because this can affect:

- the choice of type of diet for the patient
- the choice of, and dose rate of, drugs used in treatment
- the prognosis for medical or surgical intervention
- interpretation of laboratory results
- interpretation of ECG information.

Physical Examination

In man there are a number of non-invasive, objective measurements that are routinely used as indicators of nutritional status (e.g. measurement of skin fold thickness) but there is no generally accepted method for cats or dogs. This leaves us with subjective visual appraisal and palpation of skeletal muscle mass. A reduction in skeletal muscle mass might indicate energy malnutrition and/or negative nitrogen balance. Anorectic cats, or those with catabolic disease such as cardiac failure or hyperthyroidism, often lose lean body mass very rapidly. In the future non-invasive techniques using ultrasound or electrical impedance may prove useful.

It is useful to attribute a body score to individuals when assessing nutritional status (see also Chapters 8, 9 and 18 for body score methodology):

Body Score	Description
5	Gross Obesity
4	Overweight
3	Normal
2	Underweight
1	Emaciated

Body Weight Assessment

See Table 10.1.

Obesity

Obesity is associated with increased oxygen consumption which is met by increased stroke volume. Myocardial changes including hypertrophy may result and arrhythmias may occur. Respiratory efficacy is reduced in obesity and is manifest as 'pickwickian syndrome' with hypoventilation, which may predispose to the development of cor pulmonale.

Mortality increases in people with obesity in whom the development and progression of cardiac disease may be exacerbated, resulting in cardiomegaly, cor pulmonale, circulatory congestion, oedema, ascites and hypervolaemia (Van Itallie, 1980). Similar changes may be recognised in canine and feline patients. Hypertension may also be exacerbated by obesity.

Obesity may result in low voltage QRS complexes which can make ECG interpretation difficult, particularly in cases of suspected pericardial effusion or myocardial disease. It should be remembered that obesity can mask an underlying depletion of lean body mass.

Questions to Answer	Comment
Overweight ? **NB Needs to be differentiated clinically from 'apparent weight gain' because of abdominal distension due to hepatomegaly or ascites.**	Compare to published 'normal weight range' for breed and frame size; 15% greater than normal is significant. Subjective assessment : a) cannot feel ribs on palpation b) loss of 'waist' between last rib and iliac crest when viewed from above c) large fat pad at base of tail (dogs) d) large pendulous skin fold or 'skirt' in inguinal region (cats) e) large perivulval folds of skin (dogs).
Underweight ?	Compare to published 'normal weight range' for breed and frame size; 15% less than normal is significant. Subjective assessment : a) can see ribs b) can easily palpate ribs and dorsal processes of spinal vertebrae with poor muscle mass evident c) generally poor body mass on visual inspection d) may be exhibiting non-specific signs of muscle weakness. In the author's experience , the presence of cardiac cachexia is a grave prognostic indicator.
Weight gain or loss recently ?	Cardiac patients often have a history of recent weight loss that precedes or coincides with the onset of cardiac signs. Even animals that are obese when presented to the clinician may have undergone recent weight loss. Animals with cardiac disease are often in a catabolic state and/or have depressed appetites or are anorectic. They may also have impaired gastrointestinal, pancreatic or hepatic function resulting in maldigestion, malabsorption or impaired metabolism.
Has the weight change been rapid or gradual ?	In the author's experience rapid, severe weight loss is a poor prognostic indicator.

Table 10.1: *Body weight assessment.*

Reduced cardiac output accompanies many forms of cardiac disease and results in increased concentrations of circulating catecholamines which may induce a state of peripheral insulin resistance, and so confound the utilisation of blood glucose. Obesity in dogs is associated with hyperinsulinaemia and impaired glucose tolerance (Mattheeuws *et al.*, 1984) hence non-insulin-dependent diabetes mellitus should be considered a potential complication in animals with both obesity and reduced cardiac output as risk factors.

Weight Loss

Cardiac cachexia is a common finding in animals with heart disease and, in the author's experience, patients presenting with advanced cachexia have a worse prognosis. Several causes have been suggested including hypermetabolism induced by hypoxia and/or catecholamine secretion, maldigestion and/or malabsorption, and anorexia. In cats, hyperthyroidism causes hypermetabolism as well as secondary cardiac signs.

Some authors suggest that diets with a relatively low salt content may be the cause of cachexia by inducing anorexia due to poor palatability but there is no published evidence to support this (see section on sodium).

Underweight animals require nutritional support and should have their energy intake increased – by hand feeding, tube feeding or parenteral nutrition if they are anorectic. Feed the type of ration that the animal prefers or is used to (e.g. dry or moist, a favourite brand or flavour). This is often necessary in older animals in which eating behaviour patterns are very well established. Odouriferous foods are most likely to stimulate eating, and warming food may also stimulate appetite. Feed animals with depressed appetites small amounts of food frequently throughout the day.

Dramatic alterations in ECG can be expected in animals exhibiting signs of nutritional deficiency. Hypokalaemia (serum concentrations below 3.5m Eq/litre) for example, induces generalised muscle weakness and in dogs ECG changes including increased amplitude of T-waves and progressive sagging of the ST-segment.

Cardiac patients that are underweight are in a catabolic state, in which case underlying primary causes such as hyperthyroidism or other major organ failure should be screened for during the clinical work-up. On routine blood results reduced plasma albumin concentrations, the albumin:globulin ratio, transferrin concentration and total lymphocyte count may all reflect poor nutrition as well as other possible causes such as impaired hepatic function or the presence of renal disease. (See also Chapters 8 and 18 for nutritional assessment.)

Radiographic Findings

Radiographic findings may help in the nutritional assessment of the animal in the following ways:

1) Evidence of fat deposition at various sites in the body – particularly look for subcutaneous fat over the spine on lateral radiographs, falciform fat in the abdomen, pericardial fat, and mesenteric fat in the abdomen (gives contrast to serosal surface of the small intestine if present).
2) Radiographic evidence of right sided heart failure should prompt an assessment of intra-abdominal organ function, particularly hepatic, renal and gastrointestinal tract, dysfunction of which may affect normal digestion, absorption and utilisation of food. The main radiographic signs to look for are increased size (width) of the caudal vena cava, hepatomegaly, abdominal distension, and loss of soft tissue detail in the abdomen with a homogeneous 'ground glass' appearance (e.g. due to ascites). Loss of visceral detail and a homogeneous appearance is also seen in thin, underweight animals with little intra-abdominal fat to provide contrast with the soft tissue structures.
3) Lack of lean body mass is best recognised on radiographs of the proximal limbs where there should be well developed musculature of the biceps and triceps (forelimb) and of the quadriceps and hamstring muscles (hindlimb).

NUTRITION AS A CAUSATIVE OR COMPLICATING FACTOR IN CARDIAC DISEASE

Nutrition should always be considered as a potential causative factor in cardiac disease under the following circumstances:

- more than one individual in a closed population (household, kennel/cattery or litter) are affected
- the animal is fed a home-made or 'fad' diet
- the animal is not fed a 'complete' commercial pet food
- the animal receives unusual supplements to its basic ration.

Calcium

Calcium is required for normal muscle contractility, membrane permeability, myocardial function and neuromuscular transmission.

The final trigger for muscular contraction (including cardiac muscle) is an increase in cytosolic calcium concentration and defects in myocardial calcium pump function may affect cardiac performance. Findings suggest that feeding a high protein diet to rats may induce increased calcium-binding sites on the sarcoplasmic reticulum membranes (Diolulu, 1987) and this mechanism may explain the lower blood pressure and apparent protective effect against hypertension and stroke, seen in stroke-prone rats fed high protein diets.

Hypocalcaemia such as occurs in eclampsia (also called puerperal tetany or milk fever) produces hyperexcitability and, if untreated, results in tetany and death.

Cardiac arrhythmias and even cardiac arrest can be precipitated during the overzealous administration of calcium parenterally, so calcium replacement for hypocalcaemia should be given slowly and electrical activity of the heart should be monitored using an ECG throughout such treatment.

Toxicity due to a single high oral dose of calcium is unlikely. Chronic excessive intake, particularly in the presence of high phosphorus or high vitamin D intake may lead to generalised soft tissue calcification, including calcification of the myocardium.

L-Carnitine

L-Carnitine (3-OH-4-N-trimethylaminobutyrate) is a water-soluble quaternary amine which is present in many natural foodstuffs of animal origin, especially liver and muscle tissue, but very little is found in plant materials. It can be synthesised from lysine and methionine in the liver.

Cardiac myocytes depend upon the oxidation of fatty acids for their energy supply and L-carnitine facilitates transfer of activated long-chain fatty acids across the double membrane of the cardiocyte mitochondria. Carnitine also assists in the removal of toxic waste products formed within the mitochondria. Lack of free L-carnitine results in primary myocardial disease in many species including humans, turkeys, dogs and hamsters. The condition has been reported to occur in a family of Boxer dogs (Keene *et al.*, 1991), and also in unrelated Dobermann Pinschers and American Cocker Spaniels.

Recent studies suggest that myocardial free carnitine deficiency occurs in approximately 50% of dogs with dilated cardiomyopathy and that chronic rapid ventricular pacing may induce this local deficiency in the presence of normal or elevated plasma concentrations of L-carnitine (Keene, 1994).

L-Carnitine deficiency is likely to be caused by inadequate synthesis, dietary deficiency (actual or due to malabsorption), increased losses (such as renal), increased esterification of free carnitine or membrane transport defects at the level of the cardiac myocyte.

Dogs require exogenous carnitine to maintain plasma concentrations even though they can synthesise it, and in part this may be due to their limited ability to reabsorb carnitine in the kidneys.

The precise mechanism of the role of carnitine in cardiomyopathy is unknown but it is hypothesised that membrane transport defects are the probable cause, based upon the fact that myocardial deficiency (confirmed by myocardial biopsy) is associated with normal, or even high plasma concentrations of L-carnitine in 80% of cases. Primary dietary deficiency is unlikely to be the cause unless the ration consists exclusively of plant materials.

Dietary supplementation is recommended in confirmed deficiency, and up to 50% of dilated cardiomyopathy cases show a therapeutic response to L-carnitine administration at a dose of 50–100mg/kg body weight three times daily. D-Carnitine and mixtures of D- and L-carnitine are ineffective as supplements in dogs. At the doses recommended carnitine has not been reported to cause any undesirable side effects.

Chromium

Chromium deficiency has been implicated as an important factor in the aetiopathogenesis of atherosclerosis in humans.

Chromium supplementation to humans has been reported by various authors to reduce serum glucose, insulin, cholesterol, triglycerides, or total lipids – all of which may have a role in the occurrence of atherosclerosis, and chromium administration causes regression of atherosclerotic lesions in rabbits (Abraham *et al.*, 1980, 1982).

There are no published requirements for chromium in the cat or dog.

Copper

Cardiac hypertrophy, cardiac and arterial lesions, altered ECG and hyperlipidaemia are all features of dietary copper deficiency as well as degenerative heart disease and, not surprisingly, this has led to the hypothesis that relative or absolute copper deficiency may be involved in some forms of cardiovascular disease.

Copper is an integral part of many enzymes, and coenzyme concentrations have been shown to be decreased in copper-deficient tissues which could lead to the typical pathological changes seen.

The zinc:copper ratio has been suggested as a risk factor for coronary heart disease based on studies in rats (Klevay, 1975). Also, copper deficiency has been associated with decreased systemic blood pressure, and excessive dietary copper intake with increased systolic pressure (Davis and Mertz, 1987). In experimental animals and humans tachycardia and extrasystolic beats (both ventricular and supraventricular premature beats) have been reported to occur in copper deficiency.

In cattle, copper deficiency can result in 'falling down disease' in which the primary lesion is a slowly progressive myocardial degeneration which leads to acute heart failure. In copper-deficient pigs sudden cardiac failure can result due to cardiac hypertrophy, and copper-deficient chicks, pigs and guinea pigs may die of spontaneous rupture of the heart or artery due to defective connective tissues.

Copper is an essential nutrient for dogs and cats, and deficiency is often associated with anaemia –

which is a reflection of its role in normal iron metabolism. A role for copper in cardiovascular diseasc has not been reported in these species.

Magnesium

Magnesium concentrations in heart muscle and erythrocytes decrease in the presence of congestive heart failure, and there is a correlation between intracellular magnesium deficiency and potassium deficiency. Paroxysmal ventricular fibrillation occurs in human patients with hypomagnesaemia (Loeb *et al.*, 1968).

Digitalis significantly lowers serum magnesium concentrations which, in turn, predisposes patients to digitalis toxicity.

The short-term effects on the heart of hypomagnesaemia include ECG abnormalities, cardiac dysrhythmias and changed sensitivity of the heart to drugs.

Magnesium may be a protective factor against hypertension in humans, (Weinsier and Norris, 1985).

The precise role (if any) of magnesium in cardiac diseases of companion animals needs further investigation. Kittens fed a magnesium deficient diet grew poorly and developed muscular weakness, hyperirritability, convulsions, anorexia, reduced serum and bone concentrations of magnesium and calcification of the aorta. Similar signs are seen in puppies fed a magnesium deficient diet and ECG measurements are also abnormal, being similar to those seen in hyperkalaemia. In cats excessive magnesium intake has also been associated with the development of struvite crystalluria.

Both thiazide and loop diuretics promote the urinary loss of magnesium, and additional losses can result from the use of some drugs including amphotericin-B, gentamycin, tobramycin and digitalis derivatives. Single serum magnesium concentrations are an unreliable measure of magnesium status, and estimation of the magnesium content of mononuclear cells, or of bone or cardiac muscle biopsies are more sensitive. Serial measurements of serum magnesium may, however, be helpful for assessing trends in individual animals.

Selenium

Keshan Disease in humans is characterised by cardiogenic shock, cardiac enlargement, congestive heart failure, arrhythmias, ECG changes and occasionally cardiac thrombosis. It can be treated and prevented by the administration of selenium supplementation (using sodium selenite) (Yan *et al.*, 1984). Selenium deficiency has also been reported in patients receiving total parenteral nutrition without selenium.

Experimentally, selenium has profound effects on cardiac function in the dog by increasing heart rate, peripheral resistance, blood pressure and ischaemic responses to cardiotoxic drugs (Guo *et al.*, 1979).

The cardioprotective effects of selenium are thought to be mediated by reducing lipid oxidation by free radicals.

Sodium

Restriction of sodium (salt) intake has long been accepted as a useful mechanism to reduce the fluid retention that accompanies many forms of heart disease.

As cardiac output or blood pressure fall the renin-angiotensin-aldosterone cascade is stimulated and this results (amongst other things) in the retention of sodium and water - mainly through increased tubular reabsorption in the kidneys (Ross, 1987). As a result of this mechanism, extracellular and vascular fluid volume increase, thus increasing preload. There is a dilution effect on plasma protein concentration which decreases plasma oncotic pressure causing water to move from the vascular to the interstitial compartment resulting in oedema, ascites or congestion.

In support of this mechanism, aldosterone blood concentrations increase in spontaneous congestive heart failure in dogs (Bojs and Conn, 1965), and dogs in congestive heart failure, and those with asymptomatic heart disease exhibit impaired sodium excretion (Hamlin *et al.*, 1967).

Current methods of treatment for the fluid retention that occurs in heart failure include the administration of diuretics which vary in their methods of action. The most frequently used diuretic, frusemide, is a loop diuretic which blocks sodium absorption in the loop of Henle. It also promotes urinary loss of magnesium and potassium and, as with thiazides, can cause hypomagnesaemia or hypokalaemia. Hypomagnesaemia potentiates the cardiac effects of hypokalaemia. Dehydration is a common complication of the overzealous use of potent diuretics and this can result in pre-renal azotaemia. Prolonged diuresis may also lead to depletion of water-soluble vitamins.

An understanding of the haemodynamic mechanisms occurring in heart failure has led to the recommendation that dietary sodium intake be controlled to reduce preload. However, some authors have recently questioned the rationale for sodium restriction in congestive heart failure implying that it may induce hyponatraemia (Stepien and Miller, 1994). There is no evidence that hyponatraemia can be caused by dietary restriction alone, indeed sodium homoeostasis is so efficient that a ration containing only 0.0075% sodium fed to adult dogs failed to result in any side effects (Morris *et al.*, 1976). Chronic dilutional hyponatraemia may occur as a rare complication of severe congestive heart failure when it is associated with major defects in water excretion not with depletion of total body sodium (Bonagura and Lehmkuhl, 1992).

The haemodynamic changes described above are occurring in compensated heart failure and the current recommendation not to restrict dietary sodium intake until the patient is decompensated is irrational. I prefer to minimise sodium intake at the earliest possible stage in heart disease (Stage I- New York Heart Association 1964) **before** it progresses to congestive failure. There is no harm in feeding a relatively low sodium diet.

However such rations should be avoided in the presence of dehydration, chronic diarrhoea or in severely debilitated animals with or without hyponatraemia.

Clinicians frequently misinterpret the nutritional information on pet food labels and in general there is misunderstanding about the current recommendations on sodium intake in heart disease. Some authors inaccurately refer to 'severe sodium restriction' (Stepien and Miller, 1994) when feeding so-called 'low sodium' diets (Hill's Prescription Diets Canine h/d and Feline h/d; Pedigree® Low Sodium). These diets actually contain more sodium than the minimum requirements for dogs and cats, and they should not be expected to reduce total body sodium content or plasma sodium concentrations outside the normal range, particularly in heart failure when, as mentioned previously, homoeostatic mechanisms are operating to retain sodium. Overzealous use of diuretics which increase sodium excretion is more likely to predispose to the development of hyponatraemia than dietary reduction in intake of sodium using available complete foods.

Some authors have suggested that 'low salt' diets are unpalatable to veterinary patients and it is certainly true that some animals with heart disease are anorectic or resist dietary change, but there are many reasons for this:

- Anorexia due to the clinical condition of the animal.
- Behavioural programming through consuming a relatively high sodium content ration prior to the change to a "low salt" diet.
- Reluctance to accept a change in ration from a familiar type e.g. different brand/flavour, dry *versus* wet . Again, this is behavioural programming.
- Depressed appetite due to concomitant drug therapy (e.g. frusemide, digitoxin, digoxin, enalapril, and captopril).
- Depressed appetite caused by stress due to hospitalisation.

The sodium content of some table foods is given in Table 10.2.

Taurine

Taurine (2-aminoethanesulphonic acid) is a sulphonated beta-amino acid which was first associated with the occurrence of dilated cardiomyopathy in cats by Pion and co-workers in 1987. The precise mechanism by which taurine is associated with the disease has yet to be fully elucidated, but low plasma concentrations (less than 20nmoles/ml) were associated with dilated cardiomyopathy, and also (in some cases) with central retinal degeneration. The dilated cardiomyopathy was confirmed by characteristic echocardiographic changes which were reversed by supplementation with 250–500mg taurine/day.

Unlike most mammals, cats are unable to synthesise sufficient taurine to meet their metabolic needs and this, combined with an obligatory loss of taurine that occurs during bile secretion, means that a ration that is low in available taurine can result in low plasma concentrations. Canned foods implicated in the original paper by Pion *et al.* actually contained sufficient taurine after processing based on NRC recommendations for cats. However recent studies using radioactively labelled taurine have shown that during the canning process taurine present in the food can be rendered biologically unavailable. The precise mechanism for this change in bioavailability is unknown, but adequate supplementation of the ration by manufacturers prior to processing can increase availability and maintain plasma concentrations above 40nmoles/ml which is the current recommendation.

Thiamin

Thiamin (vitamin B_1, aneurin(e) or thiamine) was the first water-soluble vitamin to be discovered and it is found in cereal grains and roots. In humans thiamin deficiency results in beriberi, a condition in which both neurological and cardiac changes occur. Thiamin deficiency is reported to occur occasionally in cats and rarely in dogs.

Thiamin is an essential nutrient and important in energy metabolism particularly for the conversion of pyruvate to acetyl CoA. In thiamin deficiency energy metabolism is consequently impaired and pyruvate and lactate concentrations increase in the blood.

Cats usually develop anorexia and weight loss, initially with generalised weakness, ventroflexion of the neck (similar to that seen with hypokalaemia) called Chastek's paralysis, and ataxia. If untreated, neurological signs including seizures and mydriasis may result, and death can follow. Myocardial damage may be present at post mortem as well as the pathognomonic findings of haemorrhages in the periventricular matter of the brain.

Dogs show similar clinical signs, as well as slowing of the pulse, paresis, cramps, opisthotonos, gastrointestinal signs such as vomiting, and hypothermia.

In a recent outbreak of thiamin deficiency in a cattery in the UK cats developed signs of disease when the proprietor changed from feeding a complete cat food to feeding a complementary cat food. On analysis the canned food was found to contain inadequate amounts of thiamin.

The most likely causes of thiamin deficiency are:

- Destruction of the vitamin during the cooking or storage of canned commercial food. This can be avoided by incorporating sufficient thiamin in the food prior to processing.
- The presence of fish containing the enzyme thiaminase, particularly fresh carp and herring which contain a heat-labile thiaminase.

Less than 250mg sodium/100g	More than 250mg sodium/100g
Cereals and cereal products - most except custard powder, self-raising flour and savoury rice.	Bread - most except chapatis. Many contain over 500mg sodium /100g.
Milk and cream - except dried skimmed milk.	Breakfast cereals - most except Shredded Wheat, Sugar Puffs, Smacks, Ready Brek, Raisin Splitz, Puffed Wheat.
Yogurt - most types except Tzatziki.	Biscuits and cakes - most varieties.
Puddings and desserts - most except instant dessert powder.	Cheese - most types except fromage frais (Contrary to popular belief cottage cheese contains 380mg sodium per 100g).
Eggs and egg dishes - most except scrambled egg, omelette, quiche.	Butter and margarine.
Oils - all types.	Bacon meats - can contain over 2000mg sodium per 100g.
Raw (unsalted) meats - most contain less than 100mg sodium per 100g.	Meat products - most including beefburgers, brawn, pies, sausages, pate can contain over 1500mg sodium /100g.
Offals - most e.g. liver, kidney,tripe.	Crustaceans - crabs, lobsters, prawns.
Fresh fish - most except anchovies, kippers.	Fish products e.g. pies, fish cakes, fish fingers, salted/smoked.
Molluscs - most except cockles (3000mg sodium/100g).	Savoury snacks - most including potato crisps, corn snacks, twiglets.
Fresh vegetables - most. Potatoes, beans, lentils, peas, asparagus.	Powdered drinks - many including cocoa powder, Complan, Horlicks, drinking chocolate.
Herbs and spices - most except chilli powder and curry powder.	Soups and sauces - most including canned and packet soups. Some packet soups contain over 5000mg sodium per 100g.
Fruit - most except mixed peel and olives in brine.	
Nuts - most except salted or roasted, or pistachios.	
Sugars or preserves - most except golden syrup, toffees.	

Table 10.2: *Sodium content of foods (after McCance and Widdowson, 1991).*

Clinically thiamin deficiency can be treated by administration of thiamin, 100–200mg intravenously or subcutaneously twice daily. Prevention is by avoiding the feeding of raw fish and ensuring the feeding of a pet food with nutritional adequacy proven by feeding trials.

Vitamin D

In humans some reports suggest that increased intake of vitamin D may be associated with an increased risk of heart disease (Knox, 1973; Linden, 1974). Such a relationship has not been described in domesticated pets.

Excessive intake of vitamin D results in increased calcium absorption, hypercalcaemia and widespread calcification in soft tissues, including the myocardium.

Vitamin E

Vitamin E deficiency causes Zenker's degeneration of both skeletal and cardiac muscle. The role of vitamin

E in the body is complicated because of its intimate relationships with selenium, polyunsaturated fatty acids, antioxidants and sulphonated amino acids in the ration. Vitamin E is an important natural antioxidant and the amount needed depends upon the composition of the ration.

In dogs vitamin E deficiency causes skeletal muscle dystrophy with generalised muscle weakness.

In cats high polyunsaturated fatty acid intake such as in tuna and other fish oils, in the presence of inadequate vitamin E concentrations causes pansteatitis or yellow fat disease (NRC, 1986). This disease usually causes anorexia, lethargy, pyrexia and thoracic and abdominal pain. Local interstitial myocarditis may also be a feature of this disease (Gershoff and Norkin, 1962). The minimum requirement for cats is 30mg α-tocopherol per kg diet, but this will vary depending upon the amount of fat, selenium and other antioxidants present in the food. This minimum requirement may be trebled or even quadrupled in the presence of high dietary concentrations of polyunsaturated fatty acids.

NUTRITIONAL MANAGEMENT OF THE CARDIAC PATIENT

General Considerations

A ration should be selected that will provide sufficient energy and all essential nutrients in sufficient quantities to meet the animal's individual requirements. At the same time it should not contain excessive amounts of nutrients which may play a role in the development or progression of the underlying disease.

It is important to take into consideration concomitant disorders in other body systems, particularly reduced hepatic and renal function which often accompany heart failure.

The precise requirements for energy and other essential nutrients have yet to be determined for animals with most forms of heart disease.

Energy

Patients with heart disease are often in a catabolic state and some form of nutritional support may be necessary if voluntary food intake is depressed. For most forms of heart disease cage rest is recommended and, under such conditions, it is unlikely that energy needs will exceed published maintenance requirements for the individual.

As a general rule fat is the preferred energy source because it has very high digestibility and provides 2.25 times as much energy per gram as either carbohydrate or protein. Cats, being obligate carnivores, need more protein-calories in their ration than do dogs. Fat is also an important palatability factor for both dogs and cats, and it is a valuable source of fat-soluble vitamins.

A high fat diet would not be the best choice in the presence of metabolic complications such as hyperlipidaemia, gross obesity or fat malabsorption (due to impaired hepatic, pancreatic or small intestine function).

Obesity

Obesity should be avoided throughout life and, if present, be corrected in cardiac patients and animals predisposed to develop heart disease, such as those over 7 years of age.

As a general rule overweight animals should have their energy intake reduced to induce weight loss. Feeding only 60% of the animal's energy requirement for it's target (optimal) weight is usually needed to achieve this, hence a diet of low energy density specifically formulated for the purpose should be used (Hill's Prescription Diets Canine r/d or Feline r/d; Pedigree® Canine Low Calorie or Whiskas® Feline Low Calorie). Exceptions to this rule are when an obese animal is already losing weight because it is in a catabolic state, or the presence of concomitant compromise of gastrointestinal, pancreatic or hepatic function, in which case a highly digestible, moderate energy content diet is preferable.

Weight loss should not exceed 3% per week for dogs or 1% per week for cats. Excessive weight loss has been associated with arrhythmias - possibly due to depletion of potassium or magnesium, and rapid weight loss in obese cats can precipitate hepatic lipidosis.

Protein

Protein needs have not been determined for patients with heart disease, however protein malnutrition rapidly occurs in the presence of catabolic disease and inadequate food intake. Hypoproteinaemia may be present in cardiac disease with reduced liver function.

Excessive protein intake should be avoided in the presence of renal failure and azotaemia.

Cats with heart disease, and notably those with hyperthyroidism, have frequently lost a considerable amount of lean body mass by the time that they are presented to a veterinarian for treatment by their owner. This protein malnutrition needs to be reversed to avoid complications such as immune compromise, poor tissue healing and repair, weakness and generalised debilitation.

Vitamins

Both water-soluble and fat-soluble vitamin intake needs to be maintained and, if diuresis is being induced by the use of potent diuretics such as frusemide, it is prudent to increase water soluble vitamin intake to compensate for urinary losses.

Vitamin depletion may also occur in the presence of prolonged anorexia or fat malabsorption.

Minerals and Electrolytes

Heart disease is frequently seen in patients with advancing age and there may be concomitant problems in other major organ systems. When progressive renal disease is present particular attention needs to be paid to minimise excessive phosphorus and calcium intake because phosphorus retention is common and can lead to mineralisation in many tissues - including the heart itself.

Hypokalaemia and hypomagnesaemia are potential complications in heart disease and dietary intake needs to be adequate.

Restriction of sodium intake is discussed earlier in this chapter and also below under specific cardiac conditions.

Fibre

The presence of fibre in a ration reduces the bioavailability of many nutrients through complex physicochemical mechanisms. In heart disease there may be impaired hepatic, pancreatic or gastrointestinal function as well and so feeding a ration with a high dietary fibre content would be inappropriate.

Home-made *versus* Prepared Pet Foods

As a general rule home-made rations are inadequate for long-term feeding and they are expensive to produce. Commercially available complete pet foods are preferred by the author (Hill's Prescription Diets Canine h/d or Feline h/d; Canine k/d or Feline k/d; Pedigree® Canine Low Sodium and Whiskas® Feline Low Sodium).

Snacks or titbits containing a high salt content should be avoided (see Table 10.2).

Positive Nutritional Support

It is the author's experience that animals presenting in poor body condition have the worst prognosis irrespective of the underlying disease process and positive nutritional support is an essential component of their management. Recommended methods of providing nutritional assistance to cardiac patients include the following:

- Select the type of food that the patient is used to e.g. dry *versus* wet.
- Feed a highly digestible, nutritionally complete ration.
- Feed several small meals a day.
- Warm food (below body temperature).
- Add water to food (improves palatability for dogs).
- Hand feed.
- Tube feed - naso-oesophageal, oesophageal, gastrostomy. Naso-oesophageal tubes (8French for both cats and dogs) can be easily placed in conscious animals, but have the disadvantage that liquidised solid foods cannot be passed through them easily. Liquid diets can be passed through naso-oesophageal tubes, but they have the disadvantage of a relatively low energy content, so large volumes have to be given to meet energy requirements.
- Force feeding - is stressful and should be avoided in animals with clinical heart disease.
- Parenteral nutrition - In moribund cases total parenteral nutrition (TPN) should be considered but this should only be performed under the guidance of an experienced clinical nutritionist (see Chapter 17).

Congestive Heart Failure

Whatever the underlying cause, dietary management in congestive heart failure includes the following steps:

1) Ensure maintenance energy needs are met and ensure adequate essential nutrient intake. Avoid unnecessary excessive intake of nutrients which may play a role in the development or progression of cardiac disease. Preferably feed a diet that has been specifically formulated for animals with congestive heart disease.
2) Assess the nutritional status of the patient and correct any abnormality. If the patient is underweight increase energy intake. If the animal is obese and not already losing weight feed a low calorie diet according to manufacturer's instructions to reduce body weight. Do not exceed 3% loss of body weight per week for dogs, 1% loss per week for cats.
3) Limit dietary sodium intake to decrease preload. Feed a complete ration containing less than 0.1% sodium.
4) Ensure adequate intake of potassium, magnesium and water-soluble vitamins if animal is on diuretics or has concomitant renal disease.
5) If patient is anorectic provide positive nutritional support.
6) With advancing age the early introduction of a relatively low sodium diet will help with acceptance in later life when cardiac disease is most likely to occur. The author recommends the avoidance of rations with a relatively high sodium content i.e. over 0.75% sodium.

Cardiomyopathy

Dogs

If clinical signs of heart failure are present feed as for congestive heart failure.

Consider the possibility of L-carnitine deficiency. Feed a complete balanced ration containing adequate amounts of L-carnitine. If diagnosis of L-carnitine deficiency is suspected or confirmed by biopsy of cardiac muscle treat with 50–100mg/kg body weight three times daily.

If other presenting signs are consistent, consider the possibility of thiamin deficiency.

Cats

If clinical signs of heart failure are present feed as for congestive heart failure.

If dilated cardiomyopathy with/without central retinal degeneration is present consider the possibility of taurine deficiency. Feed a complete balanced ration containing adequate amounts of taurine. If low plasma taurine concentrations are detected supplement ration with 250–500mg taurine/day.

If other clinical signs are consistent consider the possibility of thiamin deficiency.

Hyperthyroidism

Hyperthyroidism is common in older cats. These animals have greatly increased energy requirements because they are in a hypermetabolic state. A high energy complete ration should be fed with the other characteristics of a diet suitable for congestive heart failure.

Hypertension

Many studies in humans (Law *et al.*, 1991) and experimental animals have confirmed that the consumption of high salt rations is associated with an increase in blood pressure compared to populations consuming lower amounts of salt. If hypertension is present as a complication of heart disease or hyperthyroidism (as suggested by the presence of retinal haemorrhages or retinal detachment, or on direct or indirect measurement) feed a complete ration containing less than 0.1% sodium.

Consider the possibility of concomitant renal failure in which hypertension is a common finding. If present, feed a renal failure diet containing relatively low protein, sodium and phosphorus. (See Table 10.2 for sodium content of some table foods.)

Myocardial Calcification

If myocardial calcification is detected on radiography or at post mortem consider the possibility of excessive calcium, vitamin D activity or phosphorus intake as well as other causes such as phosphorus retention in renal failure, primary or secondary hyperparathyroidism etc.

ECG Abnormalities

Consider the possible effects of obesity, rapid weight loss, dietary intake of potassium, magnesium and calcium.

Dogs with Pacemakers

L-Carnitine deficiency can be induced by chronic pacing. Feed a complete ration containing adequate amounts of L-carnitine.

REFERENCES

Abraham AS *et al.*, (1980). The effect of chromium on established atherosclerotic plaque in rabbits. *American Journal of Clinical Medicine* **33,** 2294.

Abraham AS *et al.*, (1982), The effect of chromium on cholesterol-induced atherosclerosis in rabbits. *Atherosclerosis* **41,** 371.

Bojs GE and Conn HL (1965). Distribution of body sodium, potassium and water and the excretion of aldosterone in dogs with spontaneous heart failure. *American Heart Journal* **69,** 72.

Bonagura JD and Lehmkuhl LB (1992). Fluid and diuretic therapy in heart failure. In: *Fluid Therapy in Small Animal Practice.* Ed SP Dibartola. W.B.Saunders, Philadelphia pp 529-553.

Davis GK and Mertz W (1987). Copper. In: *Trace Elements in Human and Animal Nutrition.* Ed. W Mertz. Academic Press, New York. pp 301-364.

Diolulu MA (1987) Dietary influence on hypertension and stroke. In: *Nutrition and Heart Disease.* Ed RR Watson. CRC Press. Boca Raton, FL. pp 107-112.

Ettinger SJ and Suter PF (1970). Low sodium diets and other drugs and methods indicated in cardiac therapy. In: *Canine Cardiology.* WB Saunders, Philadelphia pp 257-261.

Fox PR and Nichols CER (1988). Cardiac involvement in systemic disease. In: *Canine and Feline Cardiology.* Ed. PR Fox. Churchill Livingstone, New York.

Gershoff SN and Norkin A (1962). Vitamin E deficiency in cats. *Journal of Nutrition* **77,** 303.

Guo JA *et al.* (1979). The effect of sodium selenite on the haemodynamics of anaesthetized dog heart. *China's 3rd Conference on the Aetiology of Keshan Disease.*

Hamlin RL, Smith CR, Ross JN (1967). Detection and quantification of subclinical heart failure in dogs *Journal of the American Veterinary Medical Association* **150,** 1513-1515.

Keene BW *et al.*, (1991). Myocardial L-carnitine deficiency in a family of dogs with dilated cardiomyopathy. *Journal of the American Veterinary Medical Association* **198,** 647-650.

Keene BW (1994). Carnitine in dogs. *Proceedings of the 4th Annual Congress of the European Society of Veterinary Internal Medicine* 20-25.

Klevay LM (1975). *American Journal of Clinical Nutrition* **28,** 764.

Knox EG (1973). Ischaemic heart disease mortality and dietary intake of calcium. *Lancet* **i,** 1465.

Law MR, Frost CD and Wald NJ (1991). By how much does dietary salt reduction lower blood pressure? *British Medical Journal* **302,** 811-824.

Linden V (1974). Vitamin D and myocardial infarction. *British Medical Journal* **3,** 647.

Loeb HS, Pietras RJ, Gunnar RM, Tobin JR (1968). Paroxysmal ventricular fibrillation in two patients with hypomagnesaemia. *Circulation* **37,** 210-215.

McCance and Widdowson (1991). *The Composition of Foods 5th Edition.* Royal Society of Chemistry and Ministry of Agriculture Fisheries and Food. HMSO, Oxford.

Mattheeuws D, Rottiers R, Baeyens D, Vermeulen A (1984). Glucose tolerance and insulin response in obese dogs. *Journal of the American Animal Hospital Association* **20,** 287-293.

Morris ML, Patton RL, Teeter SM (1976). Low sodium diet in heart disease. How low is low? *Veterinary Medicine Small Animal Clinic* 1225-1227.

National Research Council (1985). *Nutrient Requirements of Dogs – Revised Edition.* National Academy Press, Washington D.C.

National Research Council (1986). *Nutrient Requirements of Cats – Revised Edition.* National Academy Press, Washington D.C.

New York Heart Association (1964). *Diseases of the Heart and Blood Vessels. Nomenclature and Criteria for Diagnosis. 6th edition.* Little, Brown and Co., Boston.

Pion PD, Kittleson MD, Rogers QR (1987). Myocardial failure in cats associated with low plasma taurine: a reversible cardiomyopathy. *Science* **237,** 697.

Ralston SL and Fox PR (1988). Dietary management, nutrition and the heart. In: *Canine and Feline Cardiology.* Churchill Livingstone, New York. pp219-228.

Ross JN Jr (1987). Chapter 11, Heart Failure. In: *Small Animal Clinical Nutrition III*, Eds LD Lewis, ML Morris and MS Hand. Mark Morris Associates, Topeka, KS. pp11.1-11.38.

Stepien RL and Miller MW (1994). Cardiovascular disease. In: *The Waltham Book of Clinical Nutrition of the Dog and Cat.* Ed JM Wills and KW Simpson, Pergamon Press, Oxford. pp353-371.

Van Itallie TB (1980) "Morbid" obesity : a hazardous disorder that resists conservative treatment. *American Journal of Clinical Nutrition* **33,** 358-363.

Weinsier RL, Norris D (1985) Recent developments in the aetiology and treatment of hypertension: dietary calcium, fat and magnesium. *American Journal of Clinical Nutrition* **42,** 1331

Yan GQ *et al.,* (1984). The role of selenium in Keshan Disease. *Advances in Nutrition Research* **6,** 203.

CHAPTER ELEVEN

The Renal Patient

Peter J. Markwell and John G. Harte

INTRODUCTION

Chronic renal failure (CRF) is a common illness in geriatric animals. It is characterised by inability of the kidneys to perform their normal functions. Renal failure is the result of a wide range of diseases which lead to the destruction of more than 75% of the functional parenchyma of both kidneys. It may thus be the result of neoplastic, immune-mediated, infectious, iatrogenic, metabolic, congenital, toxic, traumatic or obstructive processes. Renal failure can be caused by pre-renal factors, primary renal disease or post-renal factors. Pre-renal renal failure is the consequence of decreased glomerular blood flow that may be associated with hypovolaemia secondary to severe dehydration, shock, or circulatory problems secondary to heart failure. Lesions responsible for primary renal failure are shown in Table 11.1. Chronic interstitial nephritis (CIN) is the most commonly encountered primary renal lesion in CRF (DiBartola *et al.*, 1987). CIN can result from a range of renal disorders (e.g. chronic pyelonephritis (Lucke, 1982) and chronic glomerulonephritis), however, the inciting cause cannot be determined in most cases (DiBartola, 1987). Post-renal factors associated with renal failure include urethral obstruction, or primary urethral, bladder or ureteral injuries.

Congenital Lesions
Agenesis of the renal cortex
Renal polycystitis
Hydronephrosis
Acquired Lesions
Chronic interstitial nephritis
Chronic glomerulonephritis
Amyloidosis
Renal lymphosarcoma
Renal carcinoma
Polycystic renal disease
Chronic pyelonephritis
Periarteritis nodosa
Hydronephrosis
Nephrotoxins

Table 11.1: *Primary kidney lesions responsible for chronic renal failure.*

ASSESSMENT OF PATHOLOGICAL STATUS

History and Clinical Signs

Cats and dogs may present with a wide range of clinical and laboratory signs which are associated with a progressive decrease in renal function, rather than arising from specific renal lesions. The signs most commonly reported by the owner are anorexia, lethargy, polyuria, polydypsia and weight loss. Polyuria and polydypsia are reported less commonly in feline than in canine patients. The higher intrinsic urine concentrating ability of cats, and their normally unobserved micturition habits may account for this apparent difference. Vomiting and diarrhoea are reported to occur more frequently in canine than in feline patients (Krawiec and Gelberg, 1989).

Physical Examination

Observation of the animal may reveal poor body condition with muscle wasting and poor coat quality. Fifty-eight percent of cats with renal failure were underweight in one study (Lulich *et al.*, 1992). Dehydration, which may be indicated by dry mucous membranes, decreased skin turgor and sunken eyeballs, was a clinical finding in 70% of cats in the same study, and is also a common canine finding. Examination of the oral cavity may reveal uraemic stomatitis, pallor of the mucous membranes and uraemic halitosis. Oral lesions are more common in dogs than in cats with uraemia.

CRF may be associated with renomegaly, normal sized or small irregular kidneys. Renal diseases that are associated with large kidneys include renal lymphosarcoma, pyelonephritis, polycystic renal disease and feline infectious peritonitis (Crowell *et al.*, 1979; Hayashi *et al.*, 1982; Mooney *et al.*, 1987;). Morphological evaluation of small kidneys (<2.3 times the length of the second lumbar vertebra) may reveal chronic generalised nephritis, glomerular sclerosis and tubular necrosis.

Other signs considered to be manifestations of underlying hypertension secondary to renal disease include retinal detachment or atrophy of the optic fundus (Morgan, 1982). A systolic murmur may be auscultated where severe anaemia accompanies renal failure (Bonagura, 1989).

Laboratory Findings

Laboratory abnormalities in CRF reflect decreased renal function rather than renal lesions. Increased creatinine and serum urea nitrogen (SUN), hyperphosphataemia, hypo- or hyperkalaemia, hyponatraemia, metabolic acidosis, hypercholesterolaemia, hypoalbuminaemia, hypoproteinaemia and mild hyperglycaemia may be encountered.

SUN and creatinine provide crude indications of glomerular filtration rate (Figure 11.1). SUN is probably the most commonly used renal function test, but is affected by extra-renal factors, including dietary protein content, liver function and state of hydration. Serum creatinine concentration is less dependent on extra-renal factors (Ross, 1986).

Hyperphosphataemia is a common finding associated with reduced glomerular filtration rate (less than 25% of normal) in patients with CRF, reflecting the important role that the kidney plays in phosphate excretion. One of the key effects of elevated serum phosphorus is to decrease the activity of the enzyme 1-hydroxylase in the kidney, contributing towards a decrease in production of 1,25-dihydroxycholecalciferol. This in turn (together with hypocalcaemia where this occurs) results in increased serum parathyroid hormone (PTH) levels (Nagode *et al.*, 1993). It has been proposed that PTH is an important uraemic toxin, which may contribute to anaemia, neurotoxicity, promotion of soft tissue calcification and renal osteodystrophy (Ibels *et al.*, 1978; Massry, 1980). The most severe toxic injuries due to PTH may be inflicted upon the kidney due to a high concentration of PTH receptors in renal cells. High levels of PTH may promote the uptake of calcium by these cells, initially causing cell death, and eventually precipitation of calcium phosphate into tubule lumens. Hyperparathyroidism could, therefore, promote a viscious cycle of cell death leading to decreased renal ability to contribute to phosphate homoeostasis, increased PTH levels and the loss of more renal tissue (Nagode and Chew, 1992; Nagode *et al.*, 1993). Supporting data for this detrimental role of PTH are provided by some clinical studies, which have indicated possible slowing of progression of renal failure in dogs when plasma PTH was suppressed (Nagode *et al.*, 1991). More recent controlled experimental studies have, however, cast doubt on the benefits of reducing PTH (Finco *et al.*, 1994).

Hyperkalaemia is unusual in dogs and cats with mild to moderate polyuric CRF (Polzin *et al.*, 1989). However, hypokalaemia has been shown to be the commonest electrolyte abnormality in cats with CRF; in one series it occurred in approximately 30% of cases (DiBartola *et al.*, 1987). It may also occur occasionally in dogs (Polzin *et al.*, 1989). Hypokalaemia may be related to excessive urinary potassium losses and inadequate dietary potassium intake (Dow *et al.*, 1987). Muscle dysfunction is the cardinal sign of hypokalaemia, regardless of cause, although a range of clinical presentations including cervical ventroflexion, ambulatory difficulties and mild cardiac arrhythmias have been reported. Signs generally resolve within one to five days after initiating potassium supplementation (Dow *et al.*, 1987). Renal tubular acidosis is one of the most common causes of potassium depletion associated with renal disease and is due to the fundamental role that renal distal tubular potassium handling (net secretion or resorption) plays in potassium homoeostasis (Dow *et al.*, 1987; Brobst, 1988). Potassium depletion and hypokalaemia have been shown to produce a proximal tubular nephropathy in man and a medullary tubular nephropathy in dogs and rats. The mechanism for this remains as yet unexplained, but increased intra-renal ammoniagenesis may play a role (Abbrecht, 1968; Tollins *et al.*, 1987).

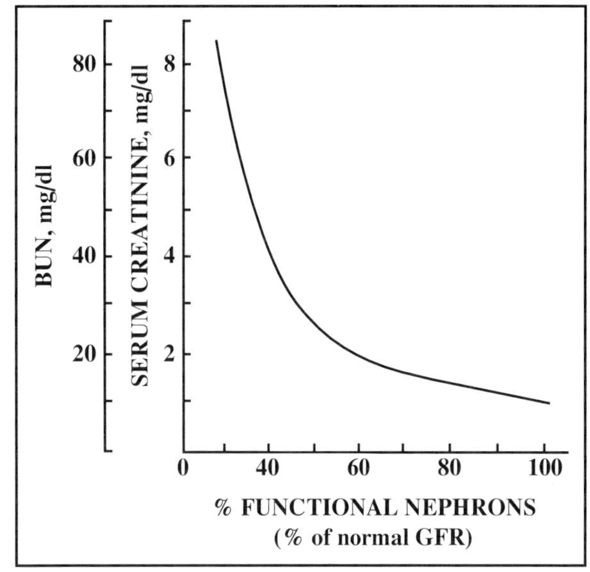

Figure 11.1: *Relationship of BUN or serum creatinine to percentage of functional nephrons. (From Chew DJ and DiBartola SP: Manual of Small Animal Nephrology and Urology, New York, Churchill Livingstone, 1986).*

Sodium homoeostasis is maintained primarily by the kidneys. In the diseased state as GFR falls, surviving nephrons increase their fractional excretion of sodium to cope with the increased load delivered to each one. In general, this response is adequate to maintain sodium balance until the condition is very advanced, although the ability of the kidney to adapt to changes in sodium intake becomes progressively narrowed (Polzin *et al.*, 1989). Hyponatraemia may occur occasionally, and is thought to result from isotonic urinary sodium losses in the face of continuing water consumption.

Normochloraemic metabolic acidosis is typical of uraemia and results from the reduced ability of diseased kidneys to excrete an effective hydrogen load (Knochel and Seldin, 1981). Typical laboratory signs of normochloraemic metabolic acidosis include low serum bicarbonate, or low carbon dioxide combining power and high anion gap values with concurrent normal serum chloride concentrations.

Hypercholesterolaemia is generally a non-specific finding in renal failure patients regardless of cause (DiBartola *et al.*, 1987). Hypoalbuminaemia and hypoproteinaemia may be masked by concurrent dehydration and are common in patients with glomerulonephritis (Nash *et al.*, 1979; Lucke, 1982).

Haematological abnormalities associated with CRF reflect the role of the kidney in erythropoiesis, decreased erythrocyte life span in uraemic conditions and the myelosuppressive effects of uraemia. In consequence, non-regenerative, normocytic, normochromic anaemia is common in patients with CRF. Typically, the cause of CRF does not influence the severity of anaemia; however, anaemia is disproportionately mild in animals with polycystic kidneys or systemic hypertension and disproportionately severe in nephrotic animals (Polzin *et al.*, 1989).

Analysis of urine from patients with CRF may reveal hyposthenuria, isosthenuria or hypersthenuria. Renal tubular disorders lead to disruption of the normal urine concentrating ability; hence, the ability to concentrate urine may be retained in the presence of azotaemia if glomerular involvement is more severe than tubular involvement. Urine specific gravity ranges of 1.020 to 1.070 have been recorded in cats with experimentally induced reductions in renal mass of as much as 75% (Ross and Finco, 1981). Persistent proteinuria in the absence of hyperproteinaemia, evidence of haematuria, or urinary tract infection is commonly seen in CRF. Severe proteinuria is less commonly observed than mild to moderate proteinuria. Glomerulonephritis, chronic tubulointerstitial nephritis, pyelonephritis, glomerular amyloidosis and renal lymphosarcoma are most commonly associated with severe proteinuria (DiBartola *et al.*, 1987). Urine protein:creatinine ratios are an accurate method of assessing 24 hour urinary protein excretion in clinically normal animals and patients with surgically induced CRF. The influence of dietary protein and the absence of haematuria or urinary tract infection should be considered when interpreting urine protein:creatinine ratios (Adams *et al.*, 1992; Bagley *et al.*, 1989). Other urinalysis abnormalities observed include the presence of urinary casts (the degree and nature of which depend on the lesions responsible for the CRF (DiBartola *et al.*, 1981) and glucosuria. Glucosuria, in the face of normal blood glucose levels, is associated with renal tubular dysfunction.

The diagnosis of CRF is usually confirmed by the presence of inadequate urine concentrating ability in the presence of concurrent azotaemia (Polzin *et al.*, 1989). Serum and urine samples should ideally be obtained concurrently, prior to treatment. A comprehensive problem-specific clinical database should be obtained on all patients presenting with a vague history and physical findings suggestive of renal failure. The key evaluations include complete blood count, serum biochemistry profile, urinalysis, abdominal radiographs and a urine culture. In geriatric cats special attention should be paid to physical and biochemical evaluation of thyroid status due to the links between hyperthyroidism and renal disease.

DIETARY STRATEGY

Dietary therapy represents a cornerstone in the management of patients with renal failure (Allen, 1989), although it is palliative, and not curative. The objectives of dietary modification may be summarised as follows:

- to meet the patient's nutrient and energy requirements
- to alleviate clinical signs of uraemia through reduction of protein catabolites
- to minimise electrolyte, vitamin and mineral disturbances
- to try to slow progression of renal failure.

The key components of dietary therapy are discussed individually below. It is, however, only one aspect of conservative medical management of chronic renal failure (CRF); additional aspects include maintenance of normal hydration through provision of unlimited access to water; avoidance of stress; administration of sodium bicarbonate, anabolic agents, and intestinal phosphorus binders; avoidance of nephrotoxic drugs; and institution of anti-hypertensive therapy (Polzin and Osborne, 1986).

Requirements

Protein

The reduced ability of the kidney to excrete both nitrogenous and non-nitrogenous protein catabolites is one of the major causes of both uraemic signs and laboratory abnormalities in animals with renal failure. Clinical studies have been reported that show restriction of dietary protein and phosphorus can reduce azotaemia, and bring about clinical benefits in both dogs (Grandjean *et al.*, 1990; Leibetseder and Neufeld, 1991; Smith *et al.*, 1994) and cats (Harte *et al.*, 1993, 1994) with CRF.

In the canine studies clear benefits were seen with regard to both clinical status and laboratory parameters, with significant reductions in serum urea and creatinine occurring within one month of starting dietary therapy. Grandjean *et al.* (1990) fed diets containing approximately 16 and 13g protein/400kcal (1674kJ) of metabolisable energy (ME), and 0.42 and 0.25% phosphorus on dry matter (DM) to dogs with average starting creatinine and urea concentrations of 1.5 to 1.7mg/dl and 87 to 76mg/dl, respectively, and noted that values for these parameters returned to within normal physiological ranges. Similar changes were not observed in a control group fed 38g protein/

400kcal (1674kJ) ME and 1.6% DM phosphorus. Leibetseder and Neufeld (1991) reported that average values of urea and creatinine, although decreasing significantly, remained just above physiological ranges. However, the dogs in this study appeared to have a greater degree of renal insufficiency (average starting values 92mg/dl and 2.3mg/dl for urea and creatinine, respectively), and the degree of protein restriction was less (22g protein/400kcal (1674kJ) ME). Whilst both of these factors may have accounted for the differences seen, comparison with preliminary data from another clinical study of the management of renal failure occurring secondarily to leishmaniasis (Smith *et al.*, 1994), suggests that the difference most probably reflected the smaller restriction of protein intake, rather than a difference in the degree of renal insufficiency.

Whilst these studies demonstrate clear benefits from restricted protein and phosphorus diets, problems associated with excessive protein restriction have been demonstrated in other studies. These observations led to a recommendation that protein intake should not be restricted to less than 1.9g/kg body weight/day (approximately 12g protein/400kcal (1674kJ) ME in the diet for a 15kg dog), unless further restriction was required to control clinical signs of uraemia (Barsanti and Finco, 1985; Polzin *et al.*, 1991). Further concerns about possible undesirable effects of low protein diets were noted in a study comparing the effects of diets providing approximately 13.6 and 27.7g protein/400kcal (1674kJ) ME. Whilst increases in body weight were noted in the dogs when fed the low protein diet, and this was thought to be a mark of improved clinical status, several unexpected effects were noted associated with this diet, including hypertension, increased serum ionised calcium and increased cholesterol (Hansen *et al.*, 1992). In reviewing this (and other studies) Kronfeld (1993) commented that these effects, together with a lack of the expected advantages of low protein diets, led him to the view that the dogs fared better on the diet with the moderate protein content.

A second benefit that has been proposed for protein restriction is slowing the rate of progression of renal disease. Evidence in support of this proposal comes from studies in partially nephrectomised (PNX) rats fed *ad libitum*. Surviving nephrons show increases in glomerular capillary pressures and flows. It has been suggested that glomerular sclerosis, and hence progression of disease occurs as a result of these sustained adaptive changes. High protein intake in the presence of renal injury contributed to the increased perfusion, and thus to eventual destruction of remnant glomeruli. Reduction of dietary protein from 24 to 6% reduced the haemodynamic changes (Brenner *et al.*, 1982; Hotstetter *et al.*, 1981). Studies in dogs suggest that it may not be appropriate to extrapolate these results to the canine species.

Results from an experimental study that followed dogs with induced renal failure fed either high, moderate, or low protein diets (approximately 54, 31 and 18g protein/400kcal (1674 kJ) ME, respectively) for up to 48 months did not support the observations made in rats. Mortality during the study was not correlated with diet, and following initial changes, there was little evidence of progression of disease in any of the groups in terms of renal function. Light microscopy revealed more renal lesions in two of four dogs fed the high protein diet, but no differences between the other two and the dogs fed the other diets. Electron microscopy findings were similar in all three groups (Bovee *et al.*, 1979; Robertson *et al.*, 1986). In addition, studies of single nephron glomerular filtration in dogs identified several differences between rats and dogs in response to renal ablation (Brown *et al.*, 1990, 1991). The most compelling evidence against a role for protein in progression was reported by Finco *et al.* (1992), who compared two phosphorus and two protein levels (16 or 32% DM) in a two year study in PNX dogs. Dietary protein (in contrast with phosphorus) did not influence either survival of the dogs, the period of stability of renal function or its rate of subsequent decline.

Summarising these data, it is evident that protein (and phosphorus) restriction is desirable in the management of CRF, as high protein diets may be associated with more severe clinical problems, laboratory abnormalities, and renal lesions. However, care should be taken to avoid unnecessarily excessive restriction of protein, because of the risks of protein malnutrition and other possible side-effects. The need to reduce protein intake as far as possible is also questionable, given the lack of evidence for progression of disease with moderate protein restriction. It seems logical, therefore, to recommend individualisation of therapy based on the severity of disease and the response of particular cases. In mild to moderate cases of renal insufficiency, clear benefits were shown for a diet containing 22g protein/400kcal (1674kJ) (Leibetseder and Neufeld, 1991), even though concentrations of urea and creatinine remained just above physiological ranges. Thus it is logical to advocate approximately this degree of protein restriction for cases with mild renal insufficiency (creatinine approximately up to 2.3mg/dl), and then adjust therapy if necessary on the basis of clinical response and laboratory measures. With more severely affected animals a greater degree of protein restriction may be required to adequately control azotaemia, although again careful observation of cases should be performed, both to assess response to diet and to monitor for the development of any undesirable effects. It is important that high quality protein sources are used in the formulation of restricted protein diets to minimise the risks of essential amino acid deficiency.

The potential risks of protein reduction in the cat's diet are much greater than for the dog. The cat is unable to down-regulate hepatic enzyme activity associated with protein catabolism even in the face of a reduction in dietary protein intake (Rogers *et al.*, 1977), thus it is particularly at risk of protein malnutrition. Controversy currently exists regarding the influence of dietary protein restriction on the progression of feline renal dysfunction (Adams *et al.*, 1994; Finco and Brown, 1989). One recent study showed that dietary protein and energy restriction limited proteinuria and glomerular injury in cats with induced renal failure, compared with a group receiving higher protein and energy intake (Adams *et al.*, 1994). However, glomerular filtration rate remained stable in both groups over the one year that the cats were followed, and the study did not differentiate between the effects of protein and energy restriction. Given the inconclusive nature of these data, it is not clear whether protein restriction will be of benefit in non-azotaemic cats with early renal disease. Protein restriction should, however, be considered for cats with azotaemia and hyperphosphataemia that persist despite good hydration. It has been suggested that uraemic cats should consume a minimum of approximately 3.3–3.8g/kg/day of high biological value protein (Osborne *et al.*, 1982). This is equivalent to approximately 19–25g protein/400kcal (1674kJ) ME depending on energy intake. Positive results in terms of both laboratory parameters and clinical status were reported in a clinical study of cats with CRF receiving a diet containing 25.8g protein/400kcal (1674kJ) (Harte *et al.*, 1993, 1994).

Phosphorus

For the reasons described above, dietary phosphorus restriction is an important part of dietary management of chronic renal failure, and may impact favourably on the progression of renal disease (Brown *et al.*, 1991; Polzin, 1987).

The most complete study of the effect of phosphorus restriction in dogs with renal failure was reported by Finco *et al.* (1992). In this study PNX dogs were fed diets containing either 16 or 32% protein, and 0.44 to 0.49 or 1.46 to 1.50% phosphorus (DM), and followed for up to two years. Survival was significantly influenced by dietary phosphorus, but not by protein. In addition, the period for which GFR was stable was significantly greater in the low phosphorus group. The results of this study provided good evidence of the benefit of phosphorus restriction in the management of CRF. It is of interest that the benefits were noted despite the fact that renal mineralisation was not influenced by diet. PTH levels, although related to diet in the early stages of the study, later tended to rise in all groups. Clearly, further studies are required to elicit fully the mechanism of action of phosphate restriction.

The benefits of phosphate restriction in cats have also been reported (Ross *et al.*, 1982). In this study the effects of phosphorus restricted (0.42% DM) and normal phosphorus (1.6% DM) diets were compared over periods up to 343 days. Serum phosphorus concentration was significantly higher in the normal phosphate group. Serum PTH levels were markedly higher after 6 weeks in the normal phosphorus group, and subsequently increased further. Serum PTH levels were only slightly higher than clinically normal controls in the low phosphorus group. Neither diet caused a significant change in renal function during the study, but the kidneys of the cats on the higher phosphorus intake showed mineralisation, fibrosis, and cell infiltration whereas those from the cats fed the phosphorus restricted diet showed little or no changes.

Based on these data it is logical to restrict dietary phosphorus to approximately 0.4% DM in diets for patients with CRF. Further control of phosphorus, or individualisation of therapy may be achieved by the use of oral phosphorus binding agents (e.g. aluminium hydroxide gel).

Calcium

Calcium *per se* does not affect the progression of renal failure, although as discussed above, a fall in blood calcium levels is a trigger for PTH release. A number of factors may contribute to hypocalcaemia, including poor gastrointestinal absorption associated with decreased levels of 1,25-dihydroxycholecalciferol and reduced intake following anorexia. Hyperphos-phataemia may also contribute through complexing ionic calcium. However, the concentrations of phosphorus needed to accomplish this process probably do not occur early in the course of disease (Nagode *et al.*, 1993). Thus, one recommendation is that calcium intake should be normal or supplemented in dogs with CRF (Bovee, 1983).

Conversely, it has been recommended that the calcium-phosphorus product in the blood should not exceed approximately 60 in the dog and 55 in man (measurements in mg/dl) (Massry, 1980), as this may promote further soft tissue calcification and lead to progression of renal damage. A further complication is the variation between individuals in the course of disease. Calcium levels in blood may be low, normal or high (Barsanti and Finco, 1985; Finco and Rowland, 1978; Lulich *et al.*, 1992; Polzin *et al.*, 1983). Calcium supplementation, which would be desirable in the presence of known hypocalcaemia, would be contraindicated in the presence of hypercalcaemia. For these reasons the clinician needs to individualise calcium supplementation to suit a particular case, and adjust it according to the response in terms of measured blood and clinical parameters.

Calcitriol

Calcitriol (1,25-dihydroxycholecalciferol) treatment, to reduce the magnitude of increased PTH, has been recommended for the management of patients with CRF after measures such as protein and phosphorus restriction and the use of phosphorus binding agents have been implemented. A once daily oral regimen at an average dose of 2.5ng/kg has been recommended for both dogs and cats. Serum biochemistry should be evaluated regularly during therapy (Chew *et al.*, 1993).

Sodium

There is controversy regarding the prevalence of hypertension amongst dogs with chronic renal disease; some reports suggest that it is between 58 and 93%, whereas others suggest a much lower figure (Cowgill and Kallet, 1983; Michell and Bodey, 1994). Although less well documented than in other species, systemic hypertension has also been reported in cats in association with chronic renal insufficiency (Morgan, 1986). Hypertension, where it occurs, may be important for two reasons. Firstly, it can result in a variety of pathophysiological consequences, including left ventricular hypertrophy, neurological abnormalities and ocular lesions; and secondly, because hypertension may contribute to the progression of renal disease. Reduction of blood pressure in animals with documented hypertension is thus a desirable goal of therapy (Ross and Labato, 1989). It has been reported that expansion of extracellular fluid volume, hypertension and oedema may occur in uraemic dogs receiving normal or high sodium intake (Cowgill, 1983). These findings suggest that the traditional recommendation to supplement sodium is not appropriate for most cases of CRF in dogs.

Conversely, severe sodium restriction should probably also be avoided. This could promote volume depletion in some dogs with CRF that are unable to adapt to varying sodium intake, and may also result in a decreased capacity to reabsorb bicarbonate, thus contributing to metabolic acidosis. However, this latter effect was not seen when diets containing 0.25% DM sodium were fed (Schmidt and Gavellas, 1977; Polzin *et al.*, 1989). For these reasons most recommendations are for diets with 'normal' to 'moderately restricted' sodium content for dogs with CRF. Suggested ranges include 0.25 to 0.8% DM (Polzin *et al.*, 1989), and 0.1 to 0.3% DM (Cowgill, 1983; Ross and Labato, 1989). In the absence of specific data relating to cats, it seems appropriate to make similar recommendations.

These levels are likely to be lower than in the normal foods that a patient may previously have been fed. This difference is one important reason for recommending gradual change over from the animal's previous diet to a restricted protein diet, because the capacity to adjust sodium excretion rapidly in response to changes in intake becomes severely impaired as renal insufficiency progresses (Cowgill, 1983).

Potassium

As noted above, urinary potassium losses in cats may lead to potassium depletion if compounded by decreased potassium intake. The dietary potassium content in the study leading to this observation was 0.34% DM (Dow *et al.*, 1987). These data suggest that this level of dietary potassium may be inadequate for many cats with CRF. However, not all cats with CRF show hypo- or normokalaemia. In a recent report of 116 cases of feline CRF, 30% showed hypokalaemia, but a further 13% showed hyperkalaemia (Lulich *et al.*, 1992). This emphasises the need for monitoring of potassium status in cats with CRF, and the possible requirement for supplementation or adjustment of intake on an individual basis. Oral supplementation is safest. Potassium gluconate, which is available in flavoured tablets and elixirs, is a more palatable supplement than potassium chloride.

Water-soluble Vitamins (B Group and C)

Polyuria is a very common clinical sign in dogs with CRF, although it may be less prevalent in cats (Lulich *et al.*, 1992). Water-soluble vitamins are excreted in urine and not stored within the body, thus the potential for development of deficiency of these vitamins exists in the polyuric animal. A tendency towards development of water-soluble vitamin deficiency has been noted in human uraemic patients, particularly in those undergoing diuresis. For this reason supplementation of diets with water-soluble vitamins may be beneficial for some dogs and cats with CRF.

Energy

It is important to minimise metabolism of protein to provide energy in uraemic patients, either from dietary or endogenous sources, as this will add to the nitrogenous waste products requiring excretion through the failing kidneys. The goal, therefore, is to meet the animal's requirements from non-protein sources of energy in the diet. Carbohydrate and fat fulfil this criterion, but of the two, fat offers advantages as it provides approximately twice the energy per gram, and aids palatability in the diet. For these reasons diets designed for the management of CRF are usually formulated with a relatively high fat content. The presence of the high fat content also increases the energy density of the diets. This allows the animal, which may have a poor appetite, to obtain its nutritional requirements from a relatively small volume of food.

The maintenance energy requirements of dogs and cats with CRF have not been established. In the absence of this information it is recommended that the standard equations for the calculation of maintenance energy requirements (see Chapter 3) are used at the commencement of dietary management, with subsequent adjustments to suit the individual case.

Feeding Strategy

Food Types

Several companies produce restricted protein and phosphorus diets formulated for the management of CRF in dogs and cats. These commercial foods have a number of advantages over home-prepared diets; in particular, the nutritional profile will be both known and consistent. In some cases these diets are designed so that they can be mixed, to provide a degree of individualisation of therapy. Formulation of home-prepared diets is possible, although considerable care is required to ensure nutritional adequacy and consistency. A series of recipes for home-prepared therapeutic diets, including one for renal failure, have been described (Donoghue and Kronfeld, 1994).

Feeding Practices

Dietary management of renal failure is often complicated by anorexia that is harmful to patients, promoting catabolic loss of body tissue. Dietary management requires a highly palatable diet which animals with reduced appetites will find acceptable despite the inherent protein and phosphorus restriction. High fat diets provide a rich source of essential fatty acids and are a highly palatable source of non protein calories.

Cases of total anorexia may respond temporarily to appetite stimulants (e.g. benzodiazepines) (Macy and Ralston, 1989), but attention must be paid to discrepancies between the nutritional requirements and actual daily intakes of anorectic patients. Where clinically appropriate more aggressive therapy such as force or tube feeding should be considered.

Practical measures to improve intake include the use of highly odorous food, the warming of food prior to feeding, the maceration of food to enhance its texture. Prompting learned feeding behaviour by using familiar feeding dishes in environments familiar to the patient and by petting and stroking may also stimulate eating. The smell of food is vital in soliciting and maintaining the patient's interest: strong meat, fish or cheese odours are often favoured by cats.

Assessment of Success

Monitoring provides an opportunity to review status and optimise therapy. The priorities in initial monitoring of the newly discharged patient are assessment of physical status (especially hydration and body weight), evaluation of key laboratory parameters (SUN, creatinine, phosphorus, potassium, packed cell volume, serum albumin and total protein) and assessment of compliance to dietary and medical therapy. The frequency of subsequent regular monitoring depends on the severity of the patient's condition. It is recommended that patients receiving protein and phosphorus restricted diets are monitored at least every six months. Regular biochemical and physical assessment of renal patients is an important and often neglected component of medical and dietary therapy. Regular monitoring allows the veterinarian to ensure that dietary and medical management remains optimal for the needs of the patient.

REFERENCES

Abbrecht PH (1968). Effects of potassium deficiency on renal function in the dog. *Journal of Clinical Investigation* **48,** 432.

Adams LG, Polzin DJ, Osborne CA and O'Brien TD (1992). Correlation of urine protein /creatinine ratio and twenty four hour urinary protein excretion in normal cats and cats with surgically induced chronic renal failure. *Journal of Veterinary Internal Medicine* **6,** 36.

Adams LG, Polzin DJ, Osborne CA, O'Brien TD and Hostetter TH (1994). Influence of dietary protein/calorie intake on renal morphology and function in cats with 5/6 nephrectomy. *Laboratory Investigation* **70,** 127.

Allen TA (1989). Management of advanced chronic renal failure. In: *Current Veterinary Therapy X: Small Animal Practice*. Ed RW Kirk. WB Saunders, Philadelphia p 1195.

Bagley RS, Center SA and Lewis RM (1989). The influence of blood contamination and lower urinary tract inflammation on the urine protein / creatinine ratio in the dog. *Journal of Veterinary Internal Medicine* **3,** 130.

Barsanti JA and Finco DR (1985). Dietary management of chronic renal failure in dogs. *Journal of the American Animal Hospital Association* **21,** 371.

Bonagura JD (1989). Cardiovascular diseases. In: *The Cat: Diseases and Clinical Management.* Ed RG Sherding. Churchill Livingstone, New York p 649.

Bovee KC (1983). The role of dietary protein in the pathogenesis and management of chronic renal failure in the dog. *Proceedings of the 7th Kal Kan Symposium*, p 27. Kal Kan, Vernon CA.

Bovee KC, Kronfeld DS, Ramburg C and Goldschmidt M (1979). Long-term measurement of renal function in partially nephrectomised dogs fed 56, 27 or 19% protein. *Investigative Urology* **16,** 378.

Brenner BM, Meyer TW and Hotstetter TH (1982). Dietary protein intake and the progressive nature of kidney disease. *New England Journal of Medicine* **307,** 652.

Brobst D (1988). Review of the pathophysiology of alterations in potassium homeostasis. *Journal of the American Veterinary Medical Association* **188,** 1019.

Brown SA, Finco DR, Crowell WA, Choat DC and Navar LG (1990). Single nephron adaptations to partial renal ablation in the dog. *American Journal of Physiology* **258,** F495.

Brown SA, Finco DR, Crowell WA and Navar LG (1991). Dietary protein intake and the glomerular adaptations to partial nephrectomy in dogs. *Journal of Nutrition* **121,** S125.

Chew DJ and DiBartola SP (1986). *Manual of Small Animal Nephrology and Urology.* Churchill Livingstone, New York.

Chew DJ, Nagode LA, Carothers MA and Steinmeyer CL (1993). Calcitriol treatment of renal secondary hyperparathyroidism in dogs and cats. *Proceedings of the 11th ACVIM Forum,* p 164. American College of Veterinary Internal Medicine, Blacksburg, VA.

Cowgill LD (1983). Diseases of the kidney. In: *Textbook of Veterinary Internal Medicine (2nd edition).* Ed SJ Ettinger. WB Saunders, Philadelphia p 1793.

Cowgill LD and Kallet AJ (1983). Recognition and management of hypertension in the dog. In: *Current Veterinary Therapy VIII.* Ed RW Kirk. WB Saunders, Philadelphia p 1025.

Crowell WA, Hubbell JJ and Riley JC (1979). Polycystic renal disease in related cats. *Journal of the American Veterinary Medical Association* **175,** 286.

DiBartola SP, Rutgers HC, Zack PM and Tarr MJ (1987). Clinicopathological findings associated with chronic renal disease in cats. *Journal of the American Veterinary Medical Association* **190,** 1196.

DiBartola SP, Spaulding GL, Chew DJ and Lewis RM (1981). Urinary protein excretion and immunopathologic findings in dogs with glomerular disease. *Journal of the American Veterinary Medical Association* **177,** 73-77.

Donoghue S and Kronfeld DS (1994). Home-made diets. In: *The Waltham Book of Clinical Nutrition of the Dog and Cat.* Eds JM Wills and KW Simpson. Pergamon Press, Oxford pp 445-449.

Dow SW, Fettman MJ, Lecouteur RA and Hamar DW (1987). Potassium depletion in cats: renal and dietary influences. *Journal of the American Veterinary Medical Association* **191,** 1596.

Finco DR and Brown SA (1989). Newer concepts and controversies on dietary management of renal failure. In: *Current Veterinary Therapy X: Small Animal Practice.* Ed RW Kirk. WB Saunders, Philadelphia p 1198.

Finco DR, Brown SA, Cooper T, Crowell WA, Hoenig M and Barsanti JA (1994). Effects of parathyroid hormone depletion in dogs with induced renal failure. *American Journal of Veterinary Research* **55,** 867-873.

Finco DR, Brown SA, Crowell WA, Duncan RJ, Barsanti JA and Bennett SE (1992). Effects of dietary phosphorus and protein in dogs with chronic renal failure. *American Journal of Veterinary Research* **53,** 2264.

Finco DR and Rowland GN (1978). Hypercalcaemia secondary to chronic renal failure in the dog and a report of 4 cases. *Journal of the American Veterinary Medical Association* **179,** 990.

Grandjean D, Paragon BM, Grandjean R, Pibot P and Foraz JL (1990). Interet d'une alimentation hypoproteique et hypophosphoree dans l'evolution post seuil critique d'une insuffisance renale chronique chez le chien. *Recueil de Medecine Vétérinaire* **166,** 865.

Hansen B, DiBartola SP, Chew DJ, Brownie C and Nagode L (1992). Clinical and metabolic findings in dogs with chronic renal failure fed two diets. *American Journal of Veterinary Research* **53,** 326.

Harte JG, Markwell PJ and Moraillon R (1993). Dietary management of feline renal disease. *Feline Medicine Symposium (in association with North American Veterinary Conference),* pp 27. Waltham, Vernon, CA.

Harte JG, Markwell PJ, Moraillon R, Gettinby GG, Smith BHE and Wills JM (1994). Dietary management of naturally occurring feline renal failure. *Journal of Nutrition* **124,** 2660S.

Hayashi T, Ishida T and Fujiwara K (1982). Glomerulonephritis associated with feline infectious peritonitis. *Japanese Journal of Veterinary Science* **44,** 909.

Hotstetter TH, Olsen JL, Rennke HG, Venkatachalam MA and Brenner BM (1981). Hyperfiltration in remnant nephrons: a potentially adverse response to renal ablation. *American Journal of Physiology* **241,** F85.

Ibels LS, Alfrey AC, Haut L and Huffer WE (1978). Preservation of function in experimental renal disease by dietary restriction of phosphate. *New England Journal of Medicine* **298,** 122.

Knochel JP and Seldin DW (1981). The pathophysiology of uraemia. In: *The Kidney, 2nd edition.* Eds BM Brenner and FC Rector. WB Saunders, Philadelphia.

Kopple JD (1984). Chronic renal failure: nutritional and nondialytic management. In: *Current Therapy in Nephrology and Hypertension.* Ed RJ Glassock. Mosby, St Louis p 252.

Krawiec DR and Gelberg HB (1989). Chronic renal disease in cats. In: *Current Veterinary Therapy, X: Small Animal Practice.* Ed RW Kirk. WB Saunders, Philadelphia p 1170.

Kronfeld DS (1993). Dietary management of chronic renal disease in dogs: a critical appraisal of dietary protein. *Journal of Small Animal Practice* **34,** 211.

Leibtseder JL and Neufeld KW (1991). Effects of medium protein diets in dogs with chronic renal failure. *Journal of Nutrition* **121,** S145-S149.

Lucke VM (1982). Glomerulonephritis in the cat. *Veterinary Annual.* Blackwell, Oxford **22,** 270.

Lulich JP, Osborne CA, O'Brien TD and Polzin DJ (1992). Feline renal failure: questions, answers, questions. *Compendium for Continuing Education for the Practising Veterinarian* **14,** 127.

Macy DW and Ralston SL (1989). Cause and control of decreased appetite. In: *Current Veterinary Therapy X: Small Animal Practice*. Ed RW Kirk. WB Saunders, Philadelphia p 18.

Massry SG (1980). Requirements of vitamin D metabolites in patients with renal disease. *American Journal of Clinical Nutrition* **33,** 1530.

Michell AR and Bodey AR (1994). Canine hypertension. *Proceedings of the 12th ACVIM Forum* 502-505.

Mooney SC, Hayes AA, Matus RE and Macewen EG (1987). Renal lymphoma in cats: 28 cases (1977-1984). *Journal of the American Veterinary Medical Association* **191,** 1473.

Morgan R (1982). Systemic hypertension in four cats: ocular and medical findings. *Journal of the American Animal Hospital Association* **22,** 371.

Morgan RV (1986). Systemic hypertension in four cats: ocular and medical findings. *Journal of the American Animal Hospital Association* **22,** 615-621.

Nagode LA and Chew DJ (1992). Nephrocalcinosis caused by hyperparathyroidism in progression of renal failure: treatment with calcitriol. *Seminars in Veterinary Surgery* **7,** 202.

Nagode LA, Chew DJ, Steinmeyer BS and Carothers MA (1993). Renal secondary hyperparathyroidism: Toxic aspects, mechanisms of development, and control by oral calcitriol treatment. *Proc 11th ACVIM Forum*, p 154. American College of Veterinary Internal Medicine, Blacksburg, VA.

Nagode LA, Chew DJ, Steinmeyer BS *et al.* (1991). Low doses of oral calcitriol retard progression of naturally occurring renal disease in the dog. In: *Vitamin D-gene regulation, structure-function analysis and clinical application.* Eds A Norman, R Bouillon, M Thomassett *et al.* De Grutyer, New York pp 879-880.

Nash AS, Wright NG, Spencer AJ, *et al.* (1979) Membraneous nephropathy in the cat: a clinical and pathological study. *Veterinary Record* **105,** 71.

Osborne CA, Polzin DJ, Abdullah S, Klausner JS and Rogers QR (1982). Role of diet in the management of feline chronic polyuric renal failure: current status. *Journal of the American Animal Hospital Association* **18,** 12.

Polzin DJ (1987). Conservative medical management of renal failure. *Proceedings of the 54th Annual Meeting of AAHA*, p 168.

Polzin DJ and Osborne CA (1986). Dietary management of canine renal failure. In: *Nephrology and Urology*. Ed EB Breitschwerdt. Churchill Livingstone, New York p 151.

Polzin DJ, Osborne CA, Hayden DW and Steven JB (1983). Influence of reduced protein diets on morbidity, mortality, and renal function in dogs with induced chronic renal failure. *American Journal of Veterinary Research* **45,** 506.

Polzin DJ, Osborne CA and Lulich JP (1991). Effects of dietary protein/phosphate restriction in normal dogs and dogs with chronic renal failure. *Journal of Small Animal Practice* **32,** 289.

Polzin DJ, Osborne CA and O'Brien T (1989). Diseases of the kidneys and ureters. In: *Textbook of Veterinary Internal Medicine (third edition)*. Ed SJ Ettinger. WB Saunders, Philadelphia p 1962.

Robertson JL, Goldschmidt M, Kronfeld DS, Tomaszewski JE, Hill GS and Bovee KC (1986). Long-term responses to high dietary protein in dogs with 75% nephrectomy. *Kidney International* **29,** 511.

Rogers QR, Morris JG and Friedland RA (1977). Lack of hepatic enzymatic adaptation to high levels of dietary protein in the adult cat. *Enzyme* **22,** 348.

Ross LA (1986). Feline renal failure. In: *Nephrology and Urology*. Ed EB Breitschwerdt. Churchill Livingstone, New York p 109.

Ross LA and Finco DR (1981). Relationship of selected clinical function tests to glomerular filtration rate and renal blood flow in cats. *American Journal of Veterinary Research* **42,** 1704.

Ross LA, Finco DR and Crowell WA (1982). Effect of dietary phosphorus restriction on the kidneys of cats with reduced renal mass. *American Journal of Veterinary Research* **43,** 1023.

Ross LA and Labato MA (1989). Use of drugs to control hypertension in renal failure. In: *Current Veterinary Therapy X: Small Animal Practice.* Ed RW Kirk. WB Saunders, Philadelphia p 1201.

Schmidt RW and Gavellas G (1977). Bicarbonate reabsorption in experimental renal disease: effect of proportional reduction of sodium or phosphate intake. *Kidney International* **12,** 393.

Smith BHE, Markwell PJ, Rodriguez-Garcia MC and Azacarte J (1994). The dietary management of canine renal failure caused by leishmaniasis. *Proceedings of the European Society of Veterinary Internal Medicine Congress* 167.

Tollins JP, Hostetter MK and Hostetter TH (1987). Hypokalemic nephropathy in the rat: role of ammonia in chronic tubular injury. *Journal of Clinical Investigation* **79,** 1447.

CHAPTER TWELVE

Chronic Hepatobiliary Disease

Hein P. Meyer and Jan Rothuizen

INTRODUCTION

Hepatobiliary diseases include all disorders affecting the parenchyma of the liver, the efferent or afferent vascular system, and the biliary tree and may be primary or secondary.

Patients with hepatobiliary disease are encountered frequently in companion animal practice. It is estimated that 2-3% of all animals presented at the University Clinic for Companion Animals in Utrecht have some kind of hepatobiliary disease. Hereditary portosystemic shunts and chronic active hepatitis, which account for the major portion of the patients with hepatobiliary diseases, occur in 2-3% of investigated breeds (Meyer *et al.*, 1995), and 0.1-1% of all clinical cases in dogs (Strombeck, 1991), respectively. Since the liver plays an essential role in the homoeostasis of the metabolism of protein, carbohydrate, and fat, nutritional support plays an essential role for many patients with longstanding liver disease.

Hepatobiliary diseases may be categorised depending on their cause (Table 12.1). Most of these disorders may lead to an increase in hepatic vascular resistance, which results in portal hypertension. Portal hypertension in turn may lead to the formation of multiple portosystemic collaterals and ascites. Irrespective of its initial cause, severe and longstanding hepatic dysfunction often leads to just a few syndromes with potentially serious metabolic consequences, i.e., **hepatic encephalopathy** and **cholestasis**. The pathophysiology of these syndromes and their respective nutritional support will be discussed in this chapter. Since the cat has some unique features with respect to metabolism and liver physiology, special attention will be given to the nutritional support of feline patients with liver disease.

HEPATIC ENCEPHALOPATHY

Hepatic encephalopathy (HE) is a commonly occurring syndrome in dogs and cats with liver disease. It is defined as a metabolic dysfunction of the brain resulting from impaired liver function (Conn, 1989). HE can be separated into an acute form due to fulminant hepatitis and a chronic form in which abnormal liver perfusion by portal blood is the essential pathogenetic factor. Fulminant hepatitis is rare in the dog and cat. Hence in these species almost all cases of HE are of the chronic form. Therefore, this discussion will only deal with chronic HE which differs pathogenically from acute HE.

The essential factors that must coexist in liver disease in order to develop chronic HE are portosystemic collateral circulation and damage to or atrophy of the liver parenchyma itself. The impaired liver function may be primary, i.e., the cause of the portosystemic shunting, or it may be secondary. In the former there is always portal hypertension leading to the formation of multiple collateral vessels between the vena portae and the vena cava or azygos. In the latter the primary disease is a single congenital portosystemic shunt.

Congenital	Hereditary portosystemic shunts Copper toxicosis Congenital liver fibrosis Portal vein hypoplasia (with or without fibrosis) Neonatal (lobular dissecting) hepatitis
Immune mediated	Chronic active hepatitis/cirrhosis Dobermann hepatitis Biliary cirrhosis (cat) Granulomatous hepatitis
Storage disorders	Lipidosis (cat) Amyloidosis
Infectious	Cholangitis (cat) Leptospirosis
Neoplastic	Metastatic Primary
Others	Toxic hepatopathy Thrombosis of the portal vein

Table 12.1: *Common hepatobiliary diseases in the dog and cat.*

Derangement	Cerebral effect
Hyperammonaemia (possibly synergism with mercaptans and fatty acids?)	Decreased glutamate Increased synaptic glutamate (?) Increased glutamine
Decreased BCAA:AAA ratio	Deranged dopaminergic neurotransmission
Increased endogenous benzodiazepines	Increased GABA-ergic tone

Table 12.2: *The pathogenesis of hepatic encephalopathy.*

Congenital portosystemic shunts (PSS) are inherited and may occur in 2–3% of the population (Meyer *et al* 1995). They may be either intrahepatic (large and giant breeds, such as the Irish Wolfhound and Bernese Mountain Dog) or extrahepatic (medium and toy breeds, such as the Yorkshire Terrier, Cairn Terrier, and Dachshund) (Rothuizen *et al.,* 1982; Maddison 1988, 1991). In hereditary PSS there is a complete diversion of portal blood via the shunts (Meyer *et al.,* 1994), thus, bypassing the liver from birth onward and depriving the liver of growth factors, oxygen, and essential nutrients. Consequently, affected animals have a severely underdeveloped liver.

Brain dysfunction in HE is essentially a neurotransmitter dysfunction. The main transmitter systems involved are glutamate, gamma-amino butyric acid and benzodiazepines (GABA/BZ), and dopamine. The complexity of all these changes may be the main reason for the still unsolved pathogenesis of HE (Table 12.2).

Hyperammonaemia and Glutamate Neurotransmission

Ammonia, which is a product of intestinal nitrogen metabolism, normally enters the liver via the portal vein. The hepatic clearance of ammonia is very efficient and under physiological conditions only minute amounts of ammonia enter the systemic circulation and thus reach the astrocytes which form a barrier between the circulation and the neurons in the brain. In the astrocytes, ammonia is incorporated into glutamate to form glutamine, which is catalysed by glutamine synthetase.

Portosystemic shunting leads to a high concentration of systemic ammonia and the reserve capacity of glutamine synthetase is exceeded (Bosman, 1991). The excess ammonia then diffuses into the neurons, where it inhibits the enzyme glutaminase which converts glutamine into glutamate. This results in depletion of the neuronal glutamate pool and increase in the cerebral glutamine concentration.

Glutamate is one of the most abundant excitatory neurotransmitters in the brain. The compromised availability of glutamate as a result of hyperammonaemia is thought to be an important factor in the deranged neurotransmission in HE (Hamberger, 1981). Lowering the concentration of ammonia in plasma and cerebrospinal fluid has been shown to be beneficial in the management of patients with HE (de Bruijn, 1986).

The GABA/BZ Receptor Complex

GABA and the GABA/BZ receptor complex is the most abundant inhibitory neurotransmitter system throughout the central nervous system. In the neuron GABA is formed from glutamate. An increased activity of GABA-containing pathways may contribute to the manifestations of HE.

Whether the increased GABA-ergic tone is actually due to an increase in GABA concentration (formed locally or derived from the gut) is disputed (Maddison *et al.,* 1987). Several studies have shown the existence of an increased concentration of endogenous benzodiazepines in humans, rabbits, and rats with HE (Mullen *et al.,* 1988; Basile *et al.,* 1991). Avoidance of the intake of benzodiazepines (both dietary or medicinal) is essential to prevent aggravation of the increased GABA-ergic tone.

Amino Acid Metabolism and Dopaminergic Neurotransmission

Impaired liver function may result in a disturbed metabolism of amino acids and carbohydrates. In health, the neutral aromatic amino acids (AAA) tyrosine, tryptophan, and phenylalanine are efficiently cleared from the portal blood by the liver. In the presence of PSS, these amino acids bypass the liver and hence systemic concentrations are high. Because of a decrease in carbohydrate metabolism and subsequent hypoglycaemia, muscles and other tissues utilise the ketogenic neutral branched chain amino acids (BCAA) leucine, isoleucine, and valine. This leads to a decreased BCAA:AAA molar ratio in the circulation (Iob *et al.,* 1970; Fischer and Baldessarini, 1971; Aguirre *et al.,* 1974; Soeters 1979). Increased concentrations of both insulin and glucagon, together with a low insulin:glucagon ratio, aggravate the decrease in plasma BCAA:AAA (Soeters and Fischer, 1986; Fiaccadori *et al.,* 1991). In both humans and dogs the normal BCAA:AAA ratio of 3–3.5 decreases to 0.6–1.2 in subjects with HE (Soeters, 1979).

Since both AAA and BCAA use the same carrier for neutral amino acids (NAA) to enter the brain (Orlowski *et al.,* 1974), a decreased availability of BCAA will lead to an increased uptake of AAA, resulting in a high concentration of AAA in the brain.

In the brain, phenylalanine (phe) can be converted to tyrosine (tyr), which is precursor for the catecholamines (dopamine, noradrenaline). In the several conversion steps from tyr to the catecholamines, the enzyme tyrosine-3-hydroxylase is the rate-limiting step. When there is an excess of AAA, the precursors accumulate and phe and tyr are abnormally decarboxylated to form ß-phenylethanolamine and octopamine, respectively. These two abnormal metabolites have been postulated to be 'false' neurotransmitters, inertly occupying the catecholamine (preferentially dopamine) receptors and thus preventing catecholaminergic neurotransmission.

Based on the literature and our own findings (Rothuizen and Mol, 1987; Meyer and Rothuizen, 1994), we hypothesise that in HE there is a blockade of the catecholaminergic neurotransmission due to 'false' neurotransmitters, and that this blockade can be reversed by the administration of an excess of branched chain amino acids.

Dietary Strategy in Hepatic Encephalopathy

From the involvement of ammonia in the pathogenesis of HE it can be deduced that protein restriction is a cornerstone in the treatment of HE (de Bruijn, 1986; Uribe 1989). However, chronic excessive protein restriction is undesirable, because patients with HE are already in a catabolic state (Rosen *et al.*, 1978; Uribe 1989). Apart from the total protein intake, the source and quality of proteins may also affect HE. Meat and blood have long been known to worsen the state of HE, whereas vegetable and milk proteins have been shown to be beneficial (Fenton *et al.*, 1966). On the other hand, the use of the latter proteins can be disputed, since they may be a major source of benzodiazepines (Bosman, 1991). Therefore, in view of the present state of knowledge, moderate protein restriction (protein content not below 11% (DM base)) at a rate of 2.1g crude protein/kg body weight/day seems most desirable (Laflamme *et al.*, 1994) for chronic treatment of patients with HE.

The possible involvement of 'false' neurotransmitters as a result of excess aromatic amino acids gives another clue for an active dietary strategy. By avoiding AAA, and instead feeding protein containing high concentrations of BCAA one could possibly restore the formation of the normal catecholaminergic neurotransmitters and prevent the further production of 'false' neurotransmitters. Several studies using high concentrations of BCAA have been performed in humans and experimental animals (Soeters, 1979) with HE, both chronic and acute. Oral or intravenous administration of BCAA normalised the BCAA:AAA molar ratio in serum and cerebrospinal fluid, but the effect on the degree of HE was variable. Of four recent reviews of clinical trials in humans, one showed a decreased mortality rate and improved mental performance during administration of BCAA (Naylor *et al.*, 1989), but the other three reported no detectable influence (Wahren *et al.*, 1983; Eriksson and Conn, 1989; Morgan 1990). A study in dogs with HE has shown a detrimental effect of the use of a high BCAA diet (Laflamme *et al.*, 1993). Further research on the applicability of this concept has to be done to establish the role of BCAA in the diet for HE.

If portal hypertension as a consequence of hepatic disease is a clinical problem, a diet with a low sodium and a high potassium content is advisable (Laflamme, 1988).

We do not recommend the use of home-made diets in such cases, because of the inconvenience and risk for introducing deficiencies in various constituents. Therefore, a low protein diet containing at least the minimum requirements of the National Research Council (NRC) (1985, 1986) for all macro- and trace elements is the best we can offer to dogs and cats with chronic liver disease at the moment (Table 12.3).

CHOLESTASIS

Cholestasis is defined as a reduction in bile flow. It may be extrahepatic, as a consequence of any obstruction in the extrahepatic bile ducts (e.g., cholangitis, chronic pancreatitis, pancreatic neoplasia) or intrahepatic. The latter may be caused by reduced clearance, metabolism or excretion of biliary constituents

	Protein (%)	Fat (%)	Carbohydrates (%)	Special requirements
HE (dogs and cats, unless lipidosis)	14–18 (2.1g CP/kg BW/day)	25	55	High digestibility, preferably high ratio BCAA:AAA[1]
HE plus ascites	14–18	25	55	High digestibility, high ratio BCAA:AAA low sodium, high potassium
Lipidosis (cats)	35–40 (75kcal[2] ME/kg BW/day)	25	30–35	Preferably high contents of taurine, arginine, carnitine, choline

Table 12.3: *Dietary recommendations in chronic liver disease.*

Contents in % of dry matter.

1 Foods that have a high ratio of branched chain amino acids to aromatic amino acids are fish, eggs and beef.

2 75kcal or 314kJ.

or by their regurgitation. Intrahepatic cholestasis may occur in all liver diseases. Bile flow is virtually never reduced so much that fat metabolism becomes compromised. Consequently, fat metabolism is scarcely disturbed in liver disease with the exception of total extrahepatic cholestasis, but this disorder nearly always requires surgical intervention. Perioperative care for such patients should include parenteral substitution of the fat-soluble vitamins (A, D, E, and K) until the extrahepatic cholestasis is relieved surgically. Hence chronic dietary management of cholestasis, which was previously advised in the form of a low fat diet (Hardy, 1983), is no longer recommended in either veterinary medicine (Bauer, 1986) or human medicine (Morgan, 1991). A balanced commercially available diet meeting the requirements of the NRC should suffice.

FELINE LIVER DISEASE

Feline liver function has several special features which make the cat less tolerant to fasting and more dependent on an adequate daily supply of amino acids than are other species (Rogers and Morris, 1978; Center, 1986; Rogers and Morris, 1991). The first reason for this is that the capacity to synthesise arginine is lower than that in other species. Arginine is an intermediate of the urea cycle, in which ammonia is converted to urea. Arginine also plays a role in the production of apoproteins, which are incorporated in very low density lipoproteins (VLDL). VLDL are the means of transporting triglycerides from the liver to adipose tissue. Marginal availability of arginine may therefore lead to hyperammonaemia, even without severe liver dysfunction or collateral circulation, and to disturbed transport of triglycerides. Second, the taurine requirement in cats is high. Taurine plays a role in VLDL production and the conjugation of bile acids. Third, carnitine availability in cats may be marginal. Carnitine is essential for the transport of long-chain fatty acids into the mitochondria, where they can be ß-oxidised. Fourth, the flexibility of aminotransferases in cats is low, which means that amino acids are being used in the Krebs cycle, even when low protein or high carbohydrate diets are given. This can at least partly explain the high protein requirement of the cat.

Feline Hepatic Lipidosis and its Dietary Support

Hepatic lipidosis is the consequence of a disruption of the balance between the supply of fatty acids and triglycerides to the liver and the ß-oxidation and removal of triglycerides (in VLDL) from the liver (Figure 12.1).

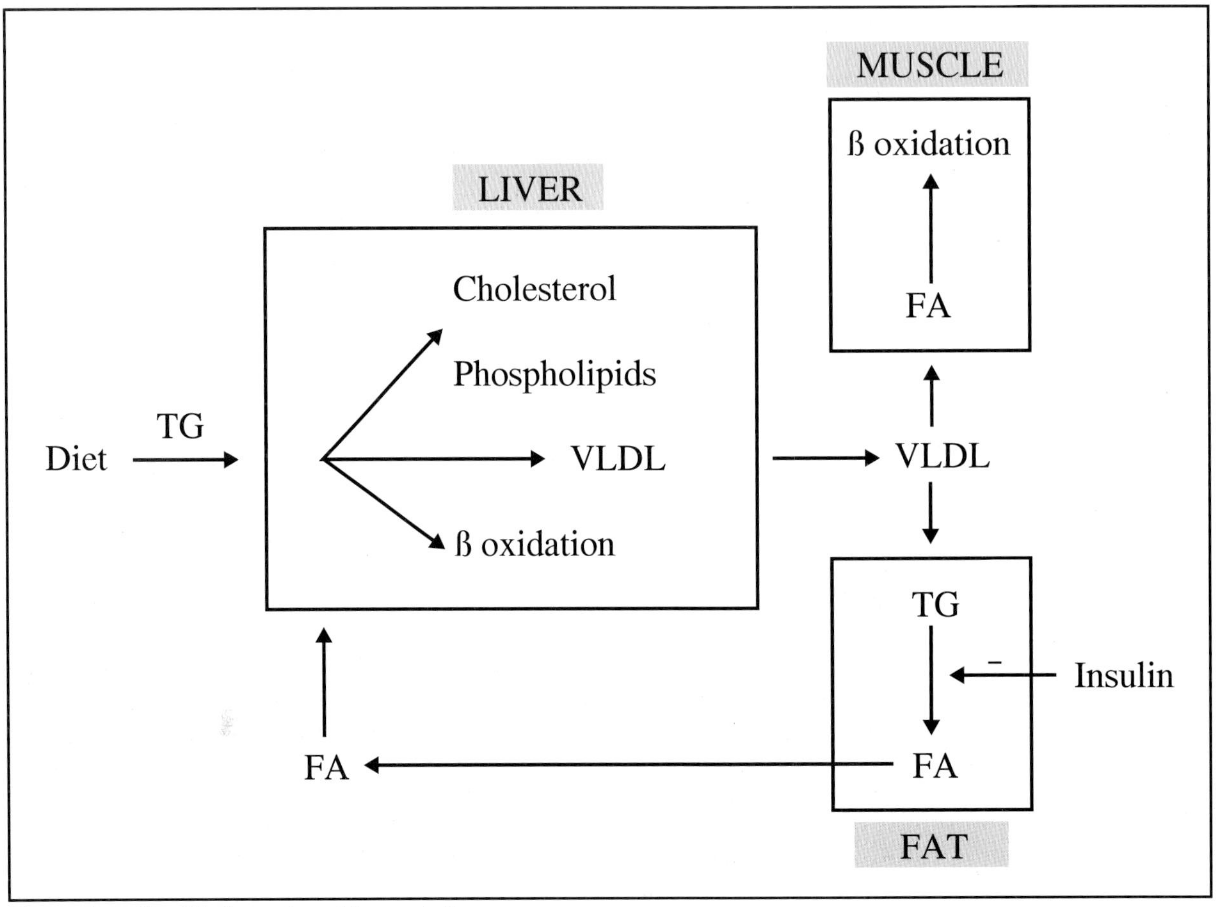

Figure 12.1: *Simplified overview of fat metabolism.*

TG triglycerides
FA fatty acids
VLDL very low density lipoproteins

From a pathophysiological point of view it is clear that the feline liver is prone to disruptions in lipid homoeostasis. In man, many factors can disturb this balance including prolonged fasting, high caloric intake, alcoholism, Cushing's syndrome, diabetes mellitus, toxins, and drugs (e.g., tetracycline). Hepatic lipidosis is especially common in the USA (Garvey, 1991). The number of patients with feline hepatic lipidosis (FHL) diagnosed in our clinic tends to increase annually. Several entities have been proposed as causes of FHL, including obesity, diabetes mellitus, hyperthyroidism, growth hormone excess, and prolonged fasting (failure to meet the high requirement for arginine, carnitine, and taurine) (Garvey, 1991; Center, 1991; Biourge *et al.,* 1993). In obesity, diabetes mellitus, hyperthyroidism, and growth hormone excess, insulin effects are diminished (either by hypoinsulinism, decreased receptor density or affinity, or by post receptor defects), leading to disinhibition of hormone-sensitive lipase. A disproportionate release of fatty acids from the adipose tissue and subsequent uptake by the liver may be one of the most important factors in the development of hepatic lipidosis.

Since any disruption in hepatic lipid metabolism can cause lipidosis, it is unlikely that there is a common cause for all cases of FHL. In many cases of FHL no underlying disorder or disturbance other than prolonged fasting can be found. These cases are as yet referred to as idiopathic FHL. The lack of appetite may be primary or secondary, since an increase in the concentration of free fatty acids causes anorexia. The clinical picture of FHL is often characterised by signs of hepatic encephalopathy and a state of prolonged fasting and debilitation. Histological examination of a percutaneous liver biopsy is essential for the diagnosis of idiopathic FHL and to exclude secondary predisposing factors leading to FHL.

Vigorous supportive care (intravenous fluid administration and the supplementation of vitamins) may be needed in serious cases. Tube feeding is essential in the management of FHL. A nasogastric tube may be well tolerated by the patient, but placement of a gastrostomy tube is better for long-term therapy (see Chapter 17). The tube can be placed under endoscopic guidance or under guidance of an orally inserted wire. Tube feeding with a liquid food (or any good quality cat food, thinned with water to make a gruel) containing sufficient high quality protein and having high caloric density is the primary goal of therapy. In particular the levels of arginine, taurine, choline, and carnitine should be high, which is the case in some specially formulated liquid diets for cats. The paradox of feeding high protein diets in cases of lipidosis with HE is explained by the functional cause of HE (i.e., arginine deficiency) in such cases. Protein overload should be avoided, however. The carbohydrate content of this diet should not be too high, since excess carbohydrates promote lipogenesis. Although therapy with high fat containing diets or lipid infusions has been advocated (Biourge *et al.,* 1990, 1993), there is no pathophysiological basis for giving diets with a supranormal fat content, since surplus lipids further expand the triglyceride overload in the liver (Morgan, 1991). The prognosis of FHL is guarded: with aggressive and longlasting therapy, for which a patient and dedicated owner is an absolute prerequisite, approximately 50% of the patients will recover fully (Biourge *et al.,* 1993, Jacobs *et al.,* 1989).

REFERENCES

Aguirre A, Yoshimura N, Westman T and Fischer JE (1974). Plasma amino acids in dogs with two experimental forms of liver damage. *Journal of Surgical Research* **16,** 339.

Basile AS, Jones EA and Skolnick P (1991). The pathogenesis and treatment of hepatic encephalopathy - evidence for the involvement of benzodiazepine receptor ligands. *Pharmacological Reviews* **43,** 27.

Bauer JE (1986). Nutrition and liver function: nutrient metabolism in health and disease. *Compendium of Continuing Education* **8,** 923.

Biourge V, MacDonald MJ and King L (1990). Feline hepatic lipidosis: pathogenesis and nutritional management. *Compendium of Continuing Education* **12,** 1244.

Biourge V, Pion P, Lewis J, Morris JG and Rogers QR (1993). Spontaneous occurrence of hepatic lipidosis in a group of laboratory cats. *Journal of Veterinary Internal Medicine* **7,** 194.

Bosman DK (1991). *Pathophysiology and therapy of hepatic encephalopathy. An experimental and clinical study* [Dissertation] University of Amsterdam, Amsterdam, The Netherlands.

Center SA (1986). Feline liver disorders and their management. *Compendium of Continuing Education* **8,** 889.

Center SA. Hepatic lipidosis (1991). In: *Consultations in Feline Internal Medicine*, 1st edition. Ed RA August. WB Saunders, Philadelphia pp 451-462.

Conn HO (1989). The hepatic encephalopathies. In: *Hepatic Encephalopathy: Management with Lactulose and related Carbohydrates.* Eds HO Conn and J Bircher. Medi-Ed Press, East Lansing, MI. pp 3-14.

de Bruijn KM (1986). *Clinical and experimental studies on ammonia metabolism and treatment forms of portal-systemic encephalopathy* [Dissertation] University of Groningen, Groningen, The Netherlands.

Eriksson LS and Conn HO (1989). Branched-chain amino acids in the management of hepatic encephalopathy - an analysis of variants. *Hepatology* **10,** 228.

Fenton JCB, Knight EJ and Hupherson PL (1966). Milk and cheese diet in portal systemic encephalopathy. *Lancet* **i,** 164.

Fiaccadori F, Pedretti G, Ferrari C, Pizzaferri P, Riggio O, Orlando N and Pezzarossa A (1991). Insulin and glucagon levels in fulminant hepatic failure in man. *Digestive Diseases and Sciences* **36,** 801.

Fischer JE and Baldessarini RJ (1971). False neurotransmitters and hepatic failure. *Lancet* **ii,** 75.

Garvey MS (1991). Feline liver disease In: *Proceedings of the XVI WSAVA Congress.* Ed J Leibetseder. Gisteldruck, Vienna, Austria pp 175-181.

Hamberger AC (1981). Regulation of glutamate biosynthesis and release by pathophysiological levels of ammonium ions. In: *Glutamate as a Neurotransmitter*. Eds G Di Chiari and GL Gessa. Raven Press, New York pp 320-356.

Hardy RM (1983) Diseases of the liver. In: *Textbook of Internal Medicine. Diseases of the Dog and Cat, 1st edition.* Ed SJ Ettinger. WB Saunders, Philadelphia, pp. 1372-1434.

Iob V, Mattson WJ jr, Sloan M, Coon WW, Turcotte JG and Child CG (1970). Alterations in plasma-free amino acids in dogs with hepatic insufficiency. *Surgery, Gynecology and Obstetrics* **130,** 794.

Jacobs G, Cornelius L, Allen S and Greene C (1989). Treatment of idiopathic hepatic lipidosis in cats : 11 cases (1986-1987). *Journal of the American Veterinary Medical Association* **195,** 635.

Laflamme DF (1988). Dietary management of canine hepatic encephalopathy. *Compendium of Continuing Education* **10,** 1258.

Laflamme DP, Allen SW and Huber TL (1993). Apparent dietary protein requirement of dogs with portosystemic shunt. *American Journal of Veterinary Research* **54,** 719.

Laflamme DP, Allen SA and Huber TL (1994). Recent advances in dietary management of hepatic diseases. *Veterinary Quarterly* **16**(suppl.), 34S.

Maddison JE, Dodd PR, Johnston JA and Farrell GC (1987). Brain gamma-aminobutyric acid receptor binding is normal in rats with thioacetamide-induced hepatic encephalopathy despite elevated plasma gamma-butyric acid-like activity. *Gastroenterology* **93,** 1062.

Maddison JE (1988). Canine congenital portosystemic encephalopathy. *Australian Veterinary Journal* **65,** 245.

Maddison JE (1991). Canine congenital portosystemic encephalopathy: a spontaneous animal model of chronic hepatic encephalopathy. In: *Progress in Hepatic Encephalopathy and Nitrogen Exchange.* Eds F Bengtsson *et al.* CRC Press, Boca Raton pp 99-104.

Meyer HP and Rothuizen J (1994). Increased free cortisol in plasma of dogs with portosystemic encephalopathy (PSE). *Domestic Animal Endorinology* **11,** 317.

Meyer HP, Rothuizen J, Ubbink GJ and Vandeningh TSGAM (1995). Increasing incidence of hereditary intrahepatic portosystemic shunts in Irish wolfhounds in the Netherlands (1984-1992). *Veterinary Record* **136,** 13-16.

Meyer HP, Rothuizen J, Van den Brom WE, Voorhout G, Van Sluijs FJ, How KL and Pollak YWEA (1994). Quantitation of portosystemic shunting in dogs by ultrasound-guided injection of ^{99m}Tc-macroaggregates into a splenic vein. *Research in Veterinary Science* **57,** 58.

Morgan MY (1990). Branched chain amino acids in the management of chronic liver disease - facts and fantasies. *Journal of Hepatology* **11,** 133.

Morgan MY (1991). Nutritional aspects of liver and biliary disease. In: *Oxford Textbook of Clinical Hepatology.* 1st edition. Eds N McIntyre *et al.* Oxford University Press, Oxford pp 1339-1388.

Mullen KD, Martin JV, Mendelson WB, Bassett ML and Jones EA (1988). Could an endogenous benzodiazepine ligand contribute to hepatic encephalopathy? *Lancet* **i,** 457.

National Research Council (1985). *Nutritional Requirements of Dogs.* National Academy Press, Washington D.C.

National Research Council (1986). *Nutritional Requirements of Cats.* National Academy Press, Washington D.C.

Naylor CD, O'Rourke K, Detsky AS and Baker JP (1989). Parenteral nutrition with branched-chain amino acids in hepatic encephalopathy - a meta-analysis. *Gastroenterology* **97,** 1033.

Orlowski MG, Sessa JP and Green JP (1974). Gamma-glutamyl transpeptidase in brain capillaries: possible site of a blood brain barrier for amino acids. *Science* **184,** 66.

Rogers QR and Morris JG (1978). Why does a cat require a high protein diet? In: *Nutrition of the Dog and Cat.* Ed RS Anderson. Pergamon Press, Oxford pp 45-65.

Rogers QR and Morris JG (1991). Nutritional peculiarities of the cat. In: *Proceedings of the XVI WSAVA Congress.* Ed J Leibetseder. Gisteldruck, Vienna, Austria pp 261-266.

Rosen HM, Soeters PB, James JH, Hodgman J and Fischer JE (1978). Influences of exogenous intake and nitrogen balance on plasma and brain amino acid concentrations. *Metabolism* **27,** 393.

Rothuizen J and Mol JA (1987). The pituitary-adrenocortical system in canine hepatic encephalopathy. *Frontiers in Hormone Research* **17,** 28.

Rothuizen J, Van den Ingh TSGAM, Voorhout G, Van der Luer RJT and Wouda W (1982). Congenital porto-systemic shunts in sixteen dogs and three cats. *Journal of Small Animal Practice* **23,** 67.

Soeters PB (1979). *Hepatic Encephalopathy : a new perspective for therapy* [Dissertation]. Maastricht University, Maastricht, The Netherlands.

Soeters PB and Fischer JE (1986). Insulin, glucagon, amino acid imbalance and hepatic encephalopathy. *Lancet* **ii,** 880.

Strombeck DR (1991). *Small Animal Gastroenterology*. Stonegate Publishing, Davis CA pp 593-628.

Uribe M (1989). Dietary management of portal-systemic encephalopathy. In: *Hepatic encephalopathy: management with lactulose and related carbohydrates*. Eds HO Conn and J Bircher. Medi-Ed Press, East Lansing, MI. pp 95-112.

Wahren J, Denis J, Desurmont P, Eriksson LS, Escoffier JM, Gauthier AP, Hagenfeldt L, Michel H, Opolon P, Paris JC and Veyrac M (1983). Is intravenous administration of branched chain amino acids effective in the treatment of hepatic encephalopathy? A multicenter study. *Hepatology* **3,** 475.

CHAPTER THIRTEEN

Gastrointestinal Problems

Edward Hall

INTRODUCTION

The gastrointestinal (GI) tract is the natural pathway by which food is ingested and digested, and nutrients are absorbed. Thus the enteral route, being the most physiological, is the preferred and most economical for feeding. When an animal is unwilling or unable to ingest food because of localised upper GI disease, and yet has a functional intestine, enteral nutrition by some form of tube feeding is indicated (see Chapters 17 and 18). However, in many GI diseases the patient can eat but digestion and absorption is impaired. Nevertheless, it is usually possible to feed enterally if a modified diet is given. Parenteral nutrition is technically difficult and expensive, and is reserved for rare cases where oral alimentation is impossible.

Dietary modification is probably as important as pharmacological intervention in the treatment of most GI diseases and indeed may be the only treatment necessary. The aim of this chapter is to demonstrate how a rational choice of diet can be made either as primary treatment or as an adjunct to moderate any symptoms. The client's desire is for their pet to be returned to normal, and thus a thorough initial investigation, a diagnosis, and rational drug and dietary therapy are important if the patient is ultimately to be returned to a regular diet.

ASSESSMENT OF PATHOLOGICAL STATUS

Clinical Examination

Good history-taking and physical examination are essential to direct further investigation along a logical and economical path and permit a rational choice of diet. The supposed cardinal signs of GI disease, vomiting and diarrhoea, may draw attention to the GI tract but disease in other organ systems may be responsible; equally, absence of these signs may result in GI disease being overlooked. In all situations, attention must be paid to the hydration status of the patient.

Questions concerning appetite, weight loss etc. are relevant to any disease but, in the context of GI disease, pertinent questions should establish a complete dietary history, the possibility of ingestion of non-food substances, and vaccination and worming history.

Clinical evaluation permits localisation of the disease process, refinement of the diagnostic procedures to be performed, and a rational choice of diet. Differentiation of regurgitation from vomiting is important. Vomiting may be an important sign of small intestinal (SI) as well as gastric disease, especially in cats. It can be useful, both diagnostically and therapeutically, if diarrhoea can be classified as SI and large intestinal (LI) in origin based on clinical signs and faecal characteristics (Table 13.1) (Burrows, 1986). Protein-losing enteropathies (PLEs) may result in ascites and/or peripheral oedema.

Laboratory Testing

The extent of any laboratory testing in GI disease is a balance between the acuteness or severity of the illness and economic considerations. A minimum database of haematology, serum biochemistry, urinalysis and faecal examination for parasites will rule out the majority of systemic causes of vomiting and diarrhoea, and suggest possible GI causes. Faecal culture is only helpful when known pathogens, such as *Salmonella* and *Campylobacter*, are found. Panhypoproteinaemia is characteristic of a PLE, but other causes of hypoproteinaemia must be excluded.

Further laboratory investigation of chronic diarrhoea in practice is limited. Serum trypsin-like immunoreactivity (TLI) concentration must always be measured to rule out exocrine pancreatic insufficiency in dogs (Williams, 1989). Assay of serum folate and cobalamin concentrations may permit detection of small intestinal bacterial overgrowth (SIBO) and proximal and distal SI disease (Batt and Morgan, 1982).

Imaging

Radiographic investigation of the chest and abdomen may be indicated in cases of regurgitation and vomiting. Plain radiographs should always be taken before any contrast study, as foreign bodies may be obscured by the contrast material. Fluoroscopic visualisation is helpful in detecting gastric disorders, but the use of graded, barium-impregnated plastic spheres to evaluate gastric emptying and intestinal transit times, and to

Sign	Small intestinal diarrhoea	Large intestinal diarrhoea
Faeces		
Volume	Markedly increased	Normal or decreased
Mucus	Rarely present	Common
Melaena	May be present	Absent
Haematochezia (fresh blood in stool)	Absent except in acute haemorrhagic diarrhoea	Fairly common
Steatorrhoea	Present with malabsorption	Absent
Undigested food	May be present	Absent
Colour	Colour variations occur	Colour variations rare; may be bloody
Defecation		
Urgency	Absent except in acute or very severe disease	Usually but not invariably present
Tenesmus	Absent	Frequent but not invariably present
Frequency	2 to 3 times normal for the patient	Usually greater than 3 times normal
Dyschezia (difficulty in defecation)	Absent	Present with distal colonic or rectal disease
Ancillary signs		
Weight loss	May occur in malabsorption	Rare except in severe colitis and diffuse tumours
Vomiting	May be present in inflammatory diseases, especially in cats	Probably occurs in ~30% of dogs with colitis
Flatulence and borborygmi	May occur	Absent
Halitosis in absence of oral disease	May be present with malabsorption	Absent unless perianal licking

Table 13.1: *Differentiation of small intestinal from large intestinal diarrhoea.*

detect partial SI obstructions has recently been reported (Guilford, 1994a). Contrast studies in malabsorption cases are usually unrewarding and have largely been superseded by endoscopy.

Endoscopy and Biopsy

Endoscopic visualisation and biopsy of lesions of the oesophagus, stomach, duodenum, ileum, and large intestine frequently permits more accurate diagnosis and more appropriate therapy but has limitations, not least the inability to reach most of the jejunum even in cats (Hall, 1994a). An exploratory laparotomy is an acceptable alternative diagnostic procedure provided biopsies are always taken. Nevertheless, in approximately half of patients with chronic SI disease, intestinal biopsies will be histologically normal (Loth *et al.*, 1990; Van der Gaag and Happé, 1990). Furthermore, common histopathological descriptions such as lymphocytic enteritis give no clue as to the underlying aetiology (Batt and Hall, 1989).

Empirical Treatment

Empirical treatment is a common approach to cases where practical or financial constraints preclude a definitive diagnosis, or where attempts at a diagnosis have failed. Furthermore, dietary trials in cases of suspected food sensitivity are, in essence, empirical. However, the empirical use of drugs can never be whole-heartedly recommended as symptoms may be masked and definitive treatment delayed, and the unjustified use of immunosuppressive drugs is potentially dangerous.

Nutritional Status

The general nutritional status of a patient with GI disease can be assessed as described in Chapters 15, 17 and 18, but in acute disease, the hydration status is often more life-threatening. In chronic diseases, assessment of protein-calorie malnutrition is based on body weight, condition score, and serum albumin concentrations. The severity of the malnutrition tends to reflect the severity and chronicity of the condition, and the need for intensive treatment with nutritional support.

Manifestations of specific nutritional deficiences secondary to malabsorption are poorly defined. Poor hair and skin condition, poor healing and susceptibility to infection may be signs of generalised malnutrition, or perhaps associated with specific deficiencies of essential fats or minerals such as zinc (see Chapter 14).

DIETARY STRATEGY

Enteral Tube Feeding

Enteral feeding by naso-oesophageal, pharyngostomy, gastrostomy or jejunostomy tubes can support the nutrition of patients with localised disease of the oropharynx, oesophagus or stomach but a functional small intestine. The composition of the food is essentially normal, but its form is modified to permit passage through a tube. Methods for tube feeding are described in Chapter 17.

Bowel Rest

The traditional, common-sense approach to the treatment of acute GI upsets is the principle of 'bowel rest' (Darrow, 1952). Food is withheld for 24 to 72 hours in order to reduce the digestive and osmotic load on the intestine and reduce the substrate available for intraluminal fermentation. Fluid and electrolyte status must be maintained, either by oral rehydration fluid or by parenteral administration.

The concept of bowel rest has recently been questioned in paediatric medicine, where cessation of feeding may have disastrous nutritional consequences; continuing to 'feed-through diarrhoea' maintains greater mucosal integrity and improves survival (Isolauri *et al.*, 1989; Snyder *et al.*, 1990). In veterinary medicine, 'feeding-through diarrhoea' will often be impossible because of concomitant vomiting. Furthermore, because the patient's nutritional status is often not as critical as in human neonates, a small short-term weight loss is acceptable to clients whereas an increased stool volume is not.

Following traditional bowel rest 'regrading', that is gradual reintroduction of food in small, frequent meals over the next week, is usually practised. A highly digestible, moderate fat, 'bland' food, such as rice and cooked eggs or boiled white meat or fish is suitable (Table 13.2). However, human studies have again shown that an immediate return to the staple diet is associated with decreased morbidity, and is less confusing for patients (Armitstead *et al.*, 1989). Since most commercial pet foods are already inherently bland, an immediate return to the patient's staple diet might be justified, but feeding a novel food may avoid the development of an acquired allergy to the patient's staple diet (Guilford, 1994c).

Primary Dietary Therapy

If the animal's normal diet is the cause of GI disease (i.e. either a true food allergy or non-immunological intolerance) then appropriate dietary modification will be curative and such treatment may be considered primary. In acute cases, temporal association of the clinical signs with the ingestion of a particular food will often result in the client voluntarily withdrawing the food. Unfortunately the association of a particular food with chronic GI disorders is often obscure; the true incidence of dietary sensitivity is unknown, and diagnostic methods are lacking (Hall, 1994b).

Timetables for diagnosis and subsequent treatment of dietary sensitivities are given in Chapter 14, but the principle is the response to elimination/exclusion diets and test meal challenges (Strombeck and Guilford, 1991). The aim is to examine the effect of a so-called 'hypoallergenic diet', consisting of single protein and carbohydrate sources not normally fed. The wheat protein gluten has been shown to be responsible for an enteropathy in Irish Setters (and probably affects individuals of other breeds); recovery on a gluten-free diet and relapse on gluten challenge confirms the diagnosis, and feeding a gluten-free diet is curative (Hall and Batt, 1992). Sensitivity to meat proteins is believed to exist, but has not been as well documented. Pet foods are traditionally beef- and cereal-based, so trials with lamb/mutton, chicken, fish, cottage cheese or tofu with rice, potato or maize are suggested. Reconstituted baby rice powder is more acceptable to cats than boiled rice grains (Guilford, 1994b).

Inflammatory bowel diseases, such as eosinophilic gastroenteritis and lymphocytic-plasmacytic enteritis, may sometimes be manifestations of dietary allergy. Elemental diets, containing only simple sugars and amino acids, have been used to treat some forms of human inflammatory bowel disease (Teahon *et al.*, 1990), but such an approach has rarely been used in small animals because of the expense and the unpalatability of the diets. Nevertheless, a trial with a hypoallergenic diet in the treatment of these patients is indicated. Studies have demonstrated a positive effect of feeding a novel protein source in feline (Nelson *et al.*, 1984) and canine colitis (Nelson *et al.*, 1988), and a recent study showed a drug-sparing effect of a chicken-and-rice diet in canine idiopathic colitis (Simpson *et al.*, 1994). However, experience suggests that some antibiotic and/or immunosuppressive therapy is usually required.

Adjunctive Dietary Therapy

Often the patient's diet is not the cause of the GI disease, but because the digestive and absorptive capacity of the gut is compromised, feeding a normal diet results in diarrhoea. Modifications to the composition of the diet, as suggested below, will not cure the disease, but may reduce clinical signs, and act as an adjunct to any drug therapy.

DOGS*						
Indications	**Characteristics**	**Protein source**[a]	**Fat**	**Carbohydrate**	**Supplements**[b]	**Substitutions**
Exclusion diet SI disease LI disease Reduced lactose	Hypoallergenic Highly digestible Low fat Gluten-free (Low fibre)	Cottage cheese[1] 6 oz[†]	Corn oil 1 tsp	Boiled white rice[2] 10 oz ± 1-6 tsp psyllium[c]	1 tsp $Ca_2(PO_4)_3$[c] 1 tsp Lo Salt[d] adult multivitamins[e]	[1] tofu 6 oz[†] [2] boiled potato 14 oz
Exclusion diet SI disease LI disease - add psyllium	Hypoallergenic Highly digestible Low fat Lactose-free Gluten-free (Low fibre)	Lamb[1] 6 oz	Nil	ditto[2]	ditto	[1] equivalent amounts of any novel protein [2] boiled potato 14 oz
Exclusion diet SI disease LI disease - add isphagula[f]	Hypoallergenic Highly digestible Low fat Lactose-free Gluten-free (Low fibre)	Rabbit[1] 6 oz	Corn oil 1 tsp	ditto[2]	ditto	[1]venison 6 oz plus 1 extra tsp corn oil [2]boiled potato 14 oz
Exclusion diet SI disease LI disease - add isphagula[c] Regrading	Hypoallergenic Highly digestible Moderate fat Lactose-free Gluten-free Low fibre	Chicken without skin[1] 6 oz	Corn oil 2 tsp	Boiled white rice[2] 8 oz	1 tsp $Ca_2(PO_4)_3$ 1 tsp Lo Salt adult multivitamins	[1]turkey w/o skin $6^1/_2$ oz or tuna 7 oz or 6 boiled eggs with 1 tsp oil only [2]boiled potato 12 oz
Exclusion diet Regrading	Hypoallergenic Highly digestible Moderate fat Lactose-free Gluten-free Low fibre	Minced beef[1] 6 oz	Corn oil 2 tsp	ditto[2]	ditto	[1]minced pork 6 oz with 1 tsp oil only [2]boiled potato 12 oz
SIBO Lymphangiectasia	Hypoallergenic Highly digestible Low fat Lactose-free	Low fat cottage cheese[1] 6 oz	Corn oil[2] 1 tsp	Boiled white rice[3] 10 oz	1 tsp $Ca_2(PO_4)_3$ 1 tsp Lo-salt adult multivitamins ± MCT oil[h]	[1]chicken w/o skin 6 oz or boiled cod 12 oz [2]safflower oil 1/2 tsp[g] [3]boiled potato 14 oz
CATS**						
Exclusion diet SI disease LI disease - add isphagula[c]	Hypoallergenic Highly digestible Gluten-free (Low fibre)	Lamb[1] 6 oz	Corn oil $^1/_2$ tsp	Baby rice 8 oz (reconstituted)	1 tsp $Ca_2(PO_4)_3$ $^1/_2$ tsp Lo-salt adult multivitamins 500 mg taurine ± liver flavouring[i] ± 1 tsp isphagula[c]	[1]chicken w/o skin 6 oz (or cottage cheese 6 oz)

Table 13.2: *Recipes for home-cooked diets for dogs with gastrointestinal disease.*

** Each canine diet provides approximately 700kcal per day, enough for an average 10kg adult dog for one day. Requirements will vary with each individual patient, and with life stage, and with severity of the disease. (Adapted from Kronfeld, 1983, 1986; Strombeck and Guilford, 1991; Batt and Burrows, 1994, Guilford, 1994.)*

*** The feline recipe provides approximately 400kcal and is adequate for an average 5kg adult cat. Requirements will vary with individual patient, with life stage and with severity of the disease. (Adapted from Kronfeld, 1983, 1986; Strombeck and Guilford, 1991; Batt and Burrows, 1994; Guilford, 1994b.)*

Notes:
Boil rice and oil with twice the volume of water and simmer for 10 minutes, then add meat and minerals and simmer for a further 10 minutes; when cool, add multivitamins. Alternatively, cook ingredients in microwave oven, and add multivitamins when cool. tsp = 5ml teaspoon.
[a] single novel protein sources are essential for exclusion diets; [b] supplements need not be given during 1–2 week exclusion trial but are essential for maintenance therapy; [c] dicalcium phosphate [$Ca_2(PO_4)_3$] may be substituted by an equal amount of bonemeal, but the diet will no longer be 'hypoallergenic'; [d] Lo Salt is KCl enriched salt substitute; [e] human adult multivitamins are preferred as many veterinary preparations contain meat and cereal extracts for flavouring; [f] low fibre is generally recommended for small intestinal (SI) disease, but addition of psyllium or other fibre may be beneficial in large intestinal (LI) disease; [g] high in polyunsaturated fatty acids; [h] gradually introduce up to 2ml/kg as a fat/calorie supplement in lymphangiectasia; [i] flavouring with $^1/_2$ oz liver (or meat stocks) may be needed for palatability, but liver must never be the sole protein source; † 1oz = 30g.

Digestibility

Mucosal brush border damage is likely to reduce the digestive and absorptive capacity of the intestine, and feeding a highly digestible diet is indicated.

Carbohydrate

Rice starch is the most digestible source of carbohydrate, and cooked rice is the preferred source in dogs with GI disease (Washabau *et al*,, 1986; Strombeck and Guilford, 1991). Cooking alters the physical state of the starch to permit hydrolysis by amylase (Gray 1992). Cats are relatively intolerant of starch compared with dogs, and protein and fat are preferred sources of energy (Rutgers, 1994).

Mucosal damage may non-specifically reduce disaccharidase activities and cause acquired intolerance to dietary sugars. Activities of lactase are relatively low in the adult intestine, especially in cats (Kienzle, 1993), and mucosal damage may result in lactose intolerance. Dairy products are probably best avoided in GI disease.

Protein

Protein should be of high digestibility and biological value; cats require a higher percentage dietary protein content than dogs. A single protein source ('hypoallergenic diet') may be used in a variety of GI diseases, and may be effective either because a true dietary sensitivity exists or because antigenic diversity is reduced. Furthermore, the possibility of acquiring an allergy to a staple dietary antigen may be precluded (Guilford, 1994c).

Fat

Reduced surface area associated with villus atrophy causes fat malabsorption, and in small intestinal bacterial overgrowth the abnormally high numbers of luminal bacteria may ferment significant amounts of fat (Batt, 1992). Reduction in dietary fat content to <15% DM is generally recommended to reduce clinical signs; more severe restriction (< 6% DM) has been suggested (Simpson *et al.*, 1993). The clinical observation that some cats with GI disease do better when fed high fat diets has not yet been substantiated (Sherding, 1989).

Lymphangiectasia results in fat malabsorption and lipoprotein loss as chylomicrons cannot be transported via lymphatics. However, medium chain triglycerides (MCTs) are absorbed directly into the portal blood and are an alternative source of fat/ calories (see later in this chapter under Food Types). MCT supplementation has been suggested for cats but is apparently unpalatable and may cause anorexia and hepatic lipidosis (Sherding, 1989).

Fibre

Previous recommendations on feeding dietary fibre to pets with GI disease have been simplistic: i.e. a low fibre diet (< 2% DM) for SI diarrhoea to improve digestibility, and a high fibre diet (>10% DM) for LI diarrhoea to normalise colonic function. Such an approach is now being discarded as the nature and function of fibre is understood. Fibre is undigestible plant material, but its historical classification into soluble and insoluble types ignores its other important property - whether it can be fermented by intestinal bacteria into short chain fatty acids. These products help fuel mucosal cells, especially colonocytes, and may modify mucosal disease. Insoluble, non-fermentable fibre, such as cellulose in wheat bran, may appear to reduce diarrhoea by its gelling action. Highly fermentable, soluble fibre, such as pectin and gum arabic, may improve apparent digestibility. Inclusion of a moderately fermentable fibre, such as beet pulp or psyllium is usually recommended (Strombeck and Guilford, 1991).

Probiotics

Probiotics are 'a live microbial feed supplement which beneficially affect the host animal by improving its microbial balance', and generally comprise lactic acid bacteria such as lactobacilli, streptococci and bifidobacteria (Fuller, 1991). Whilst some value of probiotics has been shown experimentally, their efficacy in clinical disease is questioned. The feeding of live yogurt preparations has been proposed as a simpler means of trying to achieve the same effect, although reported benefits may simply reflect supply of bacterial lactase. However, experimentally, yogurt reinforces the GI mucosal barrier and stimulates GI immunity (Isolauri *et al.*, 1993). The result may only be temporary and continual feeding may be necessary for sustained beneficial effect. Controlled studies are needed to demonstrate any potential benefit of probiotics following acute gastroenteritis or a course of antibiotics.

The 'ideal diet'

The ideal 'intestinal diet' is highly digestible but not markedly hypertonic; rapid digestion and assimilation should occur but excess small, osmotically active molecules that might cause an osmotic diarrhoea should not be present. The diet is moderately low in fat (<15% DM) to limit effects of any fat malabsorption, and lactose-free in case of lactose intolerance. If derived from a single protein source the diet may be considered 'hypoallergenic'. It should contain generous quantities of water- and fat-soluble vitamins, and essential minerals; potassium supplementation is probably important, especially in cats. Good palatability is essential if a sick animal is to eat it and, since no other source of food is likely to be given, it must be nutritionally balanced. Feeding the daily requirement in two or three divided meals reduces the load on a compromised intestine. Even more frequent feeding is unlikely to meet with owner compliance, and may abolish the normal interdigestive 'house keeping' peristaltic waves believed to sweep bacteria from the small intestine.

REQUIREMENTS

General Requirements

The nutritional requirements of patients with GI disease will be increased just as requirements are increased by any illness; an estimated 0.85 x maintenance energy requirement (MER) is a rough guide. However, a further increase may be needed to counter both the intestine's inability to digest and absorb food and its propensity to lose nutrients. Animals with a PLE may have twice the maintenance requirement. Feeding increased quantities is necessary to redress the balance, yet the GI tract will have a reduced capacity for coping. Therefore, any carbohydrate fed should be highly digestible, such as cooked rice (Strombeck and Guilford, 1991). Any protein should be of good quality and high biological value; boiled rice and eggs or cottage cheese are suitable sources. Vitamin deficiencies are likely in chronic malabsorption; oral and sometimes parenteral supplementation is necessary.

Special Requirements

The salient reasons for recommending specific diets for specific GI conditions are given below. Not all GI diseases are listed as not all need or respond to dietary modification; accurate diagnosis and specific medical and surgical treatments are recommended, rather than empirical dietary therapy. A list of the recommendations is given in the Summary Table (Appendix 1).

Diseases of the Oropharynx

If oropharyngeal disease prevents food ingestion, tube feeding can provide nutritional support.

Halitosis

Although usually associated with oropharyngeal disease, halitosis can be caused by intestinal bacterial fermentation of proteinaceous food. Lower protein, highly digestible diets may help alleviate the symptom.

Oesophageal Disease

Oesophagitis. Soft, moist food is more easily swallowed than particulate food, and avoidance of fatty and spicy foods may reduce the incidence of gastric reflux.

Oesophageal stricture / obstruction. Blending food to a fine slurry may permit passage of food into the stomach; alternatively, tube feeding by an appropriate route can be used.

Megaoesophagus. Historically animals with megaoesophagus have been fed a slurry from an elevated position, in the hope that gravity will deliver the food to the stomach without aspiration. Whilst suitable for many cases, some actually cope better with more textured food, and each patient should be assessed individually.

Gastric Dilatation/Volvulus (GDV)

An apparent association between feeding cereal-based dry foods and GDV may have falsely incriminated this food type (Burrows and Ignaszewski, 1990). Large and giant breed dogs susceptible to GDV are often fed dry food for economic reasons. Nevertheless feeding frequent small meals of a highly digestible food, and avoiding peri-prandial exercise would seem a prudent strategy.

Acute (Gastro)enteritis

Acute gastritis and vomiting often accompany acute enteritis. Complete withdrawal of food is necessary during acute vomiting, and fluid therapy is vital. Complete bowel rest followed by gradual regrading of food is often successful.

Gastric Ulceration

Withdrawal of ulcerogenic medication and treatment with anti-ulcer drugs are indicated. Feeding a homogenised, bland diet in small, frequent meals may help symptomatically.

Chronic Gastritis

Inflammation and failure of receptive relaxation in chronic gastritis result in chronic intermittent vomiting. In conjunction with drug therapy, feeding a finely ground, low fat diet in small frequent meals will improve gastric emptying. Jejunostomy tube feeding is occasionally useful in chronic gastric disease.

Borborygmus and Flatulence

The origin of these symptoms is excessive aerophagia and/or bacterial fermentation of food. Management with a diet of higher digestibility, and lower protein and fermentable fibre content may be possible, but investigation of possible underlying SIBO and mucosal disease should be considered.

Small Intestinal Bacterial Overgrowth

A reduced fat, highly digestible diet may control the symptoms of SIBO. Recurrence after successful antibiotic treatment indicates the need for investigation of underlying disease, such as a dietary sensitivity.

Dietary Sensitivity

Dietary intolerance. Non-immunological adverse reactions to food are treated with an appropriate exclusion diet. Lactose intolerance is apparently widespread, especially in cats, and dairy products can easily be avoided.

Dietary allergy. Immunologically mediated adverse reactions to food are managed by a suitable exclusion diet. Failure of owner compliance is the commonest reason for treatment failure. Immunosuppressive therapy is indicated if no suitable diet can be found either because of multiple allergies or because the animal refuses to eat it.

Gluten-sensitive enteropathy. Avoidance of gluten-containing food is required. Wheat, barley, oats and rye contain gluten or related proteins; rice, maize, potato and tapioca are gluten-free, but rice is most digestible (Strombeck and Guilford, 1991).

Protein-losing Enteropathies

It is frequently difficult to satisfy the protein and energy requirements of patients with PLE caused by severe intestinal diseases, such as inflammatory bowel disease and lymphangiectasia. The diet must include additional protein to compensate for faecal protein loss which may reach 2g/kg/day (Simpson, 1992); up to 200 % of basal requirements should be fed. Fat is usually restricted because of probable fat malabsorption. Intestinal lymphosarcoma may also cause a PLE, but anorexia and cachexia are additional nutritional complications and the prognosis is grave.

Inflammatory bowel disease: Severe inflammatory bowel disease may manifest as a PLE, but even in less severely affected cases the use of a 'hypoallergenic diet' may be beneficial. The overall antigenic load will be reduced, and in some cases the inflammatory response may actually be directed towards specific food antigens. Where no inciting agent can be identified, immunosuppressive treatment is indicated. Feeding omega-3 unsaturated fatty acids, found in marine-fish oils, may reduce inflammation (Hillier *et al.*, 1991) but controlled studies are lacking (Logas *et al.*, 1991).

Lymphangiectasia: Feeding a severely fat-restricted diet is necessary to prevent steatorrhoea, but low fat, high fibre, obesity diets are not suitable. Fat-calorie intake can be supplemented with MCT oil.

Short Bowel Syndrome

Seen following extensive intestinal resection, this syndrome has a complex pathophysiology, including SIBO, gastric hypersecretion, malabsorption and malnutrition (Williams and Burrows, 1981). Intensive pharmacological treatment and nutritional support with a low fat, highly digestible diet, supplemented with MCT oil, elemental diets and vitamins/minerals are required, although the prognosis is poor.

Idiopathic Colitis

Dietary modification with or without pharmacological therapy offers the best chance for successful management (Chiapella, 1986). Use of a single protein source, and reduced fat content may be beneficial (Simpson *et al.*, 1994). A moderately fermentable fibre, such as isphagula (e.g. isphagula husk — Isogel, Charwell; psyllium — Metamucil, Procter & Gamble), is often recommended, but wheat bran (e.g. Trifyba, Sanofi) has also been suggested (Simpson, 1992).

Irritable Bowel Syndrome

A collective term for any case demonstrating GI signs in which no organic disease can be identified, irritable bowel is unlikely to be a single disease entity. Therefore, no one diet is likely to be a panacea, although use of a low fat diet with added fibre has been advocated (Simpson, 1992).

Constipation

Any primary cause of constipation should be investigated and treated, but dietary modification can be helpful. Lactulose, a non-digestible disaccharide, acts as an osmotic laxative. Wheat bran, sterculia (Peridale, Arnolds) and methylcellulose (Celevac, Monmouth) are bulk laxatives.

FOOD TYPES

Home-cooked diets are generally used during the exclusion and challenge phases when testing for dietary sensitivities; complete control of the ingredients is possible and novel recipes can be devised. Adverse reactions to equivalent commercial diets have been reported in animals successfully managed with home-cooking (White, 1986). Suggested recipes for 'hypoallergenic diets' for dogs and cats are given in Table 13.2. Cottage cheese is often recommended as it is relatively lactose-free and contains less fat than eggs or meat, but it is not universally accepted, especially by cats.

Vitamin/mineral supplementation may not be crucial in the early diagnostic phase but is essential for maintenance. Human multivitamin products are recommended, as many veterinary preparations contain meat and cereal extracts for palatability. Taurine supplementation (500mg/every 24h) is a sensible precaution in cats. Potassium supplementation may be required in chronic diarrhoea, and addition of KCl-rich Lo Salt is a simple remedy.

MCTs are fatty acids with a C_8–C_{10} backbone, and are found naturally in coconut milk and Fractionated Coconut Oil B.P. Supplementation can more conveniently be accomplished with a pharmaceutical preparation (MCT Oil, Bristol Myers, Cow & Gate). Each ml provides approximately 8 kcal but the total dose should not exceed 20% of the animal's daily energy intake. Thus a dose of 1–2ml/kg body weight can be used in dogs, although gradual introduction is necessary as initial tolerance is sometimes poor. A more palatable 50% aqueous emulsion is available (Liquigen, Scientific Hospital Supplies) although the volume given must be doubled, and a powder containing MCTs, amino acids and vitamins/minerals (MCT Pepdite, Scientific Hospital Supplies) is also marketed.

For maintenance, home-cooking may be inconvenient and expensive, and diets may be nutritionally incomplete (Roudebush and Cowell, 1992).

Lamb-based baby foods have been suggested as a palatable choice for cats during an exclusion trial (White and Sequoia, 1989), but may be inadequate for maintenance therapy. Commercial, veterinary hypoallergenic diets (e.g. Hill's d/d, Pedigree® Selected Protein Diet) are convenient and nutritionally complete. However, no single diet is suitable for all patients and the universal use of one of these products cannot be endorsed. Indeed, after determining an animal's dietary sensitivity, it may be possible to devise an appropriate diet using ordinary commercial foods. A number of products now contain a restricted protein source and are gluten-free, but careful reading of the food label is essential to ensure that the offending food is not present in even minor quantities. Skimmed milk and yogurt contain virtually the same amount of lactose as full cream milk, but a lactose-free milk product is available if owners insist on feeding milk .

Highly digestible, restricted fat commercial diets (e.g. Hill's i/d, Pedigree® Low Fat Diet) are suitable for regrading following an acute GI upset and for adjunctive nutritional support in chronic diarrhoea. However, some restricted fat diets designed for weight reduction (Hill's r/d and w/d) have a high fibre content, and may be unsuitable for patients with GI disease because of their reduced caloric density and digestibility.

Recipes for home-cooked diets are given in Table 13.2.

Assessment of Success

Recommendations for protein-calorie requirements in GI disease are based on arbitrary assumptions with the potential for significant error. The amount of food fed has to be adjusted according to the patient's response, assessed by nutritional indices such as body weight and serum albumin concentration. If objective diagnostic criteria, such as histological abnormalities, were the basis of the diagnosis, then resolution of those criteria can be used to judge the efficacy of treatment. However, if signs resolve, clients are generally unwilling to permit repeat biopsy.

Assessment of treatment success in GI disease is usually based on improvement in clinical signs, but caution should be used when evaluating the results of empirical dietary trials. For example, cessation of diarrhoea when feeding a 'hypoallergenic diet' cannot be considered proof of a dietary sensitivity; changes in digestibility, and carbohydrate, fat and fibre content may have halted the diarrhoea despite persistence of underlying intestinal disease. Equally it is important to follow a successful exclusion trial with challenge by the original diet. Failure to reproduce signs on challenge may indicate misdiagnosis or waning of the hypersensitivity following mucosal repair, and consequently the patient is not condemned to unnecessary lifelong treatment.

REFERENCES AND FURTHER READING

Armitstead J, Kelly D and Walker-Smith J (1989). Evaluation of infant feeding in acute gastroenteritis. *Journal of Pediatric Gastroenterology and Nutrition* **8,** 240.

Batt RM (1992). Diagnosis and management of malabsorption in dogs. *Journal of Small Animal Practice* **33,** 161.

Batt RM and Burrows CF (1994). Canine gastrointestinal tract disease. In: *The Waltham Book of Clinical Nutrition of the Dog and Cat.* Eds JM Wills and KW Simpson. Pergamon Press, Oxford. pp 189-220.

Batt RM and Hall EJ (1989). Chronic enteropathies in the dog. *Journal of Small Animal Practice* **30,** 3.

Batt RM and Morgan JO (1982). Role of serum folate and vitamin B_{12} concentrations in the differentiation of small intestinal abnormalities in the dog. *Research in Veterinary Science* **32,** 17.

Burrows CF (1986). Medical diseases of the colon. In: *Canine and Feline Gastroenterology.* Eds B Jones and WD Liska. WB Saunders, Philadelphia.

Burrows CF and Ignaszewski LA (1990). Canine gastric dilatation-volvulus. *Journal of Small Animal Practice* **31,** 495.

Chiapella A (1986). Diagnosis and management of chronic colitis in the dog and cat. In: *Current Veterinary Therapy IX. Small Animal Practice.* Ed RW Kirk. WB Saunders, Philadelphia.

Darrow DC (1952). Therapeutic measures promoting recovery from the physiologic disturbances of infantile diarrhea. *Pediatrics* **9,** 519.

Fuller R (1991). Probiotics in human medicine. *Gut* **32,** 439.

Gray GM (1992). Starch digestion and absorption in nonruminants. *Journal of Nutrition* **122,** 172-177.

Guilford WG (1994a). Whats's new in gastrointestinal diagnosis? Gastroscopic food sensitivity testing and radiopaque markers. *Proceedings of the 1994 BSAVA Congress.*

Guilford WG (1994b). Feline gastrointestinal tract disease. In: *The Waltham Book of Clinical Nutrition of the Dog and Cat.* Eds JM Wills and KW Simpson. Pergamon Press, Oxford. pp 221-238.

Guilford WG (1994c). New ideas for dietary management of intestinal disease. *Journal of Small Animal Practice* **35,** 620-624.

Hall EJ (1994a). Small intestinal disease - is endoscopic biopsy the answer? *Journal of Small Animal Practice* **35,** 408.

Hall EJ (1994b). Gastrointestinal aspects of food allergy: a review. *Journal of Small Animal Practice* **35,** 145.

Hall EJ and Batt RM (1992). Dietary modulation of gluten sensitivity in a naturally occurring enteropathy of Irish setter dogs. *Gut* **33,**198.

Hillier K, Jewell R, Dorrell L and Smith CL (1991). Incorporation of fatty acids from fish oil and olive oil into colonic mucosal lipids and effects upon eicosanoid synthesis in inflammatory bowel disease. *Gut* **32,** 1151.

Isolauri E, Juntunen M, Wiren S, Vuorinen P and Koivula T (1989). Intestinal permeability changes in acute gastroenteritis: effects of clinical factors and nutritional management. *Journal of Pediatric Gastroenterology and Nutrition* **8,** 466.

Isolauri E, Majamaa H, Arvola T, Rantala I, Virtanen E and Arvilommi H (1993). *Lactobacillus casei* strain GG reverses increased intestinal permeability induced by cow milk in suckling rats. *Gastroenterology* **105,** 1643.

Kienzle E (1993). Carbohydrate metabolism of the cat. 4. Activity of maltase, isomaltase, sucrase and lactase in the gastrointestinal tract in relation to age and diet. *Journal of Animal Physiology and Animal Nutrition* **70,** 89.

Kronfeld DS (1983). Feeding cats and feline nutrition. *Compendium of Continuing Education for the Practicing Veterinarian* **5,** 419.

Kronfeld DS (1986). Therapeutic diets for dogs and cats including a simple system of recipes. *Tijdschrift voor Diergeneeskunde* **111,** 37S.

Logas D, Beale KM and Bauer JE (1991). Potential clinical benefits of dietary supplementation with marine-life oil. *Journal of the American Veterinary Medical Association* **199,** 1631.

Loth L, Leib MS, Davenport DJ and Monroe WE (1990). Comparisons between endoscopic and histologic evaluation of the gastrointestinal tract in dogs and cats: 75 cases (1984-1987). *Journal of the American Veterinary Medical Association* **196,** 635.

Nelson RW, Dimperio ME and Long GG (1984). Lymphocytic-plasmacytic colitis in the cat. *Journal of the American Veterinary Medical Association* **184,** 1133.

Nelson RW, Stookey LJ and Kazacos E (1988). Nutritional management of idiopathic chronic colitis in the dog. *Journal of Veterinary Internal Medicine* **2,** 133.

Roudebush P and Cowell CS (1992). Results of a hypoallergenic diet survey of veterinarians in North America with a nutritional evaluation of homemade diet prescriptions. *Veterinary Dermatology* **3,** 23-27.

Rutgers HC (1994). The alimentary system. In: *Feline Medicine and Therapeutics*. Eds EA Chandler, CJ Gaskell and RM Gaskell. Blackwell, Oxford.

Sherding RG (1989). *The Cat. Diseases and Clinical Management.* Churchill Livingston, New York.

Simpson JW (1992). Role of nutrition in aetiology and treatment of diarrhoea. *Journal of Small Animal Practice* **33,** 167.

Simpson JW, Anderson RS and Markwell PJ (1993). *Clinical Nutrition of the Dog and Cat.* Blackwell, Oxford.

Simpson JW, Maskell IE and Markwell PJ (1994). Use of a restricted antigen diet in the management of idiopathic canine colitis. *Journal of Small Animal Practice* **35,** 233.

Snyder JD, Molla AM and Cash RA (1990). Home-based therapy for diarrhea. *Journal of Pediatric Gastroenterology and Nutrition* **11,** 438.

Strombeck DR and Guilford WG (1991). *Small Animal Gastroenterology. 2nd edition.* Stonegate Publishing, Davis, CA.

Teahon K, Bjarnason I, Pearson M and Levi AJ (1990). Ten years' experience with an elemental diet in the management of Crohn's disease. *Gut* **31,** 1133.

Van der Gaag I and Happé RP (1990). Follow-up studies by peroral small intestinal biopsies and necropsy in dogs with chronic diarrhea. *Journal of Veterinary Medicine A* **37,** 561.

Washabau RJ, Strombeck DR, Buffington CA and Harrold D (1986). Evaluation of intestinal carbohydrate malabsorption in the dog by pulmonary hydrogen gas excretion. *American Journal of Veterinary Research* **47,** 1402.

White SD (1986). Food hypersensitivity in 30 dogs. *Journal of the American Veterinary Medical Association* **188,** 695.

White SD and Sequoia D (1989). Food hypersensitivity in cats: 14 cases (1982-1987). *Journal of the American Veterinary Medical Association* **194,** 692.

Williams DA (1989). Exocrine pancreatic insufficiency. In: *Current Veterinary Therapy X. Small Animal Practice.* Ed RW Kirk. WB Saunders, Philadelphia.

Williams DA and Burrows CF (1981). Short bowel syndrome - a case report in a dog and discussion of the pathophysiology of bowel resection. *Journal of Small Animal Practice* **22,** 263.

CHAPTER FOURTEEN

Nutrition and Skin Disorders

Richard G. Harvey

INTRODUCTION

Nutritional dermatoses, in particular those dermatoses due to absolute deficiencies of dietary nutrients, are very rarely encountered in practice (Miller, 1989; Muller *et al.*, 1989). This is undoubtedly because of the widespread use of commercially prepared, nutritionally balanced diets. Relative deficiencies of a particular nutrient, such as zinc, may be encountered occasionally, as may toxicoses such as hypervitaminosis A or pansteatitis. Dietary hypersensitivity or intolerance is a rare diagnosis, although authorities differ on the true incidence of the disorder (Walton, 1967; Carlotti *et al.*, 1990). Also pertinent to a nutrition text such as this is the use of nutritional components such as retinoids, essential fatty acids and niacinamide in the management of certain dermatoses not related to deficiency. This chapter will address these topics, principally with reference to the dog and cat.

Given that most of the nutritional dermatoses are rare, the conditions will be low on the list of any particular differential diagnosis. Since the fundamental metabolic processes of the skin are directed toward hair growth, steady-state replacement of the stratum corneum and maintenance of the epidermal permeability barrier any nutritional dermatosis that impacts on these processes will result in signs such as scale, oiliness and hair loss. Thus, there are no dermatological signs pathognomonic for a deficiency. Careful scrutiny of a thorough history and a complete physical examination may suggest that a dietary dermatosis be considered (Table 14.1) but, as in all dermatological cases, careful workup and elimination of differential diagnoses is necessary. There is no place for the snap diagnosis. If a dietary deficiency is diagnosed then the clinician should strongly advise the feeding of a commercially prepared, balanced diet rather than attempting to supplement a deficient diet (Buffington, 1987).

DIETARY DEFICIENCIES

Protein–Calorie and Essential Fatty Acid Deficiency

Protein is necessary for epidermal turnover and hair growth. It has been estimated that these processes may require as much as 30% of a dog's daily protein intake (Buffington, 1987). Protein deficiency results in hyperkeratosis, epidermal hyperpigmentation and loss of hair colour. Telogen defluxion and alopecia may result as the hair is gradually replaced by a thin, poor, lustreless coat which enters telogen (Figure 14.1). Long-term protein deficiency is unlikely to be encountered in clinical practice but may be encountered in animals maintained for prolonged periods on very low protein diets or with chronic illness such as chronic renal failure. Short-term protein deficiency may occur in animals subject to suddenly increased maintenance requirements. Bitches in late pregnancy or at peak lactation may be at risk, since owners may not realise that an increase in both quantity and quality of protein is necessary for animals at certain stages of their life. In these circumstances the growth of hair is temporarily suspended resulting in weak points in the hair shaft. As these hairs emerge from the follicle they are prone to fracture at these points of weakness, resulting in a patchy alopecia (Figure 14.2).

Poor Feeding Management	Home-produced, unbalanced diet Oversupplementation with a dietary component e.g. raw eggs or oily fish Oversupplementation with a mineral e.g. calcium Similar signs in a group of dogs fed the same diet
Signalment	Arctic breeds are susceptible to zinc deficiency
Clinical signs	Scale, crust, alopecia, pruritus
Medical history	Glucocorticoid-resistant pruritus

Table 14.1: *Pointers to the presence of a nutritional dermatosis.*

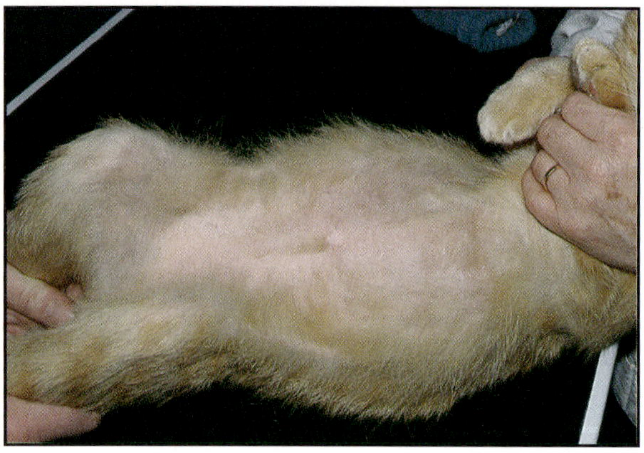

Figure 14.1: Telogen defluxion. The cat was suffering from chronic renal failure (protein-losing nephropathy). Note the alopecia on the ventral abdomen.

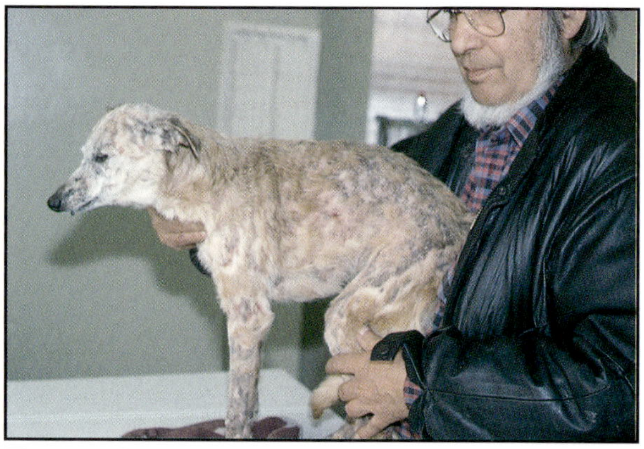

Figure 14.2: Anagen defluxion. Elderly whippet exhibiting patchy alopecia. The animal had suffered an episode of acute nephritis two months prior to the hair loss.

Diagnosis of protein deficiency is made principally by reference to the dietary history, and management requires the feeding of a balanced diet with an adequate protein content.

Essential fatty acids fulfil a number of roles in the body such as conferring fluidity on cell membranes, binding water into the stratum corneum, forming the epidermal permeability barrier, acting as antioxidants, and providing substrate for eicosanoids such as prostaglandins and leukotrienes. The essential fatty acids are derived from dietary alpha-linolenic and linoleic acid (Frankel and Rivers, 1978). In the dog these parent compounds are further metabolised by alternate desaturation and elongation into physiologically active derivatives which subserve some of the functions described above, particularly as sources of eicosanoids (Figure 14.3). Cats lack delta-6-desaturase and require linoleic and arachidonic acids in their diet (Frankel and Rivers, 1978).

Commercially prepared canned diets are adequately supplemented but the fat content of the dried type is low compared to canned and moist diets and the level of linoleic acid may fall below adequate if the food is stored for too long, particularly in a warm, damp environment (Kelly, 1992). The first cutaneous signs compatible with essential fatty acid deficiency in the dog are a dull coat accompanied by a fine scale (Lewis, 1981). Prolonged deficiency results in alopecia, a greasy skin (particularly affecting the pinnae and feet), exfoliative dermatitis and secondary pyotraumatic dermatitis. In the cat the earliest signs of a dietary deficiency do not become apparent for many months and manifest as a dry staring coat and profuse scale, later followed by varying degrees of erythema, alopecia and pruritus (Rivers and Frankel, 1978; MacDonald, *et al.*, 1984).

The diagnosis of essential fatty acid deficiency may be suggested by the clinical signs and nutritional history. Management is best achieved by feeding a balanced diet with appropriate essential fatty acid content (see Chapter 1).

Vitamin and Mineral Deficiency

Vitamin deficiencies are so rarely diagnosed that Lewis (1981) proposed that clinical signs suggestive of the deficiency of a single vitamin or mineral should raise suspicion of a genetic enzyme defect rather than a deficient diet. Suspicion of a deficiency should prompt the feeding of a commercially prepared, balanced diet. Vitamin A deficiency is unlikely in animals fed commercially prepared diets although it may occur in animals on fat-restricted diets or those with poor fat absorption (Buffington, 1987). The cutaneous signs of Vitamin A deficiency include hyperkeratosis of the epidermis and hair follicles, and also of the sebaceous glands and their ducts (Muller *et al.*, 1989). Alopecia may be noted. Individual deficiency of B-group vitamins may occur in animals on bizarre diets because dietary components inactivate specific vitamins. Thus avidin in raw egg white will bind biotin. B-group deficiency may be a risk in animals affected by chronic enteritis or in cases where prolonged antibacterial therapy has reduced the synthetic ability of enteric flora (Lewis, 1981). Signs of a non-pruritic, scaly alopecia have been reported (Muller *et al.*, 1989). Naturally occurring vitamin E deficiency has not been reported in dogs.

Zinc deficiency may reflect absolute dietary zinc deficiency although this is considered rare in animals fed high quality, commercially prepared diets. More commonly there is a relative deficiency, due to interaction with other dietary components or an inability to utilise dietary zinc. Naturally occurring zinc deficiency has not been reported in the cat. Absorption of zinc from the gut is inhibited by iron, copper and calcium, which compete with zinc for absorption. Intestinal phytate and inorganic phosphate bind zinc and thus hinder absorption (Miller, 1989; Muller *et al.*, 1989; Thoday, 1989). Individuals of many breeds of dog, particularly Siberian Huskies and Alaskan Malamutes, are predisposed to zinc deficiency (Willemse, 1992). These animals appear unable to absorb adequate zinc, even when fed a nutritionally balanced diet. Zinc deficiency may also be seen in rapidly growing animals, particularly giant

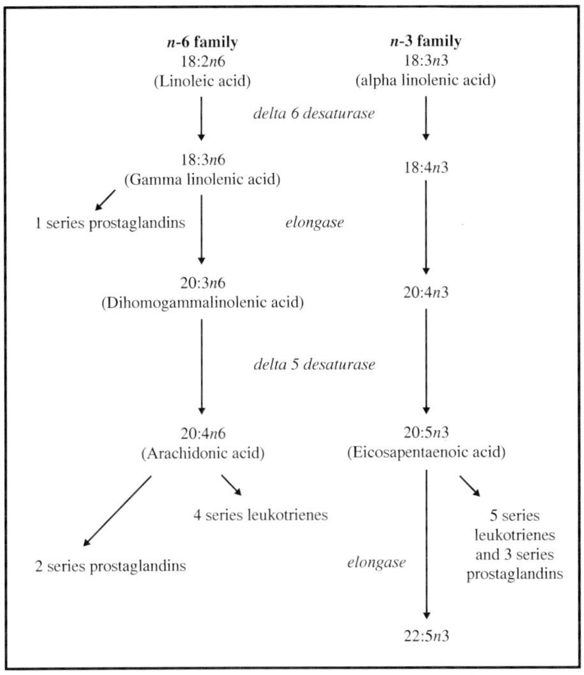

Figure 14.3: *An outline of the metabolic pathways of essential fatty acids in dogs and cats.*

Notes

*1. Cats have very little capacity to desaturate at the 6 desaturase stage (18:2*n6*-18:3*n6*).*

2. The various families of fatty acid are metabolised in parallel, by the same enzymes. The desaturase enzymes are rate limiting and, in addition, n*-3 fatty acids are preferred substrate. Thus supplementing with* n*-3 fatty acids will affect the rate of metabolism, and the concentration of final* n*-6 product. Similarly, supplementing the diet with 18:3*n6 *bypasses the rate-limiting delta 6-desaturase step and provides increased substrate for less anti-inflammatory 1 series prostaglandin. These effects are exploited in the clinical setting where combinations of* n*-6 and* n*-3 fatty acids are used to reduce inflammation.*

breeds, fed inadequate diets, or diets in which nutritional antagonism occurs, particularly due to high phytate content or oversupplementation with calcium (Muller *et al.*, 1989). In cases associated with relative dietary deficiency, or dietary binding of zinc, the cutaneous signs predominate, although polylymphadenopathy may be detected. Well demarcated areas of crusting, with an erythematous border, appear over the pressure points on the limbs and, in a more or less symmetrical manner, around the mouth and eyes (Thoday, 1989). The coat is dull and harsh and occasional areas of achromotrichia (loss of hair colour) may be noted. Metabolic inability to utilise zinc, such as lethal acrodermatitis of Bull Terriers, may result in severe systemic signs such as stunting, emaciation and immunoincompetance (Jezyk *et al.*, 1986).

The diagnosis of zinc deficiency must be based on the case history, clinical examination, dietary history (particularly the feeding of soya- or cereal-based diets), histopathological examination of cutaneous biopsy specimens and laboratory analysis of tissue zinc concentration (Thoday, 1989). The diagnostic value of leucocyte, serum or hair zinc concentration alone is minimal.

The prognosis for Bull Terriers with congenital acrodermatitis is very poor (Jezyk *et al.*, 1986) whereas the prognosis for individuals exhibiting signs of zinc-responsive dermatosis is good. Zinc supplementation with oral zinc sulphate at 10mg/kg, or zinc methionate at 1.7mg/kg, once daily with food is the treatment of choice (Muller *et al.*, 1989). Supplementation may be required for life in the Arctic breeds, and other individuals, demonstrating an inability to absorb adequate zinc from normal diets. Animals exhibiting signs consequent upon a relative dietary deficiency require a nutritionally balanced diet and oral supplementation only until the lesions have resolved.

Anaphylactoid reactions are due to mediator release not associated with allergy. The ingested food may release vasoactive substances such as tyramine, phenylethylamine or histamine.
Pharmacological reactions occur because of a specific, predictable, dose-related, pharmacological effect in the host. The classic example is caffeine, present in tea and in coffee beans. Caffeine is a CNS stimulant and in excess it produces tremor, anxiety, tachypnoea and insomnia.
Food idiosyncrasy represents an abnormal response not involving allergy or pharmacological reactions. Examples are gluten enteropathy in Irish Setters, lactose intolerance and dermatitis herpetiformis (tentatively diagnosed in one case).
Enterometabolism occurs when systemic reactions to absorbed products of colonic bacterial fermentation are observed. Thus bacterial decarboxylase may yield histamine, resulting in signs similar to those described above. However, histamine is unlikely to be absorbed through the normal gut wall, suggesting that gut damage must preclude histamine absorption (Roudebush and Guilford, 1991).

Table 14.2: *Dietary intolerance.*

DIETARY HYPERSENSITIVITY AND INTOLERANCE

Dermatological reactions to ingested food substances are rare (Muller *et al.*, 1989). The incidence of the condition has been cited as 1% of dermatological cases (Walton, 1967) or 15 % of allergic dermatoses (Carlotti *et al.*, 1990). There is no reported breed, age or sex predisposition (Walton, 1967; White and Sequoia, 1989; Muller *et al.*, 1989; Carlotti *et al.*, 1990; Rosser, 1990, 1993; Harvey, 1993b).

Cutaneous signs may be due to either dietary intolerance or dietary hypersensitivity. It is not possible to distinguish between these different aetiologies and, in practice, it is not necessary since case management is similar (Halliwell, 1992). Intolerance is a non-immunological, abnormal, physiological response

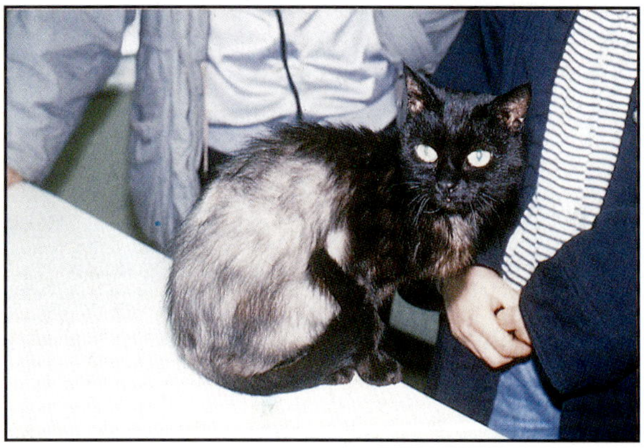

Figure 14.4: Domestic short hair cat with extensive, symmetrical alopecia due to dietary intolerance to tuna fish.

to a food (Metcalfe, 1984) and may result from a number of different mechanisms (Table 14.2). Hypersensitive reactions to dietary components have been documented in animals but are difficult to confirm in practice. It has been suggested that most cases represent Type I immediate hypersensitivity (Halliwell and Gorman, 1989).

The clinical signs of dietary intolerance and hypersensitivity vary from case to case. Although primary lesions such as oedema, erythema, papules and pustules may be seen (Walton, 1967; Muller *et al.*, 1989; White, 1986), they will often be difficult to find as secondary lesions predominate. Thus the most frequent dermatological signs of dietary hypersensitivity reflect chronic pruritus and self-trauma; excoriation, alopecia, scale, crust and secondary superficial pyoderma (Figure 14.4). In the series reported by Rosser (1990) over 80% of dogs exhibited otitis externa and 24% presented with otitis externa only. The pruritus may be regional or generalised, is typically, but not exclusively, non-seasonal and may respond to systemic glucocorticoids (Rosser, 1993; Harvey, 1993b).

The definitive diagnosis of dietary intolerance or hypersensitivity is made on the basis of elimination diets and test meal investigations (Muller *et al.*, 1989). Other investigative tests such as the intradermal injection of diluted components of the diet, ELISA or RAST testing have consistently been proven unreliable (White, 1986: Jeffers *et al.*, 1991; Kunkle and Horner, 1992). The principles of elimination diets and test meal feeding are straightforward (Table 14.3). It is important to insist on home-prepared food, at least for the diagnostic phase of the investigation, although this may be tedious, particularly if the animal is large. The temptation to use a commercially prepared diet during what may be a prolonged investigation should be resisted as a number of reports have demonstrated that they are unreliable (White, 1986; Rosser, 1990; Jeffers *et al.*, 1991). The duration of this initial, diagnostic stage should be at least 4–6 weeks although some cases may take very much longer to respond (Rosser, 1990, 1993). Some caution should be taken when feeding cats on restricted diets for prolonged periods. A diet of 100g cooked chicken and 100g boiled rice will provide adequate calories and taurine for a 4kg cat in maintenance, although it is deficient in calcium and will require supplementation (Wills and Harvey, 1994).

In most cases the identified component is a single constituent of the diet. The most commonly implicated are milk, beef and cereal. These comprise, respec-

1) Identify the components of the diet and decide on a restricted diet. The food should be home-prepared and should be composed of ingredients different from the usual diet. It should contain as few components as possible in order to minimise the risk of a false negative result. Water, a carbohydrate (boiled rice) and a source of protein (chicken, lamb, fish, soya) are required. No treats are allowed.
2) If the disease goes into remission it suggests a possible dietary intolerance. Challenge with the original diet. This serves two purposes. Firstly it helps to demonstrate a relationship between diet and disease i.e. it rules out any coincidental improvement. Secondly it gives an indication of the time for relapse to occur. This is important if challenge studies are contemplated.
3) Monitor for relapse. If no relapse occurs within 3 weeks then the improvement must be considered coincidental and dietary intolerance or hypersensitivity is not considered further.
4) If relapse occurs then reinstate the restricted diet. If the disease again goes into remission then a relationship with a dietary component is probable and challenge studies may take place.
5) Maintain on a restricted diet and challenge with individual components of the original diet. It may be appropriate to transfer the animal to a commercially prepared, balanced restricted ("hypoallergenic") diet at this stage in order to spare the owners the burden of cooking. If this is contemplated then the commercial diet should be fed as a challenge to ensure that it does not incite relapse. Individual components of the original diet are added to about 10% volume to the restricted diet for a period of 2 weeks each. A typical sequence might be milk, cheese, egg, fish, flour, mixer biscuit, beef, commercial canned food and any titbits or treats that are offered.
6) Advise on a balanced diet for long-term control.

***Table 14.3:** Guidelines for the use of elimination diets.*

tively, 57%, 61% and 79% of incriminated components in the four published studies in which they were identified (Walton, 1967; Carlotti *et al.*, 1990; Jeffers *et al.*, 1991; Harvey, 1993b). In these situations it is often possible to obtain a commercially prepared, balanced diet which lacks the incriminated substance. Some owners may not wish to proceed beyond Stage 4 of the elimination diet regimen (Table 14.3) i.e. confirming that the animal is asymptomatic on the restricted diet, and in these situations mineral and vitamin supplements will be required for maintenance.

DIETARY THERAPEUTICS

Essential Fatty Acids

Idiopathic defects in keratinisation characterised by varying degrees of scale, crust, oiliness and alopecia (Figure 14.5) are frustrating to manage, often requiring regular shampoo therapy. Campbell *et al.*, (1992) recently reported that oral supplementation with 1.5ml/kg sunflower oil for 30 days was beneficial. Clinical signs improved and the serum and cutaneous concentration of arachidonic acid decreased, suggesting that the sunflower oil had anti-inflammatory properties. Dietary supplementation with sunflower oil should be part of the treatment protocol for these dogs.

Canine atopy may respond to treatment with essential fatty acids. Scarff and Lloyd (1992) and Bond and Lloyd (1992) reported a double blind placebo-controlled study in which significant reduction in erythema and an overall improvement in clinical condition was reported. More recently Bond and Lloyd (1994) have shown that the use of essential fatty acid supplements reduces the amount of prednisolone required to control the clinical signs of atopy in dogs. Although more expensive than systemic glucocorticoids the complete lack of side effects in the vast majority of dogs makes this the medical treatment of choice in many instances. Some 30–40% of dogs can be sufficiently well controlled to obviate the requirement for systemic glucocorticoids, although a lag period of up to 12 weeks may be necessary before the full clinical impact of supplementation is noted (Figures 14.6 and 14.7).

Feline allergic dermatoses such as flea bite hypersensitivity and atopy may respond to supplements of essential fatty acids, particularly those containing linoleic acid (Harvey, 1992, 1993a; Miller *et al.*, 1993). The lack of side effects makes this method of control particularly attractive for long-term treatment of some feline dermatoses (Figures 14.8 and 14.9).

Vitamins A, B and E

Vitamin A-responsive dermatosis is a rare condition almost entirely confined to Cocker Spaniels (Ihrke and Goldschmidt, 1983). There may be a greasy coat, loss of hair, mild to moderate pruritus and secondary pyoderma. The condition is characterised by focal areas of

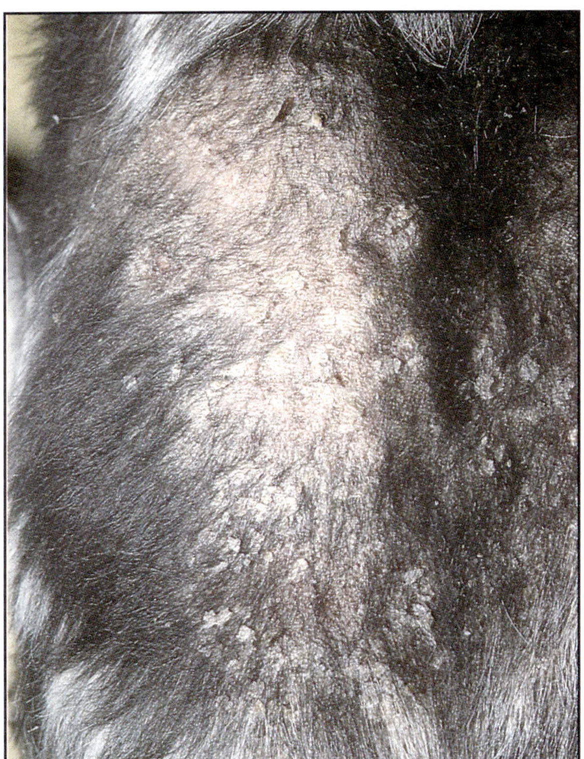

Figure 14.5: *Extensive alopecia, scale and crust along the dorsum of a Cocker Spaniel with a defect in keratinisation (primary seborrhoea). Dietary supplementation with sunflower oil may bring about some improvement.*

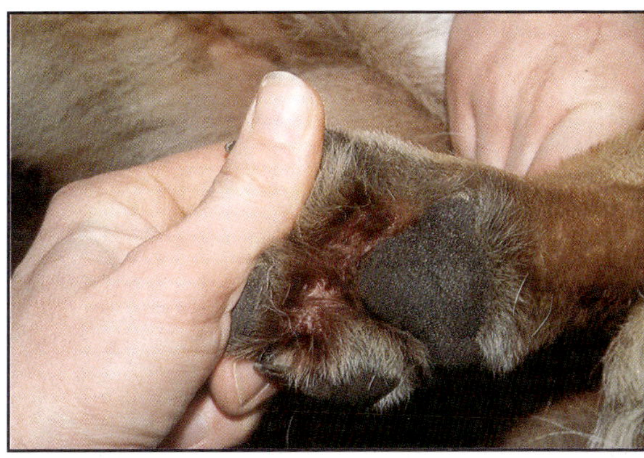

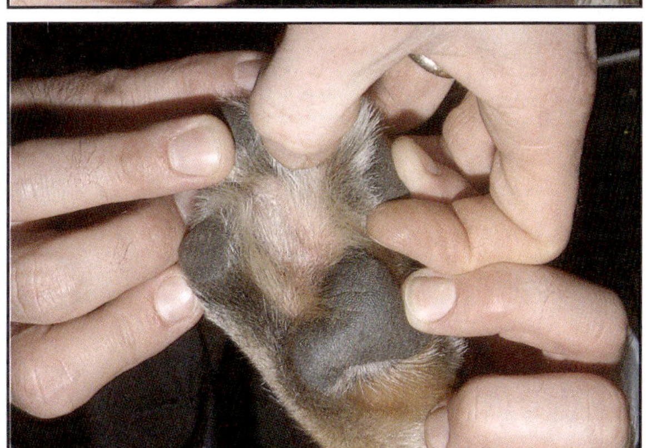

Figures 14.6 *and **14.7:** Plantar interdigital regions of a Boxer with atopy. In **Figure 14.6** the erythema is readily apparent. After 8 weeks of dietary supplementation with a commercial fatty acid supplement (Efavet Regular) there was a marked improvement in the dog's condition and the interdigital erythema had resolved (**Figure 14.7**).*

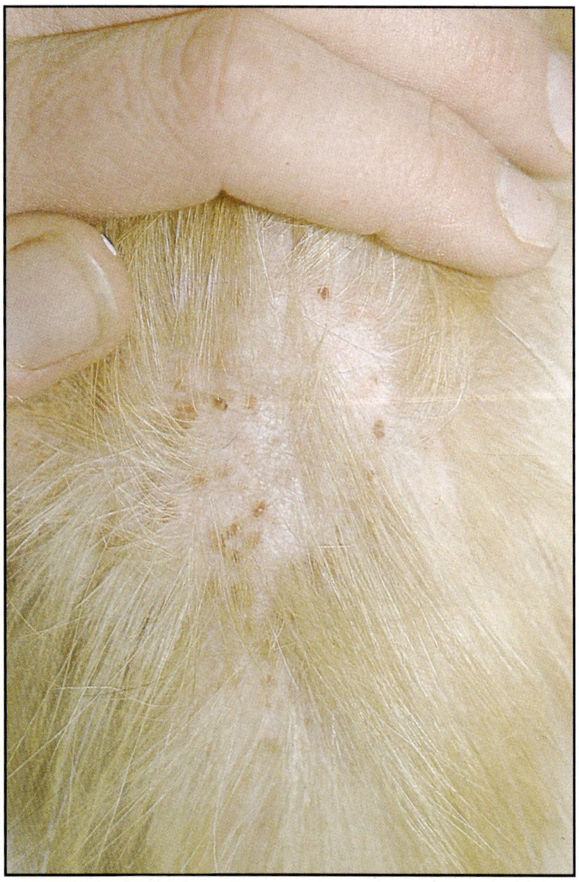

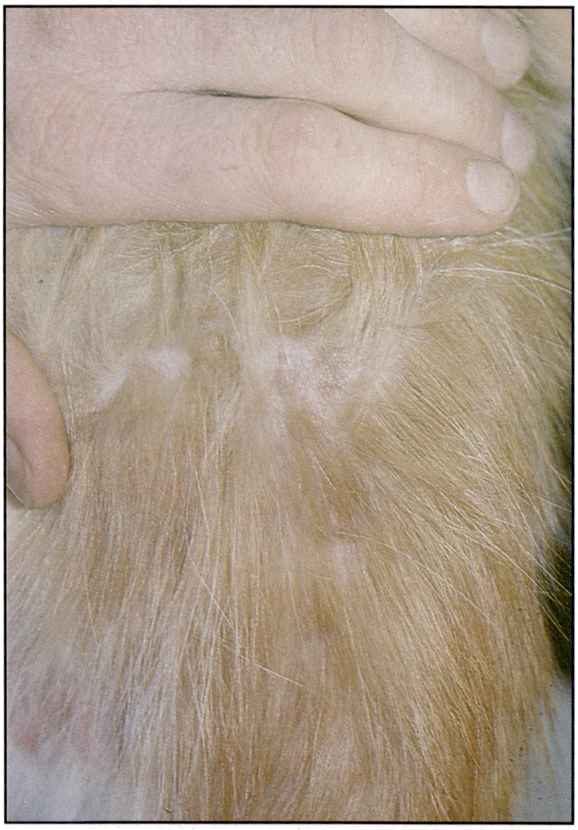

*Figures 14.8 and 14.9: Feline papulocrustous dermatitis (miliary dermatitis). In **Figure 14.8** the erythematous, crusted papules are readily apparent. After 6 weeks of dietary supplementation with a commercial fatty acid supplement (Efavet Regular) the lesions had resolved **Figure 14.9**.*

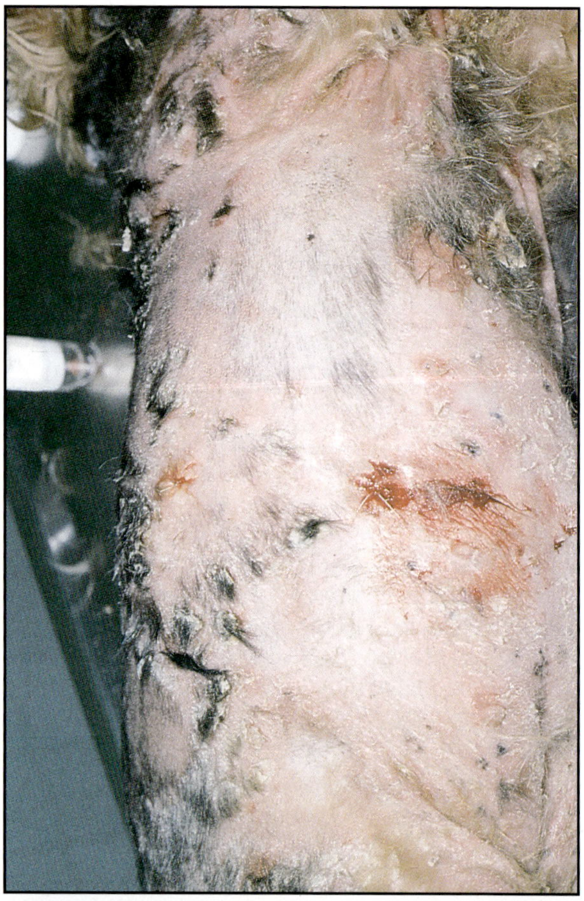

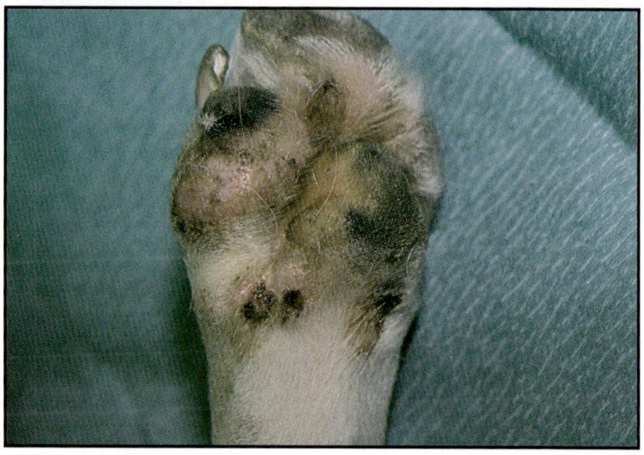

*Figures 14.10 and 14.11: Two conditions which may respond to retinoid therapy. In **Figure 14.10** the ventral neck of a 13-year-old Yorkshire Terrier with mycosis fungoides is illustrated and in **Figure 14.11** the chronically affected foot of a Bull Terrier is shown.*

follicular plugging with plaque-like accumulations of keratin. Histopathological examination of these areas reveals a markedly disproportionate follicular hyperkeratosis. There is no evidence that affected animals are fed diets deficient in vitamin A but the lesions slowly resolve with doses of 10,000 IU vitamin A daily.

Retinoids are synthetic vitamin A derivatives which exert marked effects on the skin, particularly keratinisation. Power and Ihrke (1992) reported a study of the oral administration of etretinate in the management of idiopathic defects in keratinisation (primary seborrhoea). Cocker Spaniels, in particular, showed dra-

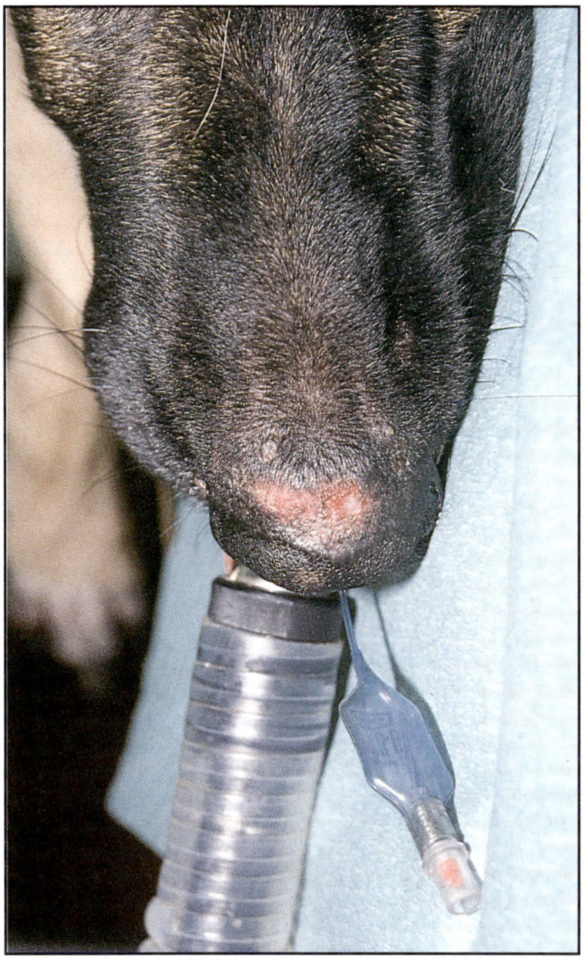

Figure 14.12: Discoid lupus erythematosus in a German Shepherd Dog. This condition may respond to niacinamide and tetracycline.

matic improvements with respect to the scale, crust and alopecia although the associated otitis externa did not respond. Other conditions which are reported to show a favourable response to retinoids include some cases of chronic pododermatitis and mycosis fungoides (Figures 14.10 and 14.11).

Granulomatous sebaceous adenitis is an uncommon disease featuring a progressive scaling and alopecia. Many cases progress to a generalised, patchy dermatosis which is frequently refractory to treatment. Stewart *et al.* (1991) reported that isotretinoin was effective in the management of granulomatous sebaceous adenitis in two Hungarian Vizslas although this has not been the experience of clinicians using the drug in other breeds.

Other dermatoses characterised by defects in keratinisation such as feline acne, Schnauzer comedone syndrome and congenital lamellar ichthyosis have been reported to respond to treatment with retinoids (Kwochka, 1989). There is a single case report of a dog with multiple intracutaneous cornifying epitheliomata which resolved when the dog was treated with isotretinoin (Henfrey, 1991). Retinoids are highly teratogenic and, at present, are restricted to hospital pharmacies.

Niacinamide (the amide of niacin) has been used in combination with oxytetracycline in the treatment of discoid lupus erythematosus (Figure 14.12). A dose of 500mg tid in conjunction with 500mg tetracycline tid was given to dogs weighing less than 10kg whilst those weighing more than 10kg were given 250mg of each drug tid and a 40 % excellent response rate was recorded in 20 dogs (White *et al.*, 1992).

Vitamin E is the generic name for a group of compounds which function as anti oxidants and free-radical scavengers. Naturally occurring vitamin E deficiency has not been reported in dogs but megadoses of vitamin E have been reported to be of benefit in the management of canine discoid lupus erythematosus and acanthosis nigricans (Scott *et al.*, 1983; Scott and Walton, 1985). Reports from other clinicians are less favourable.

REFERENCES

Bond R and Lloyd DH (1992). Double blind comparison of olive oil and a combination of evening primrose oil and fish oil in the management of canine atopy. *Veterinary Record* **131,** 558-560.

Bond R and Lloyd DH (1994). Combination of concentrated essential fatty acid and prednisolone therapy in the management of canine atopy: an open study. *Veterinary Record* **134,** 30-32.

Buffington CA (1987). Nutrition and the skin. *Proceedings of the 11th Annual Kal Kan Symposium for the Treatment of Small Animal Diseases* pp. 11.

Campbell KL, Uhland CF and Dorn GP (1992). Effects of sunflower oil on serum and cutaneous fatty acid profiles in seborrhoeic dogs. *Veterinary Dermatology* **3**(1), 29-35.

Carlotti DN, Remy I and Prost C (1990). Food allergy in dogs and cats: a review and report of 43 cases. *Veterinary Dermatology* **1**(2), 55-62.

Frankel T and Rivers JPW (1978). The nutritional and metabolic impact of gamma-linolenic acid (18:3*n*6) on cats deprived of animal lipid. *British Journal of Nutrition* **39,** 227.

Halliwell REW (1992). Management of dietary hypersensitivity on the dog. *Journal of Small Animal Practice* **33,** 156.

Halliwell REW and Gorman NT (1989) Nonatopic skin diseases. In: *Veterinary Clinical Immunology*. WB Saunders, Philadelphia, pp. 258-261.

Harvey RG (1992). The effect of varying proportions of evening primrose oils and fish oil on cats with miliary dermatitis. *Veterinary Record* **133,** 208.

Harvey RG (1993a). A comparison of evening primrose oil and sunflower oil for the management of papulocrustous dermatitis in cats. *Veterinary Record* **133,** 571.

Harvey RG (1993b). Food allergy and dietary intolerance in dogs: a report of 25 cases. *Journal of Small Animal Practice* **34,** 175.

Henfrey JI (1991). Treatment of multiple intra-cutaneous cornifying epitheliomata using isotretinoin. *Journal of Small Animal Practice* **32,** 363.

Ihrke PJ and Goldschmidt MH (1983). Vitamin A responsive dermatosis in the dog. *Journal of the American Veterinary Medical Association* **182,** 687-690.

Jeffers JG, Shanley KJ and Meyer EK (1991). Diagnostic testing of dogs for food hypersensitivity. *Journal of the American Veterinary Medical Association* **198,** 245.

Jezyk PF, Haskins ME, Mackay-Smith WE and Patterson DF (1986). Lethal acrodermatitis in bull terriers. *Journal of the American Veterinary Medical Association* **188,** 833.

Kelly NC (1992). Practical evaluation and feeding of dog foods. *In Practice* **14,** 8.

Kunkle GA and Horner S (1992). Validity of skin testing for diagnosis of food allergy in dogs. *Journal of the American Veterinary Medical Association* **200,** 677.

Kwochka KW. Retinoids in Dermatology. (1989). In *Current Veterinary Therapy X.* Ed RW Kirk. WB Saunders, Philadelphia. pp. 553.

Lewis LD (1981). Cutaneous manifestations of nutritional imbalances. *Proceedings of the 48th Annual Meeting of The American Animal Hospital Association* pp. 263.

MacDonald ML, Anderson BC, Rogers QR, Buffington CA and Morris JG (1984). Essential fatty acid requirements of cats: Pathology of essential fatty acid deficiency. *American Journal of Veterinary Research* **45,** 1310.

Metcalfe DD (1984). Food hypersensitivity. *Journal of Allergy and Clinical Immunology* **73,** 749.

Miller WH (1989). Nutritional Considerations in Small Animal Dermatology. *Veterinary Clinics of North America: Small Animal Practice,* **19,** 497.

Miller WH, Scott DW and Wellington JR (1993). Efficacy of DVM Derm Caps Liquid in the management of allergic and inflammatory dermatoses of the cat. *Journal of the American Animal Hospital Association* **29,** 37.

Muller GH, Kirk RW and Scott DW (1989). *Small Animal Dermatology,* 4th edn. W.B. Saunders, Philadelphia.

Power HT and Ihrke PJ (1992). Use of etretinate for treatment of primary keratinisation disorders (idiopathic seborrhoea) in cocker spaniels, West Highland white terriers and Basset hounds. *Journal of the American Veterinary Medical Association* **201,** 419.

Rivers JPW and Frankel TL (1978). Fat in the diet of cats and dogs, In: *Nutrition of the Dog and Cat. Proceedings of the International Symposium on the Nutrition of the Dog and Cat.* Ed RS Anderson. Pergamon Press, Oxford.

Rosser EJ (1990). *Proceedings, 6th Annual General Meeting, American Academy of Veterinary Dermatology and American College of Veterinary Dermatology, San Francisco;* p 47.

Rosser EJ (1993). Diagnosis of food allergy in dogs. *Journal of the American Veterinary Medical Association* **203,** 259-262.

Rosser EJ (1993). Food allergy in the cat: a prospective study of 13 cats. In: *Advances in Veterinary Dermatology, Volume 2.* Eds PJ Ihrke, IS Mason and SD White. Pergamon Press, Oxford pp. 33-39.

Roudebush P and Guilford WG (1991). A preliminary survey of histamines in pet foods and pet ingredients. *Proceedings of the American College of Veterinary Dermatology and the American Association of Veterinary Dermatology.* pp. 53-54.

Scarff DH and Lloyd DH (1992). Double blind, placebo-controlled, crossover study of evening primrose oil in the treatment of canine atopy. *Veterinary Record* **131,** 97.

Scott DW and Walton DK (1985). Clinical evaluation of oral vitamin E for the treatment of primary canine acanthosis nigricans. *Journal of the American Animal Hospital Association* **21,** 345.

Scott DW, Walton DK, Manning TO, Smith CA and Lewis RM (1983) Canine lupus erythematosus II: Discoid lupus erythematosus. *Journal of the American Animal Hospital Association* **21,** 481.

Stewart LJ, White SD and Carpenter JL (1991). Isotretinoin in the treatment of sebaceous adenitis in two Vizslas. *Journal of the American Animal Hospital Association* **27,** 65.

Thoday KL (1989). Diet-related zinc-responsive skin disease in dogs: a dying dermatosis? *Journal of Small Animal Practice,* **30,** 213.

Walton GS (1967). Skin responses in the dog and cat to ingested allergens. *Veterinary Record* **81,** 709.

White SD (1986). Food hypersensitivity in 30 dogs. *Journal of the American Veterinary Medical Association* **188,** 695.

White SD, Rosychuck RAW, Reinke SI and Paradis M (1992). Use of tetracycline and niacinamide for treatment of autoimmune skin disease in 31 dogs. *Journal of the American Veterinary Medical Association* **200,** 1497.

White SD and Sequoia D (1989). Food hypersensitivity in cats; 14 cases (1982-1987). *Journal of the American Veterinary Medical Association,* **194,** 692.

Willemse T (1992). Zinc-related Cutaneous Disorders, In: *Current Veterinary Therapy, XI.* Ed RW Kirk. WB Saunders, Philadelphia.

Wills JM and Harvey RG (1994). Diagnosis and management of food allergy and intolerance in dogs and cats. *Australian Veterinary Journal,* **70,** 322-326.

CHAPTER FIFTEEN

The Exocrine Pancreas

David A. Williams

EXOCRINE PANCREATIC INSUFFICIENCY

Assessment of Pathological Status

Diagnosis

Exocrine pancreatic insufficiency (EPI) in dogs is easily and reliably diagnosed by immunoassay of serum trypsin-like immunoreactivity (TLI) in most cases. The serum concentration of TLI reflects the functional mass of exocrine pancreatic tissue and is therefore subnormal when the acinar cells are lost as a result of acinar atrophy or end-stage chronic pancreatitis. In those rare circumstances in which there is obstruction to the flow of pancreatic juice into the small intestine, such as may occur when there is a mass lesion in the head of the pancreas, serum TLI will likely be misleadingly normal. Diagnosis of deficient exocrine secretion can be confirmed in these circumstances by assay of faecal proteolytic activity, preferably using either an azoprotein method or radial enzyme diffusion into agar gels containing casein substrate. In affected dogs there is usually negligible proteolytic activity in all faecal specimens produced, while dogs with normal pancreatic function will have appreciable activity in most samples (Williams, 1994).

While not as common as in dogs, EPI does occur in cats and has traditionally been diagnosed by assay of faecal proteolytic activity as described above. An assay for feline TLI has recently been developed in the author's laboratory, but at present is only available from that laboratory (GI Laboratory, Purdue University, 1248 Lynn Hall, West Lafayette IN 47907-1248, USA — Fax 317-496-1796). Serum TLI is stable and samples do not require special packing in order to be shipped. Specimens from outside the USA should be labeled 'USDA Import Permit Number 20731'.

Nutritional Status

Canine and feline EPI is frequently associated with malabsorption of cobalamin (vitamin B_{12}), tocopherol (vitamin E), retinol (vitamin A), and occasionally of vitamin K (Williams, 1994). Cobalamin status is usually determined by assay of serum concentration using a species-validated competitive binding radioassay. Serum tocopherol and retinol concentrations are usually assayed by high performance liquid chromatographic methods valid in all species. Vitamin K deficiency is supported by observation of prolonged prothrombin and activated partial thromboplastin times. Normalisation of coagulation times after administration of vitamin K_1 (2.5mg/kg SC q 12 h for 24–48h) confirms that vitamin K deficiency was responsible for the abnormal test results.

Dietary Strategy

The major objective for treating EPI is to re-establish near normal absorption of protein and calories so that weight loss is reversed and there is a gradual return to normal body weight. Provision of an alternative source of pancreatic digestive enzymes is of paramount importance. Dietary components that may inhibit digestive enzyme activity, such as some forms of fibre, should be avoided. Minimising dietary fibre will also reduce stool volume. Sufficient food must be given to compensate for the fact that the efficiency of absorption does not return to normal following optimal enzyme replacement. Correction of additional specific nutrient deficiencies may also be required.

Requirements

Energy

Since enzyme replacement therapy does not normalise nutrient absorption, the full caloric value of ingested food is not available to the patient (Washabau *et al.*, 1986; Pidgeon and Strombeck, 1982). Affected animals will therefore require approximately 10–15% more food for maintenance than is required by normal animals. The amount of food given should therefore be adjusted accordingly to maintain an ideal body weight.

Nutrients

Subnormal serum cobalamin concentrations can be normalised by parenteral administration of 100–250μg of cyanocobalamin once weekly for 6–8 weeks; oral supplementation is ineffective. Repeated injections may be required every 6 months or so to maintain normal serum cobalamin concentrations. Serum tocopherol concentrations can be normalised by oral administration of 100–400IU of α-tocopherol. Serum retinol concentrations should be monitored carefully if retinol supplementation is given since ideal replacement doses for patients with exocrine pancreatic insufficiency are not well defined, and the possibility of excessive supplementation with resultant toxicosis exists.

Special Needs

Most dogs and cats can be successfully managed by supplementing each meal with pancreatic enzymes present in commercially available dried pancreatic extracts. Numerous formulations of these extracts are available (tablets, capsules, powders, granules) and their enzyme contents and bioavailabilities vary widely (Roberts, 1989; Dimagno *et al.,* 1993). Addition of 2 teaspoons of powdered pancreatic extract per 20kg of body weight to each meal is generally an effective starting dose. This can be mixed with a maintenance dog food immediately prior to feeding.

As soon as clinical improvement is apparent owners can determine a minimum effective dose of enzyme supplement that prevents return of clinical signs. This varies slightly between batches of extract, and also from dog to dog, probably reflecting individual variation in extrapancreatic digestive reserve. Most affected dogs require at least one teaspoonful of enzyme supplement per meal, but lower doses may be adequate in cats and small dogs. One meal per day is sufficient in some dogs, while others continue to require two. Commercial dried pancreatic extracts are expensive and when available, substitution of 3-4oz (90-120g) per 20kg of body weight of chopped raw ox or pig pancreas obtained from animals certified as healthy following appropriate post mortem inspection, is a more economical alternative (Westermarck, 1987). Pancreas can be stored frozen at -20°C for at least 3 months without loss of enzyme activity.

While administration of pancreatic enzymes with food is generally successful, only a small proportion of the oral dose of some enzymes, particularly of lipase, is delivered functionally intact to the small intestine, and fat absorption does not return to normal (Pidgeon and Strombeck, 1982; Grendell, 1983). Pancreatic lipase is rapidly inactivated at the acid pH encountered in the stomach, while trypsin and some other pancreatic proteases, although relatively acid resistant, are susceptible to degradation by gastric pepsins (Grendell, 1983). In human beings only 35% of trypsin and 17% of lipase ingested with a meal can be recovered intact from the duodenum (Dimagno *et al.,* 1993). Numerous attempts have been made to increase the effectiveness of enzyme supplementation. These include pre-incubation of enzymes with food prior to feeding, supplementation with bile salts, neutralisation or inhibition of secretion of gastric acid, and use of enteric-coated preparations.

Pre-incubation of food with enzyme powder for 30 minutes prior to feeding does not improve the effectiveness of oral enzyme treatment in promoting fat absorption in dogs with ligated pancreas ducts (Pidgeon and Strombeck, 1982). This is not surprising since optimal lipase activity will not be achieved unless the enzyme is in solution at the appropriate pH and temperature and in the presence of appropriate concentration of colipase and bile acids, conditions which are unlikely to be encountered in the feeding bowl.

Gastric acid secretion may be reduced by administration of histamine type 2 (H2) receptor antagonists. Cimetidine at a dosage of 300mg/20kg body weight given with food mixed with pancreatic enzymes does improve fat absorption in dogs with ligated pancreatic ducts, but does not decrease faecal wet or dry weight (Pidgeon and Strombeck, 1982). The routine use of H2 blockers in the treatment of EPI cannot be recommended given the expense of the drug and the fact that so many patients respond well when treated with enzymes alone (Pidgeon and Strombeck, 1982). Oral antacids such as sodium bicarbonate and aluminium or magnesium hydroxide are inexpensive but do not increase the effectiveness of enzyme therapy either in experimental canine EPI or in human patients with chronic pancreatitis. Indeed, it is possible that the use of antacids may be detrimental since although they may increase the quantity of pancreatic lipase reaching the small intestine, they may also inhibit gastric lipase activity. The latter probably accounts for the considerable residual fat absorption in dogs with EPI (Carrière *et al.,* 1993; Balasubramanian *et al.,* 1992; Borgström, 1993).

Enteric-coated preparations have been formulated in an attempt to protect orally administered enzymes from gastric acid (Marvola *et al.,* 1986). In man these preparations have generally proved to be no more effective than non-enteric coated extracts (Dimagno *et al.,* 1993). A survey of canine patients with EPI showed enteric-coated preparations are often actually ineffective or less effective than powdered pancreatic extract (Hall *et al.,* 1991). This may reflect selective retention of enteric-coated particles in the stomach, or perhaps rapid intestinal transit preventing adequate enzyme release in the upper small intestine. Similar mechanisms may explain the ineffectiveness of an uncrushed tablet formulation of pancreatic enzymes, while in contrast the same formulation was effective when crushed prior to feeding (Pidgeon and Strombeck, 1982).

It is possible that in the future enzyme preparations containing acid-resistant fungal lipase may prove to be useful. An experimental study in dogs showed such a preparation to be effective (Griffin *et al.,* 1989). Whether this or any other method of increasing enzyme delivery to the small intestine will benefit those dogs with suboptimal weight gain remains to be seen. Such animals usually do not improve after either increasing the dose of enzymes above 2 teaspoonfuls per meal or giving cimetidine, suggesting that factors other than enzyme delivery to the small intestine are involved (Williams, 1994).

Canine EPI is almost always associated with small intestinal bacterial overgrowth, which in itself may cause fat malabsorption. While in most cases this overgrowth is a subclinical finding, in a few patients with EPI the response to other therapy is suboptimal until bacterial overgrowth is treated. Oxytetracycline (10–20mg/kg PO q 12h for 4 weeks) and tylosin (10mg/kg PO q 12h for 4 weeks) are effective antibiotics.

Food Types and Feeding Regimen

Food Types

Clinical studies in man and experimental studies in the dog show that fat absorption does not return to normal despite appropriate enzyme therapy (Pidgeon, 1987; Pidgeon and Strombeck, 1982; Dimagno *et al.*, 1993). Dogs appear to compensate by eating slightly more than usual, and as with any individual dog it is necessary to regulate the amount of food given in order to maintain ideal body weight.

In order to overcome residual digestive deficits, the feeding of a highly digestible, low fibre diet has been advocated. A non-blinded clinical study found that owners considered that their dogs generally did better (reduced flatulence and borborygmi, decreased faecal volume and frequency of defecation) when fed a commercial highly digestible diet compared to previously fed home-cooked or regular maintenance diets, but there was no difference in appetite, drinking, colour or consistency of faeces, or in coprophagy (Westermarck *et al.*, 1990). Results of experimental studies to evaluate highly digestible diets have shown consistent reductions in faecal weight, but have not shown consistent benefit with regard to fat digestibility, probably because different studies were not comparable with regard to variables such as feeding patterns and the use of gastric acid modifiers that might affect digestibilities of different diets (Pidgeon, 1987; Williams, 1992). Some types of dietary fibre have been shown to impair pancreatic enzyme activity *in vitro*, and high fibre diets probably should be avoided (Dutta and Hlasko, 1985; Isaksson *et al.*, 1982). Highly digestible diets may be of particular value in promoting caloric uptake in those dogs with EPI that do not regain normal body weight.

A low fat content diet has been used successfully in the long-term management of canine EPI, but has not been shown to be superior to a regular diet (Simpson *et al.*, 1994). Low fat diets may prove marginal in supplying calories to those rare patients that have difficulty regaining body weight. Such patients may benefit from medium chain triglyceride supplementation. Some medium chain triglycerides are absorbed intact, and they are hydrolysed more readily by gastric lipase than are long chain triglycerides; their absorption is not completely independent of pancreatic enzymes, however, and they are probably not as well absorbed in EPI as commonly accepted (Caliari *et al.*, 1993).

Feeding Regimen

Two meals a day are usually sufficient to promote weight gain. Larger dogs (20kg) will generally gain 0.5–1.0kg per week, and diarrhoea and other clinical signs such as polyphagia and coprophagia often resolve within 4–5 days. Costs of enzyme replacement are minimised by feeding a single daily meal, and following return to normal body weight many patients do well when maintained on such a regimen.

Assessment of Success / Reappraisal Over Time

Assessment of Success

Body weight should return to normal over the 2–4 month period following institution of enzyme replacement therapy; patients should appear clinically normal once body weight stabilises near to ideal body weight. Faecal volume and consistency should normalise over the first week of treatment, while polyphagia, if present, usually diminishes within 1–2 weeks.

Reappraisal over Time

Even though body weight and faecal characteristics may normalise following treatment, and vitamin K deficiency has only been reported in untreated patients with EPI, subnormal serum cobalamin and tocopherol concentrations can persist or even develop insidiously over several months. Suspected deficiencies can be investigated by assay of serum concentrations as described above.

ACUTE AND CHRONIC PANCREATITIS

Assessment of Pathological Status

Diagnosis

There is no ideal test or combination of tests for the diagnosis of pancreatitis in either dogs or cats, and in the absence of direct examination of pancreatic tissue, the diagnosis can only be tentative (Williams, 1994). Nonetheless, careful evaluation of the entire clinical picture, including history, findings on physical examination, and serum pancreatic marker enzymes and pancreatic ultrasonographic abnormalities, will in many instances give a high degree of confidence in the presumptive diagnosis.

Nutritional Considerations in the Aetiology of Pancreatitis

The exocrine pancreas is highly responsive to changes in nutritional substrates present in the diet, and it has been reported that pancreatitis is more prevalent in obese animals (Williams, 1994). There is evidence that low protein–high fat content diets induce pancreatitis, and that pancreatitis is more severe when induced in dogs being fed a high fat content diet, and less severe when induced in lean dogs (Simpson, 1993; Williams, 1994). Malnutrition has also been reported to cause pancreatic inflammation and atrophy in human patients, and pancreatitis has been observed after re-feeding following a prolonged fast, particularly in extremely malnourished individuals (Pitchumoni and Scheele, 1993). Supplementation of the diet with the amino acid analogue ethionine induces pancreatitis in several species, including dogs and cats (Simpson, 1993; Williams, 1994; Walker *et al.*, 1993).

Hyperlipoproteinaemia, often grossly apparent, is common in dogs with acute pancreatitis, and may develop secondary to pancreatitis as a result of abdominal fat necrosis, or may be a cause of the disease. Some familial hyperlipoproteinaemias of human beings are associated with frequent episodes of pancreatitis that respond to control of serum triglyceride levels (Pitchumoni and Scheele, 1993; Guzman *et al.*, 1985) and the clinical impression of a high prevalence of pancreatitis in the Miniature Schnauzer dog in the USA may be related to underlying idiopathic hyperlipoproteinaemia (Williams, 1994). There is also anecdotal evidence that pancreatitis in dogs often develops following a fatty meal. It is not known why hyperlipoproteinaemia might cause pancreatitis, but it has been suggested that toxic fatty acids are generated within the pancreas by the action of lipase on abnormally high concentrations of triglycerides in pancreatic capillaries (Guzman *et al.*, 1985; Pitchumoni and Scheele, 1993).

Dietary Strategy

Overstimulation of pancreatic secretion may be an important factor in the aetiology of some cases of pancreatitis, and so foods that are potent stimulators of pancreatic secretion are best avoided in the recovery phase of acute pancreatitis, as well as in those patients with chronic pancreatitis.

The treatment of acute pancreatitis involves maintenance of fluid and electrolyte balance while withholding food and water, thereby allowing the pancreas to rest and recover from the inflammatory episode (Leach *et al.*, 1992; Banks, 1993). While there is no definitive proof that withholding food and water is beneficial in facilitating recovery from pancreatitis, many affected patients are anorexic or vomit if fed, and so a period of food deprivation is probably advisable. If any oral intake is allowed, or when food and water are re-introduced, small amounts of foods that are not potent stimulators of pancreatic secretion are advisable, that is, avoidance of high fat or protein content foods.

Requirements

Energy and Nutrients

Energy balance and nutrient supply are usually not of significance in the short-term management of acute pancreatitis, and so food can usually be withheld safely for 2 to 4 days. In obese animals it is advisable to feed a low fat content diet at below maintenance requirements following recovery from the acute phase of pancreatitis, at least until ideal body weight is reached.

While the prognosis is poor for those patients that repeatedly cannot tolerate food, total parenteral nutrition may be beneficial by sustaining such patients while the digestive system is rested for 7–10 days (Banks, 1993). This may prove to be particularly useful in cats, which are at risk of developing hepatic lipidosis if calories are withheld for too long a period of time.

In many patients a single episode of pancreatitis occurs, and all that is necessary in the way of long-term therapy is to avoid feeding meals with an excessively high fat content. In other patients repeated bouts of pancreatitis occur and it may be beneficial to feed a moderately or severely fat-restricted diet permanently. In spite of this, some animals experience recurrent disease (Pidgeon, 1987).

Special Needs

Oral pancreatic enzyme supplements may decrease the pain that accompanies chronic pancreatitis in human beings, probably by feedback inhibition of endogenous pancreatic enzyme secretion. It is not known if they are of similar value in dogs or cats, but there is evidence for inhibition of pancreatic secretion mediated by intraluminal pancreatic enzymes in dogs (Shiratori *et al.*, 1989; Hosotani *et al.*, 1986). However, there is also evidence in human beings that pancreatic enzyme extracts given at clinical dosages and with food do not inhibit, but rather stimulate pancreatic secretion (Mossner *et al.*, 1989). Despite these contradictory observations, a trial period of enzyme therapy may be warranted in individuals with chronic or recurrent signs attributable to pancreatitis.

Food Types and Feeding Regimen

Small amounts of water should be offered after the patient has stopped vomiting. If there is no recurrence of clinical signs, food may be gradually re-introduced. The diet should have a high carbohydrate content (rice, pasta, potatoes) since protein and fat are more potent stimulants of pancreatic secretion and may therefore be more likely to promote a relapse. If there is continued improvement, gradual introduction of a low fat content maintenance diet should be attempted. Another period of food deprivation should be instituted if signs of pancreatitis recur (Pidgeon, 1987).

Assessment of Success and Reappraisal Over Time

Response to therapy is best judged by resolution of clinical signs or anorexia, vomiting and depression. In some patients serum pancreatic marker enzymes remain elevated in spite of apparent clinical recovery. The significance of this is not known but it would seem prudent in such cases to be particularly careful to attempt to avoid excessive pancreatic stimulation by feeding a low fat content, and perhaps protein-restricted, diet.

REFERENCES

Balasubramanian K, Zentler-Munro PL, Batten JC and Northfield TC (1992). Increased intragastric acid-resistant lipase activity and lipolysis in pancreatic steatorrhoea due to cystic fibrosis. *Pancreas* **7,** 305.

Banks PA (1993). Medical management of acute pancreatitis and complications. In: *The Pancreas: Biology, Pathobiology and Disease*. Eds VLW Go, Ep Dimagno, JD Gardner, E Lebenthal, HA Reber and GA Scheele). Raven Press, New York.

Borgström B (1993). Luminal digestion of fats. In *The pancreas: biology, pathobiology and disease*. Eds VLW Go, EP Dimagno, JD Gardner, E Lebenthal, HA Reber and GA Scheele. Raven Press, New York.

Caliari S, Benini L, Bonfante F, Brentegani MT, Fioretta A and Vantini I (1993). Pancreatic extracts are necessary for the absorption of elemental and polymeric enteral diets in severe pancreatic insufficiency. *Scandinavian Journal of Gastroenterology* **28,** 749.

Carrière F, Laugier R, Barrowman JA, Douchet I, Priymenko N and Verger R (1993). Gastric and pancreatic lipase levels during a test meal in dogs. *Scandinavian Journal of Gastroenterology* **28,** 443.

Dimagno EP, Layer P and Clain JE (1993) Chronic pancreatitis. In: *The Pancreas: Biology, Pathobiology and Disease*. Eds VLW Go, EP Dimagno, JD Gardner, E Lebenthal, HA Reber and GA Scheele. Raven Press, New York.

Dutta SK and Hlasko J (1985). Dietary fiber in pancreatic disease: Effect of high fiber diet on fat malabsorption in pancreatic insufficiency and in vitro study of the interaction of dietary fibers with pancreatic enzymes. *American Journal of Clinical Nutrition* **41,** 517.

Grendell JH (1983). Nutrition and absorption in diseases of the pancreas. *Clinics in Gastroenterology* **12,** 551.

Griffin SM, Alderson D and Farndon JR (1989). Acid-resistant lipase as replacement therapy in chronic pancreatic exocrine insufficiency: a study in dogs. *Gut* **30,** 1012.

Guzman S, Nervi F, Llanos O, Leon P and Valdivieso V (1985). Impaired lipid clearance in patients with previous acute pancreatitis. *Gut* **26,** 888.

Hall EJ, Bond PM, Mclean C, Batt RM and Mclean L (1991). A survey of the diagnosis and treatment of canine exocrine pancreatic insufficiency. *Journal of Small Animal Practice* **32,** 613.

Hosotani R, Kogire M, Inoue K, Suzuki T, Chowdhury P, Rayford RL and Tobe T (1986). The effect of exclusion of pancreatic juice on plasma cholecystokinin and pancreatic exocrine secretions in dogs. *Digestive Diseases and Sciences* **31,** 1134.

Isaksson G, Lundquist I and Ihse I (1982). Effect of dietary fiber on pancreatic enzyme activity in vitro. The importance of viscosity, pH, ionic strength, adsorption, and time of incubation. *Gastroenterology* **82,** 918.

Leach SD, Gorelick FS and Modlin IM (1992). New perspectives on acute pancreatitis. *Scandinavian Journal of Gastroenterology* **27**(Suppl. 192), 29.

Marvola M, Heinamaki J, Westermarck E and Happonen I (1986). The fate of single-unit enteric-coated drug products in the stomach of the dog. *Acta Pharmaceutica Fennica* **95,** 59.

Mossner J, Wresky HP, Kestel W, Zeeh J, Regner U and Fischbach W (1989). Influence of treatment with pancreatic extracts on pancreatic enzyme secretion. *Gut* **30,** 1143.

Pidgeon G (1987). Exocrine pancreatic disease in the dog and cat. *Companion Animal Practice* **1,** 67.

Pidgeon G and Strombeck DR (1982). Evaluation of treatment for pancreatic exocrine insufficiency in dogs with ligated pancreatic ducts. *American Journal of Veterinary Research* **43,** 461.

Pitchumoni CS and Scheele GA (1993). Interdependence of nutrition and exocrine pancreatic function. In: *The Pancreas: Biology, Pathobiology and Disease*. Eds VLW Go, EP Dimagno, JD Gardner, E Lebenthal, HA Reber and GA Scheele. Raven Press, New York.

Roberts IM (1989). Enzyme therapy for malabsorption in exocrine pancreatic insufficiency. *Pancreas* **4,** 496.

Shiratori K, Jo YH, Lee KY, Chang TM and Chey WY (1989). Effect of pancreatic juice and trypsin on oleic acid-stimulated pancreatic secretion and plasma secretin in dogs. *Gastroenterology* **96,** 1330.

Simpson KW (1993). Current concepts of the pathogenesis and pathophysiology of acute pancreatitis in the dog and cat. *Compendium of Continuing Education for the Practicing Veterinarian* **15,** 247.

Simpson JW, Maskell IE, Quigg J and Markwell PJ (1994). Long term management of canine exocrine pancreatic insufficiency. *Journal of Small Animal Practice* **35,** 133.

Walker NI, Winterford CM, Williamson RM and

Kerr JFR (1993). Ethionine-induced atrophy of rat pancreas involves apoptosis of acinar cells. *Pancreas* **8,** 443.

Washabau RJ, Strombeck DR, Buffington CA and Harrold D (1986). Use of pulmonary hydrogen gas execretion to detect carbohydrate malabsorption in dogs. *Journal of the American Veterinary Medical Association* **189,** 674.

Westermarck E (1987). Treatment of pancreatic degenerative atrophy with raw pancreas homogenate and various enzyme preparations. *Journal of Veterinary Medicine A* **34,** 728.

Westermarck E, Wiberg M and Junttila J (1990). Role of feeding in the treatment of dogs with pancreatic degenerative atrophy. *Acta Veterinaria Scandinavica* **31,** 325.

Williams DA (1992). The pancreas: exocrine pancreatic insufficiency. In: *Veterinary Gastroenterology*. Ed NV Anderson. Lea and Febiger, Philadelphia.

Williams DA (1994). Exocrine pancreatic disease. In: *Textbook of Veterinary Internal Medicine*. Eds SJ Ettinger and EC Feldman. WB Saunders, Philadelphia.

CHAPTER SIXTEEN

Canine and Feline Diabetes Mellitus

David B. Church

DIABETIC STATUS

The syndromes known as diabetes mellitus are characterised by clinically significant glucose intolerance and an absolute or relative lack of insulin. Although the associated disturbances in protein and lipid metabolism are intimately involved in producing the clinical signs, abnormalities in carbohydrate metabolism are more readily quantified. Consequently, various methods of quantifying abnormal carbohydrate metabolism have become the standard means of diagnosing diabetes mellitus, particularly in its earlier stages or milder forms.

Animals with very mild glucose intolerance may not have sufficient impairment of nutrient metabolism to produce overt abnormalities. Clinically significant glucose intolerance usually is associated with fasting hyperglycaemia. Animals whose glucose intolerance is only revealed by a glucose tolerance test are unlikely to have a clinically overt problem with carbohydrate, lipid or protein metabolism. They may, however, have prolonged postprandial hyperglycaemia, particularly if their diet contains nutrients with a high glycaemic index.

All diabetics have some reduction in the production/release of insulin. This may be an absolute or relative deficiency. In the latter case hormonal or tissue factors modify insulin requirements resulting in increased amounts of insulin being required to achieve normal nutrient homoeostasis. This 'insulin resistance' may expose an inherent weakness in the insulin secreting capacity of the animal. Consequently, clinically significant diabetes mellitus may result from some form of tissue insulin insensitivity combined with impaired insulin secreting capacity. The chronic increased insulin demand may result in 'islet exhaustion' and an absolute insulin deficiency.

As insulin deficiency progresses, the pancreas becomes unable to maintain plasma glucose at normal levels, even between meals. Consequently, the 'subclinical' diabetic patient starts to develop the traditional clinical signs which characterise the diabetic syndrome, typically signs of malutilisation. Patients present with polydipsia and polyuria, weight loss, increased appetite and normal faecal volume. The persistent hyperlipidaemia and altered lipid metabolism results in hepatomegaly while chronic hyperglycaemia will rapidly produce cataracts in dogs. In a small proportion of cases clinical evidence of peripheral neuropathy can be detected.

The presence of glucosuria is strongly suggestive of significant glucose intolerance due to an absolute or relative insulin deficiency. The demonstration of marked ketonuria suggests an absolute insulin deficiency is more likely, as insulin's most potent action is the inhibition of peripheral lipolysis, a necessary process for the generation of clinically significant ketonuria. Although chemical urinalysis can be helpful in evaluating insulin secreting capacity, the condition is best confirmed by demonstrating fasting hyperglycaemia. Further assessment of pancreatic endocrine activity and peripheral insulin resistance often requires more detailed hormonal and tissue receptor evaluations.

Since insulin resistance with concurrent reduced insulin secreting capacity may result in clinically significant glucose intolerance, some diabetics may have residual insulin secreting capacity. Consequently it is wise to consider determining plasma insulin concentrations in most diabetic patients. It is important to collect this sample before any therapy is performed as a high proportion of patients receiving insulin develop antibodies which may interfere with standard assay techniques.

This pre-treatment plasma insulin concentration must be interpreted carefully due to the phenomenon of glucose toxicity. There appears to be a proportion of diabetics where prolonged hyperglycaemia decreases B-cell sensitivity of plasma glucose levels. This decreased sensitivity results in decreased insulin production in response to normal insulinogenic stimuli. Interestingly, this decreased capacity to respond to high plasma glucose concentrations may be corrected by a relatively short period of insulin supplementation. As a result, some animals which present with clinically significant glucose intolerance and hypoinsulinaemia may require less and less exogenous insulin over the first six months of their disease.

This decreasing insulin requirement may be enhanced by the improving insulin tolerance which occurs over the first few weeks of insulin therapy. Any animal deprived of insulin for any significant period will develop some degree of peripheral insulin resistance, probably due to reduced intracellular concentrations of glycolytic enzymes. Consequently, during the first week or two of insulin therapy the same dose of insulin is likely to be progressively more effective in lowering plasma glucose levels.

DIETARY STRATEGY

The basic strategy in managing diabetes mellitus is to achieve relatively stable blood glucose levels which are neither markedly hyper- nor hypoglycaemic. This can be attained by matching the 'glucose-lowering' effect of insulin with the 'glucose-raising' effect of the meal. Given most animals are fed twice daily, this countering of insulin's hypoglycaemic effects with a meal's hyperglycaemic effects is usually best achieved by administering intermediate-acting insulin twice daily. The effects of insulin on plasma nutrient levels can then be balanced by feeding a meal of standardised caloric density and nutrient composition shortly after each insulin administration.

The cornerstone of long-term diabetic management is consistency. The type of insulin used should be chosen to produce a consistent change in plasma glucose over time. To this end, insulins of intermediate duration given twice daily are more likely to produce a reproducible change in plasma glucose levels than longer acting insulin preparations given once daily. These intermediate insulins are usually lente or isophane preparations in dogs and protamine-zinc or lente preparations in cats. The author prefers to use porcine or human lente insulin twice daily in both species. When these insulins are used the meal is generally given 1–2 hours after insulin.

It is important for both clinician and owner to remember that keeping the feeding regimen consistent is just as important as administering constant amounts of insulin. The quantity, caloric density and constituents of the diet as well as the time of feeding should all be standardised. It is imperative the owners understand completely their obligations and the food and insulin regimens established are compatible with the normal routine of the household.

Energy and Nutrient Requirements

The diabetic animal has similar caloric requirements to normal animals. Consequently it is usually acceptable to calculate energy needs from standard tables for dog and cat caloric requirements (see Chapter 3). Some diabetic patients will require significantly less than this amount to maintain adequate body weight and some will require more. Usually the larger the patient the less calories per kilogram body weight required.

To maximise insulin's efficacy, nutrients should be absorbed and metabolised during the time insulin is acting maximally. Assuming consistent gastric emptying, this coordination is usually achieved if meals are given shortly before this period of maximum insulin activity. As a result, the timing of the meal or meals will depend on the type of insulin used and its usual pharmacokinetic characteristics.

Most diabetic patients require around 1.5 units of insulin per kg body weight per day. Generally, administering shorter duration insulins twice daily produces a more reliable effect than longer acting or 'biphasic' insulins given once daily (Church, 1982). When a twice daily insulin regimen is employed, meals can be given 1–2 hours after insulin administration; optimising coordination between the effects of the meal and insulin. When the less reliable once daily insulin regimens are used, the meals have to be given prior to the presumed peak activity time or times.

Whatever the type of insulin, meals for diabetic patients need to be consistent. Food must be given at a set time after insulin and the caloric content must be standardised. Furthermore, as the diabetic's food consumption will be regulated and the opportunity for 'snacks' severely curtailed, it is important to ensure the recommended diet is complete and balanced.

Commercial processed canned and dry pet food preparations are convenient as their caloric content is relatively predictable and consistent.

Also, with the wide variety of commercial dog and cat foods available, it is not difficult to recommend a variety of different tasting products which provide a complete diet. Consequently processed commercial foods can be used as the only dietary source, although this may not be an attractive or even optimum option in all cases.

Not all owners are comfortable about feeding commercial processed food. In addition, not all animals find processed foods highly palatable, particularly if they have not previously been part of the animal's diet. Palatability is particularly important when using relatively short duration insulins. With these insulins in particular, it is vital that all the offered food is consumed within a short space of time. Consequently, some diabetic dogs and cats need to be stabilised on standardised portions of their usual diets. In this situation it is of course important that the veterinarian ensures the diet is both balanced and complete.

Whatever the form of calories fed to the diabetic patient, the timing and the caloric content must remain consistent. Any changes in the dog's diet can only be made if the overall caloric content remains unchanged.

Food Types and Feeding Regimen

Although the composition of the diet for diabetic patients may be quite variable, it is important to realise that foods with the same available carbohydrate and fibre content can produce variable hyperglycaemic responses. Factors such as the nature and quantity of complex carbohydrates, fat content, protein content, food form and nutrient–nutrient interactions all have effects on the glycaemic response to a particular food

(Jenkins and Jenkins, 1987). As a result, more consistent diabetic control may be attained by using only food with similar hyperglycaemic effects. Unfortunately, these is very little information on the glycaemic effects of various foods in diabetic dogs and cats. However, some experimental evidence exists to suggest that modification of dietary fibre may help minimise post-prandial hyperglycaemia and possibly decrease overall insulin requirements.

Improved diabetic control has been implied when diabetic dogs are fed a diet high in complex carbohydrates (Blaxter *et al.,* 1990; Nelson *et al.,* 1994a). These complex carbohydrates or polysaccharides are digested relatively slowly, resulting in delayed and reduced postprandial hyperglycaemia in normal and diabetic dogs and people. This effect has been used to improve diabetic control in people (Atkins *et al.,* 1987; Jenkins and Jenkins, 1987) and there is now some experimental evidence of similar benefits in diabetic dogs (Blaxter *et al.,* 1990; Graham *et al.,* 1993; Nelson *et al.,* 1994a).

This type and amount of dietary fibre should be standardised. Different sources of dietary fibre may have different effects on post-prandial hyperglycaemia, insulin requirements and gastrointestinal irritation (Atkins *et al.,* 1987; Maskell and Graham, 1993). The so called 'viscous fibre' sources such as guar (a fibre source which absorbs water to produce a viscous gum) may be more potent in lowering post-prandial hyperglycaemia than non-viscous fibre sources such as wheat bran (Atkins *et al.,* 1987). However dogs and cats tolerate higher dietary levels of wheat bran than guar (Maskell and Graham, 1993) and probably higher levels of both than people (Blaxter *et al.,* 1990). Consequently, when using dietary fibre as a means of modifying diabetic control, it is important to use sufficient quantity and type to reduce post-prandial hyperglycaemia and insulin requirements without compromising palatability or gastrointestinal function.

Unfortunately, the amounts and proportions of viscous and non-viscous dietary fibres required to minimise insulin requirements and improve control for feline and canine diabetics are not known. There is some evidence that feeding diabetic dogs a diet with around 40g dietary fibre/1000kcal could lower insulin requirements and improve diabetic control (Maskell and Graham, 1993). This level of fibre is seen in a number of commercial dog foods including WALTHAM Pedigree® Canine High Fibre Diet and Hill's® r/d and w/d diets.

Currently there are only preliminary controlled experimental data evaluating the efficacy of increased dietary fibre in improving diabetic control in cats (Nelson *et al.*, 1994b). However, circumstantial evidence from the author's clinical experience suggests improved diabetic control may be achieved in some cats by adding similar proportions of wheat bran and guar to standard commercial or home-prepared meals. It should be remembered that this fibre will be less intimately associated with the food and may be separated by a fastidious eater. Furthermore, inadvertent dilution of certain dietary nutrients is possible when adding significant amounts of fibre to any diet. This possibility should be avoided by starting with a balanced and complete diet and ensuring the cat is receiving an adequate caloric intake.

Because of the tendency for diabetics to develop hyperlipidaemia and lipid related complications, diets high in fat should be avoided.

Reappraisal

There are many means by which diabetic control may be evaluated. A crude but effective method is simply to monitor water consumption and body weight. In almost all adequately controlled diabetic patients there should be a substantial reduction in daily water consumption. There are other reasons for polydipsia which may invalidate this as a marker of diabetic control but in those patients where it can be used it is a simple screening test for adequate diabetic management. Body weight is also a simple but valuable aid in assessing adequacy of caloric intake as well as subsequent utilisation.

A less convenient but more sensitive estimate of control are serial blood glucose estimations. These are performed throughout the day and generally help evaluate the adequacy of insulin's duration and dose as well as the interaction between the meal and insulin. Since some animals may not eat in hospital, the owner should feed the animal before presenting it for serial blood glucose estimations.

Unfortunately, the stress and excitement of hospitalisation and multiple venipunctures can be severe in some animals, producing artefactually high serial blood glucose levels. In these anxious individuals, urine glucose monitoring may provide a more accurate reflection of diabetic control. Unfortunately, numerous factors besides average blood glucose concentrations can alter urine glucose concentrations. This inherent variability combined with a lack of sensitivity minimises its general value. Furthermore, most well stabilised diabetics do not have significant glucosuria.

Alternative ways of assessing diabetic control involve measurement of fructosamine or glycosylated haemoglobin. Both accumulate through non-enzymatic binding of glucose molecules to amino groups of specific molecular sites on serum proteins or haemoglobin molecules respectively. Because this modification occurs slowly and largely irreversibly, at a rate dependent on the average glucose concentration, measurement of fructosamine or glycosylated haemoglobin provides an estimate of the mean blood glucose level for the preceding 5–7 days (Reusch and Hoyer-Ott, 1994).

REFERENCES

Atkins TW, Al-Hussary NAJ and Taylor KG (1987).

The treatment of poorly controlled non-insulin-dependent diabetic subjects with granulated guar gum. *Diabetes Research and Clinical Practice* **3,** 153.

Blaxter AC, Cripps PJ and Gruffydd-Jones TJ (1990). Dietary fibre and postprandial hyperglycaemia in normal and diabetic dogs. *Journal of Small Animal Practice* **31,** 229.

Church DB (1982). Canine diabetes mellitus: some therapeutic considerations. In: *The Veterinary Annual* 22nd issue. Eds GSG Grunsell and FWG Hill. Scientechnica, Bristol. p235.

Graham PA, Maskell IE and Nash AS (1993). The effects of feeding a commercially produced high fibre diet on postprandial hyperglycaemia in naturally occuring diabetic dogs. *Proceedings of the 36th Annual BSAVA Congress April 1993. Birmingham.* p195.

Jenkins DJA and Jenkins AL (1987). The glycemic index, fiber, and the dietary treatment of hypertriglyceridemia and diabetes. *Journal of the American College of Nutrition* **6,** 11.

Maskell IE and Graham P (1993). Diabetes mellitus in the dog: the role of complex carbohydrates and practical clinical management. *WALTHAM International Focus* **3,** 11.

Nelson R, Duesberg C, Ford S, Davenport D and Neal L (1994a). Dietary insoluble fiber and glycemic control of diabetic dogs. *Proceedings of the 12th Annual Veterinary Medical Forum of the American College of Veterinary Internal Medicine June 1994 San Francisco* p 993.

Nelson R, Scott-Moncrieff C, Devries S, Davenport D and Neal L (1994b). Dietary insoluble fiber and glycemic control of diabetic cats. *Proceedings of the 12th Annual Veterinary Medical Forum of the American College of Veterinary Internal Medicine June 1994 San Francisco* p 996.

Reusch C and Hoyer-Ott M (1994). Glycated hemoglobin and fructosamine: studies of in-vitro glycolisation. *Proceedings of the 12th Annual Veterinary Medical Forum of the American College of Veterinary Internal Medicine June 1994 San Francisco* p 993.

CHAPTER SEVENTEEN

Intensive Care – Nutritional Support

Andrew G. Torrance

INTRODUCTION

Most critical patients have an increased requirement for nutrients and lack appetite or have an inability to eat. The resulting protein–energy malnutrition damages the immune system, impairs healing, depresses vital organ function and affects the chances of recovery. The objective of nutritional support is to avert protein–energy malnutrition by providing a formula of fuels and other nutrients in proportions which can be used by the patient with maximal efficiency and to deliver this formula with minimal discomfort.

PATHOPHYSIOLOGY

Most of the available information on the effects of critical illness upon nutritional status in dogs and cats has been extrapolated from human patients and laboratory animal models of trauma and sepsis. Although there are some specific differences in nutritional requirements between these species it is accepted that the responses to critical disease are fundamentally the same.

When a normal dog is starved there is a decrease in metabolic rate coupled with an increase in fat oxidation and a reduction in protein catabolism. The effects of these changes are to conserve the function of the remaining tissue mass and to consume fat stores slowly. When an animal is subjected to stresses such as trauma, sepsis or burns, in the initial shock phase there is often a reduction in metabolic rate which is rapidly superceded by a hypermetabolic state once intravascular volume and tissue perfusion are restored. The hypermetabolic state is characterised by increased oxygen consumption and energy expenditure and depends upon the severity of injury. It probably represents an attempt by the body to provide adequate glucose to optimise the host defences and wound repair at the privileged site of injury. Increased secretion of the counter-regulatory hormones, glucagon, catecholamines, cortisol, and growth hormone, antagonises the effects of insulin and induces hyperglycaemia, degradation of tissue protein to provide substrate for gluconeogenesis, and increased fat oxidation. Glucose oxidation is increased but oxidation is less efficient and the overall contribution of glucose to energy expenditure is reduced. Glycogen stores become depleted rapidly. The increase in metabolic rate is sustained by fat oxidation with continuing glucose wastage.

Stress Starvation

In 'simple starvation' fat oxidation is accompanied by ketogenesis and reduced protein degradation. When starvation and hypermetabolism occur at the same time ('stress starvation') protein degradation for gluconeogenesis is not suppressed and may accelerate. There are no protein stores in the body and substrates for gluconeogenesis are obtained at the expense of tissue structure and function. Breakdown of peripheral muscle can sustain the patient for a while before more vital functions are affected. Organ systems which depend upon rapid cell turnover such as the gut and the immune system are very vulnerable and the combination of depressed immune function and failure of the gastrointestinal mucosal barrier has grave consequences for the patient. Gut associated lymphoid tissue becomes depleted and there is a reduction in IgA secretion. Bacterial translocation from the gut lumen through the compromised mucosa into the portal blood increases. The reticuloendothelial system in the liver is also impaired and thus more bacteria and toxins of gut origin find their way into the systemic circulation leading to sepsis and endotoxaemia.

In the later stages of protein–energy malnutrition hypoproteinaemia develops.

Consequences of hypoproteinaemia:

- Reduced capillary oncotic pressure
- Less resistance to fluid loss from areas of injury. Delayed wound healing
- Oedema
- Localised infection.

Protein–energy malnutrition can be a major contributing factor in multiple organ failure and ultimately in the patient's demise.

Patients suffering from stress starvation are relatively intolerant of glucose and use it inefficiently as an energy source. The hypermetabolic state is supported primarily by fat oxidation and protein breakdown. Fat and protein are therefore particularly important energy sources for the critical patient and should be emphasised when formulating diets for the critical care of small animals.

ASSESSMENT OF NUTRITIONAL STATUS

Although the physiology of stress starvation is quite well understood, there are few objective methods available for determining the nutritional status of a patient in critical care. The consequence of this is that nutritional support is guided by a series of estimates based upon the basal or maintenance energy requirements of groups of normal dogs and cats multiplied by disease factors. Such estimates are wildly inaccurate (20–110%) when applied to the individual critical patient. Until simple, non-invasive methods for tracking nutritional status are developed, the provision of nutritional support is essentially arbitrary and the clinician is reliant upon close monitoring of the patient to determine the success or failure of the nutritional support measures.

Dietary history and a good physical examination by an experienced clinician provide the most useful information regarding the body condition of a patient. Serial determination of body weight, once fluid deficits or water retention have been accounted for, gives an objective index of nutritional status. More objective assessments of energy expenditure and protein catabolism can be obtained by performing calorimetry and nitrogen balance studies but these are time consuming and technically quite demanding in veterinary patients and more appropriate for the research setting than the intensive care unit. In human hospitals objective assessments are made using anthropometric measurements and nutritional markers. The diversity of dog breeds is such that measurements cannot be validated although such measurements could be devised for cats. The assessment of bloodborne nutritional markers is an emerging field, although few of the markers in current use have been shown to be sufficiently specific or sensitive (Hill, 1994). Albumin has been used but tends to decrease at such a late stage of malnutrition that it is not a sensitive marker and it also lacks specificity because medical syndromes resulting in hypoalbuminaemia, such as protein-losing nephropathy, hepatic failure and protein-losing enteropathy, are quite commonly present in the critical patient. Other nutritional markers include prealbumin, transferrin, fibronectin, retinol binding protein and insulin-like growth factor 1 (IGF1). These have not been validated for veterinary patients.

Overfeeding is a potential complication of nutritional support and may result in liver dysfunction due to fat or glycogen infiltration, aggravated glucose intolerance, azotaemia, increased energy expenditure and oxygen demand. In critical care, weight gain is generally not the goal of nutritional support as this might lead to oversupplementation of protein and energy in animals whose organs of excretion are compromised. Prevention of weight loss is the more realistic goal.

Nutritional support can be provided via the GI tract (enteral) or by intravenous infusion (parenteral). Parenteral nutrition is less physiological than enteral, technically more demanding and has less margin for error in calculating nutrient requirements. The enteral route is usually selected unless the gut is non-functional or there is a specific contraindication such as intractable vomiting due to pancreatitis. Parenteral nutrition will be discussed in more depth later in the chapter.

The safest starting point for enteral nutritional support is to estimate the quantity of food using the maintenance energy requirement (MER) multiplied by an illness factor which depends upon the severity of the disease.

MER = 110 x [Body Weight (kg)]$^{0.75}$ kcal/day
(460 x [Body Weight (kg)]$^{0.75}$ kJ/day)

Suggested illness factors are 0.5–0.9 for hospitalisation, 1.0–1.2 for minor surgery or trauma, 1.2–1.5 for major surgery or trauma, 1.5–1.7 for sepsis or neoplasia and 2.0 for burns and head trauma.

IER = MER x illness factor

Quantity of food to feed = IER/caloric density of the food.

After bringing the patient's daily intake up to the calculated amount over a 2–3 day period the effectiveness of nutritional support must then be assessed by close monitoring of the patient's progress, weight gain and physical condition.

ENTERAL DIETS FOR CRITICAL CARE

The ideal diet for critical care should be highly palatable, readily digestible and have a high energy density. This ensures that animals with poor appetite and reduced food capacity can acquire sufficient energy from a relatively small food intake. Since many critical patients require enteral tube feeding, the diet should be liquid. Fuel sources in the diet must be tailored to the patient's requirements. In most cases this means providing a relatively high percentage of energy as protein and fat rather than carbohydrate.

Macro-nutrient levels in critical care diets
(as % energy content of diet)

	Protein	*Fat*	*Carbohydrate*
Dog	20–25	50–55	25–26
Cat	25–37	41–50	22–25

The diet should contain adequate quantities of trace minerals and vitamins. Specific nutrients which are particularly important to the dog and cat in critical care include glutamine, arginine and zinc.

Glutamine

Glutamine is the major substrate for the increased gluconeogenesis which occurs in stressed dogs. Although not normally considered to be an essential amino acid, glutamine becomes conditionally essential in animals suffering from stress starvation. Glutamine is an important fuel for rapidly dividing cells and deficiency leads to gut mucosal atrophy and compromise of the mucosal barrier to bacterial translocation. Glutamine is too labile to be included in parenteral nutrition solutions and this may be the cause of the gut atrophy seen in animals receiving total parenteral nutrition. Glutamine is supplemented in many of the available enteral diets and high doses of glutamine have a trophic effect on the gut mucosa.

Arginine

Arginine is an essential amino acid in dogs and cats and deficiency can lead to failure of the urea cycle and hyperammonaemia. Standard human enteral diets are relatively deficient in arginine and may cause hyperammonaemia in small animal patients. Arginine also stimulates the immune system and has improved the survival time of septic patients.

Zinc

Zinc plays an important role in protein and nucleic acid metabolism and promotes wound healing. Deficiency of zinc for 1 week in animals receiving an enterotomy was associated with reduced collagen synthesis within the wound and hypoalbuminaemia (Iriyama *et al.*, 1982). This suggests that trace elements should be provided even when only short-term nutritional support is anticipated.

Critical care diets suitable for tube feeding include Pedigree® Canine and Whiskas® Feline Instant Concentration Diets (WALTHAM), a/d (Hill's) and Reanimyl (Virbac).

Methods for Administering Nutrition

Voluntary intake is obviously to be encouraged, but most critical patients are either inappetant or unable to take food and are rarely able to meet their nutritional needs without support. Experienced veterinary nurses always have an armoury of methods for enhancing voluntary intake including patiently assisting feeding with a syringe, warming, wetting and cooking food to make it more appetising and using additives to improve the food's odour. Baby foods are often very appetising to small animals but should not be used exclusively because they have an inappropriate balance of nutrients. Forced feeding is not recommended in the critical patient because of the risks of increasing patient stress and of aspiration. Chemical enhancement of appetite using benzodiazepines is also only a short-term measure and rarely results in a patient achieving an adequate intake of nutrients. Sometimes an intravenous bolus of diazepam (Valium 1-2mg IV) will initiate voluntary intake which is then sustained in cats.

In many critical patients the only way to control food intake completely and ensure that the patient has the best chance of recovery is to use a tube feeding method. Numerous tube feeding methods have been described including pharyngostomy, oesophagostomy, naso-oesophageal, gastrostomy and enterostomy tubes. This author favours the naso-oesophageal tube for short-term nutritional support and the percutaneous gastrostomy tube for long-term support. There has been recent interest in the oesophagostomy tube in the USA and enterostomy tube feeding may be an alternative to total parenteral nutrition in patients with pancreatitis and gastric causes of vomiting.

Naso-Oesophageal Tubes

Contraindications include unconscious patients and disease or dysfunction of the nares, pharynx, larynx, swallowing reflex, oesophagus and stomach. Termination of the tube in the oesophagus and not the stomach reduces the risk of reflux oesophagitis.

Local anaesthetic drops are instilled into the selected nostril (Figure 17.1). A 5-10 French Gauge long PVC or silicone infant feeding tube is then measured against the patient, to extend from the external nares to the 9th rib-space in cats and the 7th rib-space in dogs (Figure 17.2). The lubricated tube is inserted into the nostril and directed ventrally and medially into the ventral meatus (Figure 17.3). In dogs, entry into the ventral meatus may be facilitated by pushing the external nares dorsally once the tube is in contact with the nasal septum. The tube is advanced towards the pharynx and into the oesophagus until the marker tape is positioned against the external nares. A small volume of saline is injected down the tube to induce a cough should the tube have entered the trachea instead of the oesophagus (Figure 17.4). A further check on tube location is then performed by injecting 5-10 ml of air and auscultating the stomach for

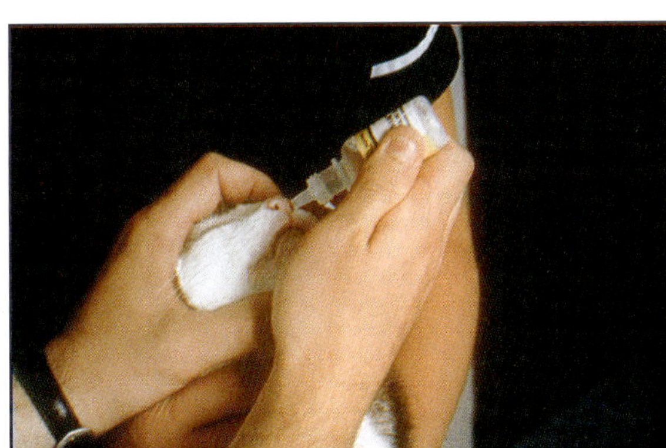

Figure 17.1: *Anaesthetic administered.*

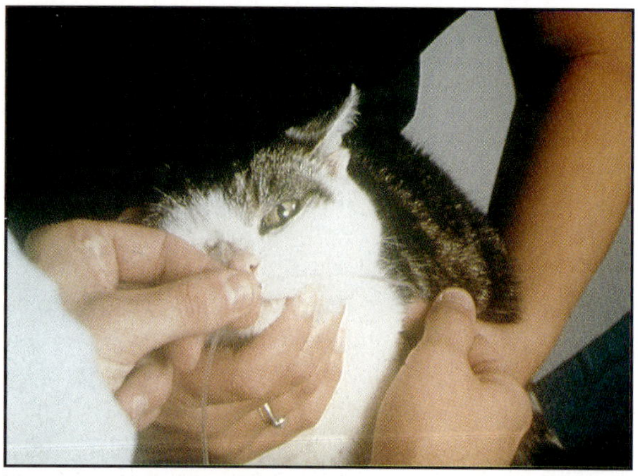
Figure 17.2: Measuring the tube.

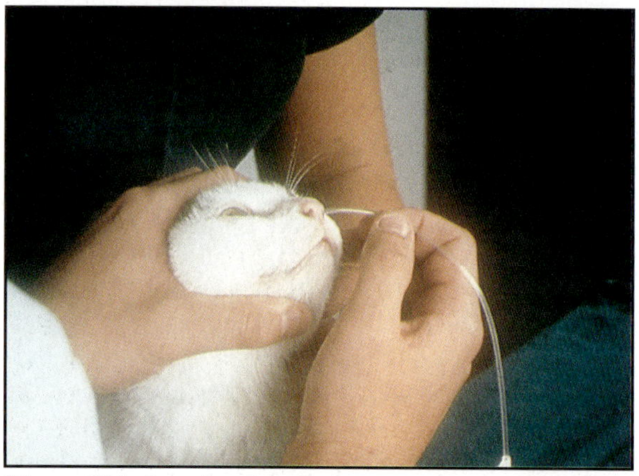
Figure 17.3: Inserting the tube.

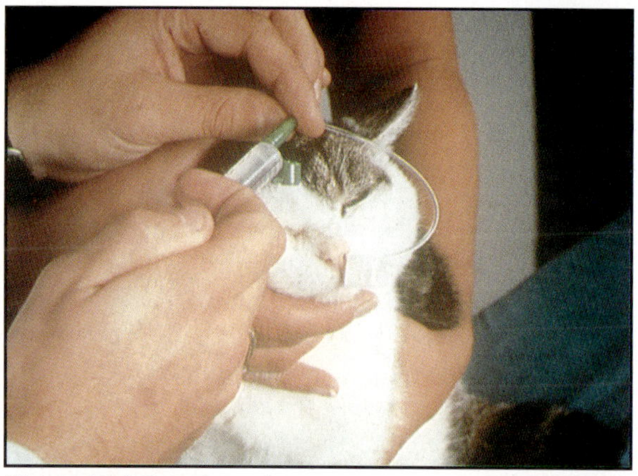
Figure 17.4: Injecting saline.

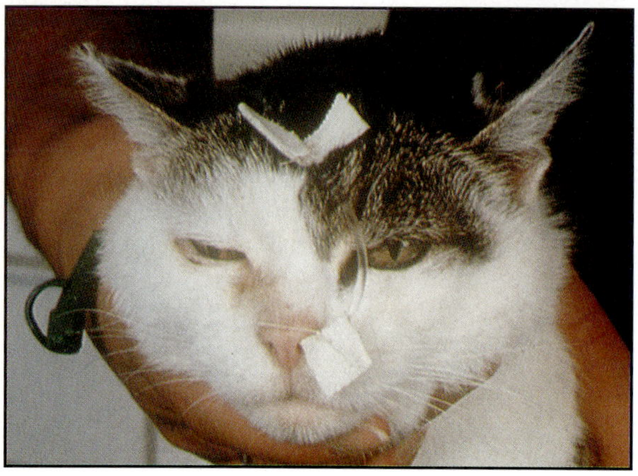
Figure 17.5: The tube is secured.

borborygmus. When you are satisfied that the tube is in the correct position, the tape is either sutured or glued with a fast acting adhesive to the external nares. Tape butterflies are then used to secure the tube with sutures or glue up the middle of the nose and between the eyes to the top of the head (Figure 17.5). An Elizabethan collar may be necessary to prevent the patient from interfering with the tube.

The tube can be used for continuous infusion of liquid diet or more commonly for feeding in intermittent boluses. In the latter case the position of the tube should be checked before each bolus of food is administered. Naso-oesophageal tubes have a narrow bore and completely liquid diets should be used. Commercial liquid enteral diets are suitable. Complications of naso-oesophageal tubes are rare but include rhinitis, epistaxis, reflux or vomiting, tube aspiration, diet aspiration or oesophagitis with stricture formation.

Percutaneous Gastrostomy Tubes

Percutaneous gastrostomy tubes can be placed endoscopically or blindly using the ELD gastrostomy tube applicator. Both methods require general anaesthesia.

Endoscopic tube placement

Purpose-made human gastrostomy tubes are usually too expensive for veterinary use and tubes for small animals are made from alternative cheaper materials. Mushroom-tipped urological catheters (16–20 French, Bard urological catheter) are useful for this purpose and can be prepared as follows: the flared end and the small nipple on the mushroom tip are removed and a short length of the tube (3cm) is then cut from the end and divided into two pieces of equal length. A small incision is made through the centre of each piece and then one of the pieces is threaded down the tube until it lies flush with the mushroom tip. This acts as the internal stent (stopper) and the second piece will subsequently be used as the external stent (stopper) for holding the tube in position (Figures 17.6a and b).

Tube placement requires two operators. The patient is placed in right lateral recumbency. An area behind the left costal arch is clipped and prepared aseptically. The endoscope is passed into the stomach which is then inflated and the left abdominal wall is transilluminated to ensure that the spleen is not trapped between the gastric and abdominal walls. The assistant depresses the abdominal wall with a finger and this is visualised with the endoscope, then the finger is moved until a suitable insertion point is identified with the endoscope. A 16 or 18 gauge, over-the-needle catheter is then pushed firmly through the body wall and into the gastric lumen. The stylet is removed and 3 metric monofilament nylon suture is inserted through the catheter into the stomach lumen. The end of the suture is caught with the endoscopic biopsy forceps. The endoscope is then slowly withdrawn from the stomach and suture is fed from outside the abdominal wall until

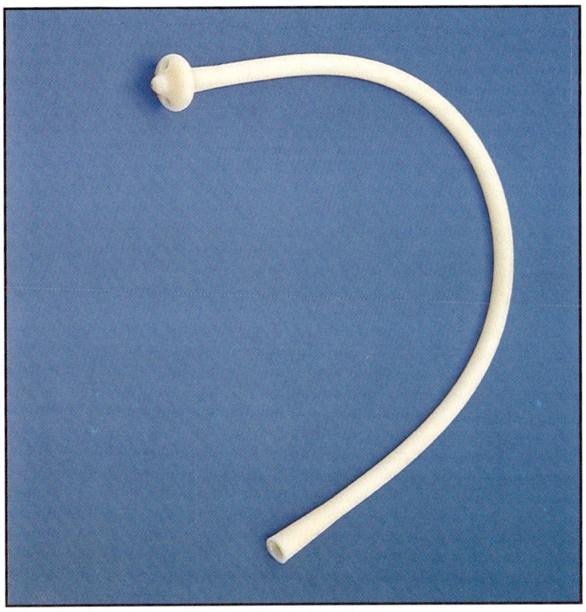

Figure 17.6a: *Mushroom-tipped catheter.*

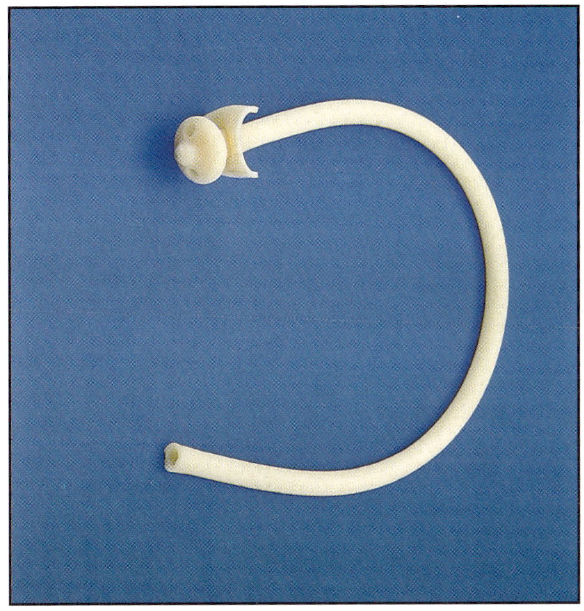

Figure 17.6b: *Tube with stent.*

it is drawn out through the mouth. The catheter is then threaded off the suture leaving a long length of suture entering the abdomen behind the costal arch, passing into the gastric lumen, up the oesophagus and out of the mouth. A hard plastic pipette tip is threaded onto the suture exiting the mouth with the sharp tip towards the patient. The suture is then passed through the end of the tube with a needle and secured carefully with multiple knot ties. The end of the tube is then drawn into the pipette tip. The suture emerging from behind the costal arch is then gently retracted, drawing the tube down the oesophagus and into the stomach. The second operator follows the tube down the oesophagus with the endoscope. The exit point of the suture is very carefully enlarged with a scalpel blade until the sharp end of the plastic pipette tip appears through the abdominal wall. As soon as it appears it is grasped with a haemostat to take the pressure off the suture and the exit point is further enlarged with a scalpel blade until the tube can be gently pulled out. The tube is pulled out until the mushroom tip and stent fit snugly against the gastric mucosa and then the second stent is threaded down the tube to secure it. The second stent should not be placed too tightly against the abdominal wall because the exit wound will swell during the healing period. The end of the tube is then capped and secured against the body wall with a tape butterfly and a suture. A light bandage can then be used to hold the tube against the abdominal wall and to prevent patient interference.

Feeding through the tube is usually delayed for 24 hours after placement and then started at 1/3 of the daily requirement in 6–8 feeds/day. The quantity fed is increased to the full daily requirement over 2–3 days. The tube should be carefully flushed after each feeding and if it becomes blocked, warm water, pancreatic enzyme solution or cola are usually effective in relieving the obstruction. Keep a note of the quantity of flush solution that has entered the stomach. The volume of liquid diet given in each bolus should be judged for each individual patient but should not exceed 50ml/kg per feed. Percutaneous gastrostomy tubes should be left in position for at least 5 days before removal to ensure that sufficient adhesions have developed between the stomach and the body wall. Complications are very rare but include splenic laceration, mild gastric haemorrhage, pneumoperitoneum, vomiting, aspiration pneumonia, inadequate gastric emptying, tube migration and infection of the stoma. Animals with oesophageal dysfunction have a relatively high incidence of aspiration pneumonia associated with gastrostomy tube feeding (Simpson and Elwood, 1994).

The ELD Gastrostomy Tube Applicator

This is quite a simple instrument for blind percutaneous placement of gastrostomy tubes, and is now commonly used for oesophagostomy tube placement. It comes in two sizes, one for cats and small dogs, and another for larger dogs. The instrument consists of a curved aluminium stomach tube with a sharp internal steel stylet operated by a spring loaded plunger (Figure 17.7). The anaesthetised patient is placed in right lateral recumbency and the instrument is passed through the mouth and into the stomach (Figure 17.8). The operator holds the handle of the instrument with the spring loaded plunger in the left hand and uses the curvature to push the end of the instrument against the gastric wall on the left side. The end of the instrument is then located with the right hand and isolated between the fingers to ensure that the spleen is not trapped between the gastric wall and the body wall (Figure 17.9). The plunger is then depressed and the sharp stylet appears through the abdominal wall (Figure 17.10). Monofilament nylon suture is tied through a hole in the end of the stylet

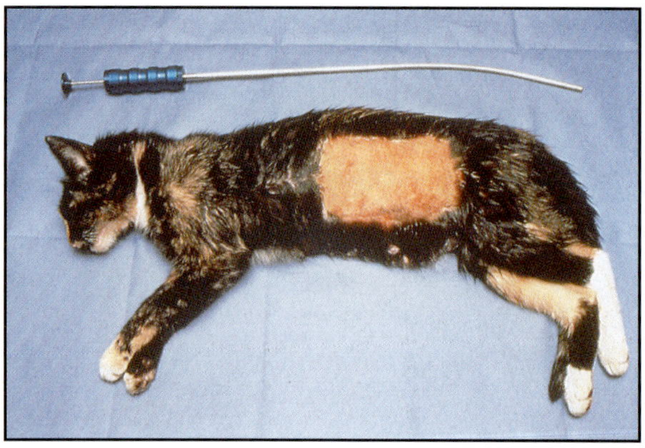

Figure 17.7: *Stomach tube.*

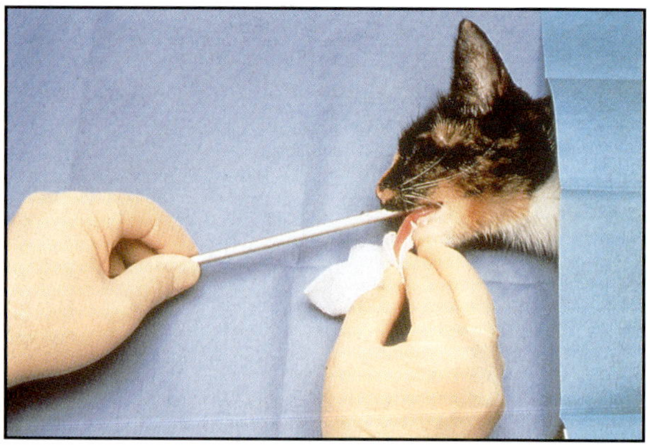

Figure 17.8: *Passing the tube.*

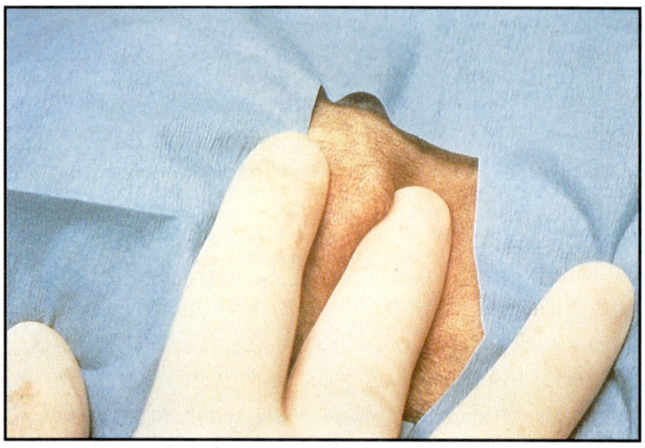

Figure 17.9: *Locating the end of the tube.*

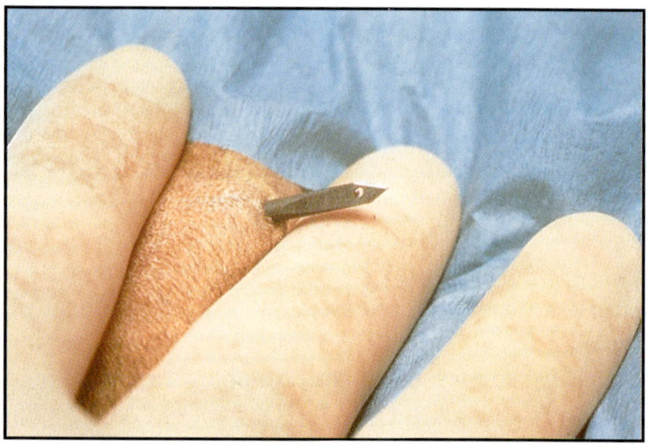

Figure 17.10: *The stylet pierces the abdominal wall.*

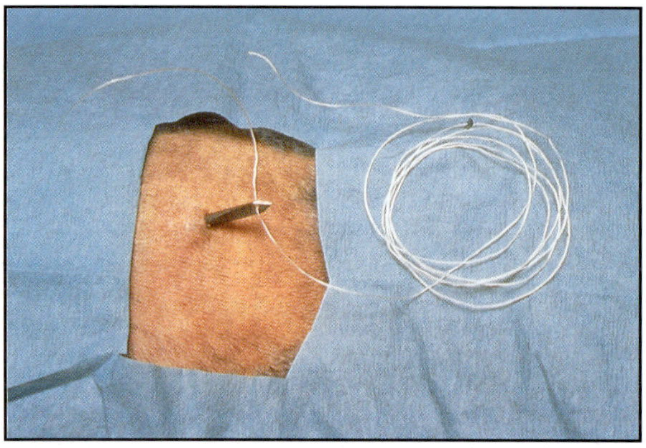

Figure 17.11: *Attaching nylon suture.*

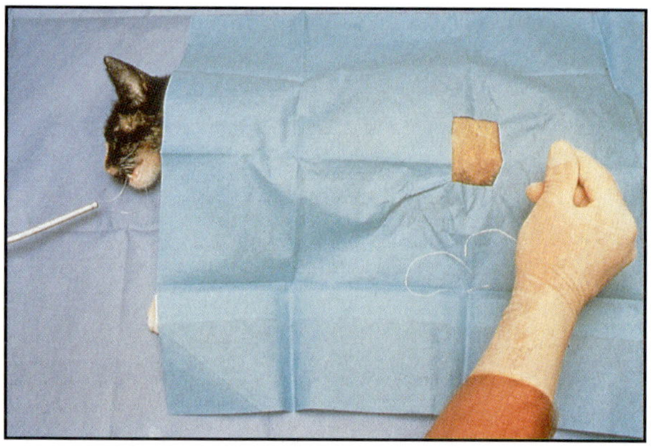

Figure 17.12: *Suture extending through mouth.*

(Figure 17.11) which is then retracted by the spring into the instrument within the gastric lumen. The instrument is then withdrawn and the suture fed through the body wall until it extends from behind the costal arch, through the stomach and oesophagus and out of the mouth (Figure 17.12). From this point on the tube placement is the same as that described above, although the snug fit of the mushroom tip of the feeding tube against the gastric mucosa cannot be confirmed endoscopically. This technique was evaluated recently in 15 cats and was found to be safe, rapid and effective and indicated when endoscopic or surgical gastrostomy is not feasible (Marks *et al.*, 1994).

Another blind gastrostomy technique was described recently which requires no special equipment at all (Fulton and Dennis, 1992). A lubricated vinyl tube is passed through the mouth into the stomach until the gastric end is seen to displace the abdominal wall. The tube is then grasped through the abdominal wall and manoeuvred so that the open end of the tube is pushed against the abdominal wall 2-3cm caudal to the end of the left 13th rib. A small skin incision is made over the lumen of the tube and a 14-16 gauge over-the-needle catheter introduced. The location of the catheter within the end of the tube is verified by waggling the needle and feeling the sides of the tube. The stylet is then removed and a guide wire made from a banjo string is introduced and pushed up the lumen of the tube until it emerges at the mouth end of the tube. Monofilament nylon suture is attached to the wire outside the abdominal wall and pulled through into the stomach lumen, up the oesophagus and out of the mouth. From this point onwards the procedure is the same as the method described above. Limitations to this technique include all those for the endoscopic technique with the addition of obesity. The method has been assessed in 6 dogs and 14 cats where it was found to be as successful as the endoscopic method.

Contraindications for gastrostomy tubes

- Nutritional support anticipated for <5 days
- Intractable vomiting
- Severe gastric or intestinal dysfunction
- Pancreatitis
- Ascites

Oesophagostomy Tubes

Percutaneous and surgical methods for oesophagostomy tube placement have been described by Crowe (1990). Experimental investigations in 12 cats and clinical trials in 50 patients (dogs and cats) showed that the only major complication was infection at the oesophagostomy site where the tubes exit the skin. This must be controlled by meticulous daily cleaning. The tubes were well tolerated and simple to place. None of the experimental animals or clinical patients developed oesophageal stricture or a persistent oesophagocutaneous fistula.

Enterostomy Tubes

Percutaneous enterostomy tubes can be placed by passing them through a percutaneous gastrostomy tube and guiding the end of the tube through the pylorus with the endoscope. This technique may be useful in animals with moderate gastric or oesophageal dysfunction where gastric emptying is impaired and there is likelihood of aspiration pneumonia. This technique is unlikely to have application in pancreatitis or in inflammatory conditions of the stomach because of the necessity for placing a gastrostomy tube first. Specific indications based upon clinical application have not been reported yet (Simpson and Elwood, 1994). Enterostomy tubes are quite commonly placed surgically, often following major procedures on the stomach. Feeding through an enterostomy tube has to be controlled carefully to avoid osmotic overload and diarrhoea. Continuous low volume infusion of a liquid enteral diet is the preferred method. Animals with pancreatitis that require long-term nutritional support may benefit from a jejunostomy tube although there is some pancreatic secretion associated with feeding. Total parenteral nutrition is not associated with significant pancreatic secretion and is therefore the preferred method if the infusion can be maintained in the long term.

PARENTERAL NUTRITION

Parenteral nutrition is only used when enteral methods are not possible and a period of starvation exceeding 5 days is anticipated. In total parenteral nutrition all the nutrients required by a patient for maintenance are given intravenously. Energy is usually provided in the form of 50% dextrose and/or 20% lipid emulsion and protein as amino acid solution. Both dextrose and amino acids are hyperosmolar and if given into a peripheral vein cause thrombophlebitis. Consequently most parenteral nutrition is given via a central vein. Long saphenous vein catheters with the tip of the catheter reaching the caudal vena cava, and jugular catheters, are favoured. This increases the risk of inducing systemic sepsis with contaminated feeding solutions and emphasises the need for aseptic catheter placement, sterile mixing of feeding solutions and careful management of the fluid giving sets.

Glucose intolerance is a feature of most critical patients and the reliance on 50% glucose solutions for providing energy makes overfeeding likely. It is therefore mandatory that the input of feeding solutions is carefully controlled using an infusion pump and that the glycaemic status of the patient is monitored carefully. Lipid emulsions have many advantages as a source of energy in total parenteral nutrition (TPN) but cannot be used exclusively because of the risk of hyperlipidaemia and reticuloendothelial dysfunction.

Lipid emulsions:

- are isotonic
- have higher energy density than glucose solutions
- can be infused through a peripheral catheter (this has enabled the recent development of peripheral total parenteral nutrition in some human hospitals)
- can become unstable when mixed directly with 50% dextrose due to the low pH of the solution and a specific mixing order of ingredients must be followed
- increase the risk of introducing sepsis because they support bacterial growth where 50% dextrose does not.

The other ingredients necessary for TPN are balanced electrolytes, trace minerals and vitamins. Combined solutions of amino acids and balanced electrolytes are available and are the most convenient and safe way for administering appropriate electrolyte concentrations. Multivitamin solutions can be added to the TPN and provide adequate concentrations of all the vitamins except vitamin K which should be administered by weekly injection in long-term parenteral nutritional support. In most cases energy is provided as a mixture of glucose and lipid emulsion and the order of mixing is:

1) amino acids and electrolytes
2) dextrose and minerals
3) lipid emulsion
4) vitamins.

Large volumes of fluids are required to achieve the appropriate level of nutritional support using parenteral solutions. This can be a serious disadvantage because many critical patients are retaining water due to renal or heart disease and the risk of fluid overload is increased. Other complications of TPN include sepsis, phlebitis and metabolic abnormalities such as hyperglycaemia and electrolyte imbalances. Reports of sepsis associated with TPN have been quite rare presumably because the risks of contamination in mixing and administration have been taken very seriously. When sepsis occurs it is often the consequence of bacterial translocation across the gut rather than contamination of the catheter or feeding solutions. As discussed earlier, TPN is associated with gut mucosal atrophy due to the absence of labile glutamine in the feeding solutions. Recently this problem has been addressed using more stable substrates for glutamine synthesis and some improvements in the mucosal barrier have been observed but parenteral glutamine is unlikely to supplant the value of intraluminal glutamine provided in high concentrations in enteral diets.

Hyperglycaemia and glucosuria rarely are clinically significant problems in dogs receiving TPN except in those with inflammatory pancreatic disease.

TPN Worksheet For Dogs

1) Basal Energy Requirement (BER) = 70 x [weight (kg)]$^{0.75}$ = ... kcal[1]/day

2) Illness Energy Requirement (IER) = 1.25–2.0 (depending upon disease) x BER

   IER = ... x BER = ... kcal[1]/day

3) Protein requirements:
   = 4g/kg in adult dogs
   = 6g/kg in dogs with extraordinary protein loss
   = 1.5g/kg in dogs with renal or hepatic failure

   Protein requirements = ... g/day

4) Volumes of nutrient solutions required:

   a) 8.5% amino acid solution = 85mg protein/ml
      To supply .... g of protein need .... ml

   b) 20% lipid solution = 2kcal/ml (8.4kJ/ml)
      To supply 40–60% of IER (........... kcal[1]) need .... ml

   c) 50% dextrose solution = 1.7kcal/ml (7.1kJ/ml)
      To supply 40–60% of IER (........... kcal[1]) need .... ml
      (Use half this volume on the first day and increase to full volume on the second day if no glucosuria)

5) Total volume of TPN solution = ... ml
   Administer at .... ml/hr (4ml/kg/h)

6) Electrolyte requirements:
   Dependent upon patient status and products selected (mixed with amino acids)

7) Vitamin requirements:
   Administer 0.5mg vitamin K/kg BW SC on the first day and weekly. Add 3ml/10kg/day of multivitamins (up to 10ml) to TPN solution.

Table 17.1: *TPN worksheet for dogs.*

[1] *Multiply your answer by 4.184 to transfer the units from kcal to kJ.*

Cats are much more susceptible to hyperglycaemia and must be monitored carefully. When compounding TPN for cats, the protein-derived calories must be subtracted from the estimated caloric needs to avoid overfeeding with glucose and lipid. If glucosuria occurs, the glucose content of the feeding solutions should be halved and if this does not control the problem, insulin therapy should be considered. Hypokalaemia is the most common electrolyte abnormality in TPN because the administration of glucose accelerates intracellular movement of potassium. Most electrolyte abnormalities can be corrected readily by changing the electrolyte composition of the solutions but close monitoring is required. Lipaemia commonly occurs during the first few days of TPN administration but if it becomes persistent the lipid content of the solutions should be decreased.

The most common reported complications of TPN in veterinary patients are those related to the mechanics of administration. These include catheter occlusion, line disconnection or breakage, and inability to replace a catheter when the first one is lost or removed intentionally. Mechanical complications are best prevented by using meticulous catheter placement and maintenance techniques and by closely supervising patients receiving TPN. Close monitoring is critical and suggested monitoring protocols are shown below:

Monitoring protocols for TPN patients

Vital signs	2–4 x per day
Urine glucose	1–2 x per day
Body weight	Every 24–48 hours
Packed cell volume	1 x per day
Total protein	1 x per day
Serum electrolytes	Every 24–48 hours
Biochemical profile	Twice weekly
Haematology	Twice weekly

TPN Worksheet For Cats

1) Basal Energy Requirement (BER) = 70 x [weight (kg)]$^{0.75}$ = ... kcal[1]/day

2) Illness Energy Requirement (IER) = 1.4 x BER = ... kcal[1]/day
   (Provide as protein and non-protein calories)

3) Protein requirements:
   = 6g/kg in adult cats
   = 3.5g/kg in cats with renal or hepatic failure
   Protein requirements = ... g/day

   Protein calories = 4kcal/g (17kJ/g) = ... kcal[1]
   Non-protein calories = IER - protein calories = ... kcal[1]

4) Volumes of nutrient solutions required:

   a) 8.5% amino acid solution = 85mg protein/ml
      To supply .... g of protein need .... ml

   b) 20% lipid solution = 2kcal/ml (8.4kJ/ml)
      To supply 50% of non-protein calories (........... kcal[1]) need .... ml

   c) 50% dextrose solution = 1.7kcal/ml (7.1kJ/ml)
      To supply 50% of non-protein calories (........... kcal[1]) need .... ml
      (Use half this volume on the first day and increase to full volume on the second day if no glucosuria)

5) Total volume of TPN solution = ... ml
   Administer at .... ml/hr (4ml/kg/h)

6) Electrolyte requirements:
   Dependent upon patient status and products selected (mixed with amino acids)

7) Vitamin requirements:
   Administer 0.5mg vitamin K/kg BW SC on the first day and weekly. Add 3ml/day of multivitamins to TPN solution.

Table 17.2: *TPN worksheet for cats.*

[1] *Multiply your answer by 4.184 to transfer the units from kcal to kJ*

Compounding and Administering TPN

The all-in-one system of compounding is favoured because it simplifies administration and monitoring of TPN. All the ingredients are mixed in one bag following the mixing protocol described above. Mixing must be performed aseptically. This can be achieved by mixing in a laminar flow hood or by using containers with a filtered venting system. Injection ports should be swabbed with 70% isopropyl alcohol prior to penetration with needles or transfer sets and air must not be injected into vials to facilitate removal of their contents. Most hospitals have TPN mixing facilities and it may be easier to specify the required ingredients and have the TPN delivered ready-mixed.

The placement and care of the TPN catheter is the most important aspect of the whole technique. Long, through-the-needle, percutaneous, single lumen, polyurethane or silicone catheters are adequate if placed with careful asepsis. The catheter must then be dedicated to TPN and not used for anything else such as drug administration or blood sampling. Line breakage should be avoided at all costs.

On the first day of TPN administration the fluids should be mixed with half the calculated requirement of 50% dextrose. If glucosuria does not develop, the full quantity is administered on the second day. When taking a patient off TPN the glucose concentration should be gradually decreased over 2-3 days to prevent rebound hypoglycaemia. Calculation of the energy requirements and the proportions of nutrients for each patient is best done using daily work sheets (Table 17.1 and 17.2). Unlike the calculations for enteral feeding the basal energy requirement (BER), rather than the maintenance energy requirement (MER), is used as the basic energy unit to avoid overfeeding. The worksheets shown are standard for TPN administration in dogs and cats (Lippert and Armstrong, 1989).

ACKNOWLEDGEMENT

I would like to thank Virbac for permission to use Figures 17.1 to 17.5.

REFERENCES

Crowe DT (1990). Nutritional support of the hospitalised patient: an introduction to tube feeding. *Compendium on Continuing Education for the Practicing Veterinarian* **12,** 1711.

Fulton RB and Dennis JS (1992). Blind percutaneous placement of a gastrostomy tube for nutritional support in dogs and cats. *Journal of the American Veterinary Medical Association* **201,** 697.

Hill RC (1994). Critical Care Nutrition. In: *The Waltham Book of Clinical Nutrition of the Dog and Cat.* Eds JM Wills and KW Simpson. Pergamon Press, Oxford pp 39-61.

Iriyama K, Mori T, Takenaka T, Teranishi T and Mori H (1982). Effect of serum zinc level on amount of collagenhydroxyproline in the healing gut during total parenteral nutrition: an experimental study. *Journal of Parenteral and Enteral Nutrition,* **6,** 416.

Lippert AC and Armstrong PJ (1989). Parenteral nutritional support, In: *Current Veterinary Therapy X.* Eds RW Kirk and JD Bonagura. WB Saunders, Philadelphia.

Marks SL, Rishniw M, Henry CJ and Kanaly ST (1994). Blind Percutaneous Gastrostomy: a new technique. *Proceedings of the 12th Annual Veterinary Medical Forum of the American College of Veterinary Internal Medicine*, No 31, pp 150.

Simpson KW and Elwood CM (1994). Techniques for enteral nutritional support, In: *The Waltham Book of Clinical Nutrition of the Dog and Cat.* Eds JM Wills and KW Simpson. Pergamon Press, Oxford pp 63-74.

CHAPTER EIGHTEEN

Feeding the Sick Animal

Bryn Tennant

INTRODUCTION

In sick animals the clinical picture may be complicated by inadequate or by inappropriate nutrition, giving rise to associated nutritional diseases. These may be diet-induced where dietary nutrients are imbalanced with respect to the patient's physiological status, or nutrient sensitive disease where nutrient requirements are affected by a variety of clinical problems such as renal, hepatic, cardiac or intestinal diseases.

Adjunctive nutritional therapy in disease management requires a nutritional support plan describing the nutrient make-up of the diet and the amount to be fed. This entails assessment of the metabolic state of the animal, an estimation of protein and energy requirements, diet selection, and close patient monitoring.

It is important to consider nutritional support for all sick animals, not solely for the critically ill. However, previously well nourished patients, with acute medical or surgical problems of anticipated short duration will generally resume eating upon resolution of their disease and are usually not candidates for nutritional support.

As few laboratory indicators of malnutrition are used clinically in animals, diagnosis is often based on subjective criteria such as dietary history and physical examination: corroborative evidence of poor nutritional status may be obtained by laboratory estimation of plasma proteins, packed cell volume (PCV), haemoglobin concentration and leucocyte count. These parameters may also be affected by disease other than malnutrition. Conversely normal values do not rule out malnutrition.

NUTRITIONAL HISTORY

When assessing a patient's nutritional requirements the history should include:

- The type and quantity of food and fluid consumed, including supplements
- The frequency of feeding
- Who feeds the animal
- The presence of any food aversions or food intolerances
- Changes in food or fluid intake; if inappetant or anorexic for 3 days then consider nutritional support
- Type of and amount of exercise
- How appropriate is the present diet
- Recent dietary changes
- The use of drugs, particularly catabolic drugs (e.g. prednisolone) or drugs that promote anorexia (e.g. digoxin, cytotoxic drugs)
- Current body weight *versus* usual body weight
- Age
- Changes in urine output
- Changes in gastrointestinal function, e.g. the presence of signs related to nausea, vomiting, diarrhoea or abdominal pain, which may increase nutrient losses
- The presence of chronic disease processes, which may increase nutrient requirements
- Previous gastrointestinal problems
- Recent trauma or surgery
- Abnormalities of the special senses (taste, sight, smell)
- The animal's social status and the presence of other animals
- The animal's productivity level; growth, pregnancy, lactation and exercise.

PHYSICAL EXAMINATION

Physical examination attempts to assess the amount of body fat and the extent of loss of lean body mass (e.g. muscle, heart, liver). Each patient should be given a body condition score based on the following system:

Body Condition Scoring System

1) Extremely thin, with marked muscle wastage in the lumbar region, and from the limbs and head and very little subcutaneous fat.
2) Thin, some muscle wastage and little body fat.
3) Optimal body weight, no evidence of muscle atrophy, plentiful subcutaneous fat, hour-glass appearance and ribs palpable but not necessarily visible.
4) Excess body fat, ribs not palpable.
5) Obese, gross amounts of subcutaneous fat.

Body weight gives some idea of nutritional status. A recent weight loss of greater than 10% or a body weight of less than 80% of normal are indicative of malnutrition. However, in many critically ill patients, body weight per se may be a poor indicator due to water retention.

Many sick animals are anorectic or inappetant. Anorexia is a complete lack of appetite with no desire to eat whereas inappetance is a reduced appetite. In many cases, the reduction in nutrient intake is associated with disease processes which increase nutrient requirements, e.g. metabolic conditions, pyrexia, sepsis, pain, surgery or trauma. As a consequence protein-energy malnutrition (PEM) develops (Dowe *et al.*, 1989). Protein-energy malnutrition may also develop in patients who consume an inappropriate diet for their physiological state, e.g. low protein diet in the face of increased protein requirements. Inadequate protein intake (protein malnutrition) leads to a loss of lean body mass. Although this is most obvious from skeletal muscle, protein loss from heart and intestines carries with it the greater risk of serious complications. Dogs with marked loss of muscle probably have a severe negative nitrogen balance and require immediate nutritional support. Reduced energy intake (energy malnutrition) is characterised by loss of adipose tissue. The incidence of PEM in veterinary medicinc is unknown, but it ranges from 25 to 65% of human trauma patients (Bistrian *et al.*, 1974, 1976: Wilcutts, 1977). It is one of the major causes of morbidity and mortality in metabolically stressed patients. Three types of PEM exist (Haider and Haider, 1984):

- Acute PEM is associated with low serum proteins, while muscle mass and fat stores are maintained. It arises as a consequence of inadequate protein intake, increased protein catabolism, an imbalance in protein and carbohydrate intake or a combination of factors. Immunoincompetence often results from acute PEM.
- Chronic PEM results from chronic undernutrition and is accompanied by loss of skeletal muscle and fat stores, while serum protein levels may be maintained within normal limits.
- Mixed PEM is the most severe form of PEM and results from stress or trauma on chronically malnourished animals. It is characterised by a combination of the above signs with depletion of skeletal muscle mass, fat stores and serum protein concentrations.

Malnutrition, if not present on admission, may develop during hospitalisation for a variety of reasons (Table 18.1). Every sick animal must be assessed to determine the likelihood of developing PEM and if the risk is high, nutritional support must be instituted (Table 18.2). The provision of nutrition at an early stage of the disease process is essential, as malnutrition results in immunoincompetence, depletion of energy stores, weakness, delayed wound healing, sepsis and organ failure within three to seven days. A complication of malnutrition is bacterial translocation and overgrowth (BTOG) (Schlichtig and Ayres, 1988). The intestinal mucosa and gut associated lymphoid tissue act to prevent systemic bacterial invasion. Stress (burns, haemorrhage, endotoxins) and malnutrition promote degradation of the intestinal mucosa and reduce the production of secretory IgA. Bacteria are

- Failure to record daily weight
- Failure to observe, measure and record the amount of food consumed
- Delay of nutritional support until the patient is in an irreversible state of depletion
- Withholding food for diagnostic procedures
- Failure to recognise and treat increased nutritional needs brought about by injury or illness
- Failure to appreciate the role of nutrition in the prevention of and recovery from infection; unwarranted reliance on drugs
- Prolonged administration of glucose and electrolyte solutions
- Rotation of staff at frequent intervals and diffusion of responsibility for patient care
- Inadequate postoperative nutritional support
- Limited availability of laboratory tests to assess nutritional status

Table 18.1: *Practices that may adversely affect the nutritional status of sick animals.*

- Decreased food intake, or anorexia for >3 days
- Current body weight <80% of normal
- Recent weight loss of >10%
- Poor body condition e.g. easily depilated hair, cracked/split nails, non-healing wounds, oedema, ascites and muscle atrophy
- Increased nutrient losses from diarrhoea, wounds, renal disease or burns
- Increased needs due to trauma, surgery, infection, hypoalbuminaemia (albumin <15g/l), anaemia, lymphopenia, pyrexia or neoplasia
- Use of drugs that promote catabolism (e.g. corticosteroids) or anorexia (e.g. digoxin, chemotherapeutic drugs)

Table 18.2: *Indications for nutritional support.*

then able to overgrow within the gut lumen and breach the enteric barrier. The resulting bacteraemia/ endotoxaemia is often fatal. Provision of food enterally helps to maintain the integrity of the gut mucosa, as food in the intestinal lumen is trophic for the mucosa, and enterocytes derive much of their nutrition from the gut lumen. The amino acid glutamine is particularly interesting. It is a non-essential amino acid in normal animals. However, in metabolically stressed animals it is used for gluconeogenesis by many tissues including the intestinal mucosa. During periods of stress and reduced food intake, synthesis of glutamine may not be sufficient to meet demands. A reduction in glutamine availability to the intestinal mucosa has been suggested to be responsible in part for intestinal mucosal degradation (Souba, 1991). The optimal glutamine intake to maintain mucosal integrity is not known. It remains to be seen whether glutamine supplementation is necessary. Rich sources of glutamine include wheat gluten. Parenteral nutritional support is less effective in preventing BTOG, because of the absence of the trophic effects of food in the intestinal lumen.

Dietary Strategy

The objectives of feeding a sick animal are to:

- meet the animal's requirement for water
- provide fat and carbohydrate to meet the animal's energy requirements, thereby reducing gluconeogenic drafting of endogenous amino acids
- satisfy protein requirements
- provide nutrients for the normal maintenance of the gastrointestinal mucosa i.e. glutamine and glucose.

Initially, pre-existing fluid or acid-base deficits should be corrected, and only subsequently should the requirements of other nutrients be addressed. As diets are used to support or to spare the workload of failing organs, the nutrient requirements of sick animals often differ from those of their healthy counterparts. Unfortunately, the nutrient requirements of ill animals are unknown.

Energy and Protein Requirements

Approximate maintenance energy requirements (MER) of

1) Healthy dogs: MER (kcal)* = 125 x ($W^{0.75}$)
   or MER (kcal) = 2 x ([30 x W] + 70).
2) Cats: MER (kcal)* = 91–98 x ($W^{0.75}$)
   or MER (kcal) = 70–90 kcal/kg BW/day

To estimate the illness energy requirement (IER) of sick animals, the MER must be multiplied by an illness factor (Tables 18.3 and 18.4). Note that for

Reason	**Illness energy requirements (IER)**
Dog:	
Hospitalisation	MER x 0.65
Minor surgery/trauma	MER x 0.65-0.75
Major surgery/trauma	MER x 0.75-0.85
Neoplasia	MER x 0.75-0.9
Severe infections/sepsis	MER x 0.85-0.9
Major burns	MER x 1
Cat (for any reason):	MER x 1

Table 18.3: *Approximate energy requirements of sick dogs and cats.*

Dogs: *MER (kcal)* = 125 x body weight$^{0.75}$ [kg] or*
MER (kcal) = 2 x ([30 x body weight] + 70) for dogs weighing 2-45kg.
Cats: *MER (kcal)* = 91-98 x body weight$^{0.75}$ [kg] or*
MER (kcal) = 70-90 kcal/kg BW/day.

cats the MER equals the IER irrespective of the disease process. The proportion of energy derived from fat, protein and carbohydrates by critically ill animals is not known. At the present time it is recommended that fats should provide 40–70% of IER as they are more efficiently used by those organs essential for survival (e.g. heart, muscle, liver) than carbohydrate. High-fat diets are also desirable for patients with respiratory failure as fat metabolism results in a lower respiratory quotient (less carbon dioxide produced per unit of oxygen used) than does glucose, thereby decreasing the workload of the lungs. Carbohydrate should provide 10–30% of the IER, unless there is severe pulmonary dysfunction when it should be lowered.

Protein is primarily required for anabolism, although, during times of stress it is also used for energy production. To ensure that the maximal amount of protein is available for tissue maintenance and repair, and that it is not required for energy production, sufficient energy must be available from carbohydrate and fat. The optimal protein requirements for sick animals are unknown. Available information suggests that, for healthy dogs protein should supply 20–22% of IER (5-6g protein/100kcal (418kJ) metabolisable energy (ME)), for dogs with increased protein requirements protein should supply 24–30% of IER (6–8g/100kcal (418kJ ME) and for cats, protein should supply 28–40% of IER (8–10g protein/100kcal (418kJ) ME). Protein intakes should be reduced in patients with renal or hepatic disease to a minimum of 3g protein/100kcal (418kJ) ME for dogs and 5g protein/100kcal (418kJ) ME for cats. Insufficient protein will result in poor healing, contribute to the development of hypoalbuminaemia and lead to loss of lean body mass. Conversely excessive protein requires additional energy expenditure by the body in order to excrete the excessive nitrogen. If signs of protein malnutrition persist in animals fed adequate

* *1kcal = 4.184kJoule.*

Body weight (kg)	Illness energy requirements (kcal)[1]				
	IF = 0.65	IF = 0.7	IF = 0.75	IF = 0.85	IF = 1.0
2	153	165	177	200	236
4	257	277	297	337	396
6	349	376	403	456	537
8	433	466	500	566	666
10	512	551	591	669	787
15	694	747	800	907	1067
20	861	927	993	1125	1324
25	1017	1096	1174	1331	1565
30	1167	1256	1346	1525	1795
35	1310	1410	1510	1712	2015
40	1447	1559	1670	1893	2227
45	1581	1703	1824	2068	2432
50	1711	1843	1974	2238	2632
55	1838	1979	2121	2403	2828
60	1962	2113	2264	2565	3018

Table 18.4: *Illness energy requirements for dogs related to body weight and illness factors.*

Illness energy requirement = (125 x body weight$^{0.75}$) x IF. IF = Illness factor.

[1] *1kcal = 4.184kJ.*

protein, then increasing carbohydrate and/or fat intake may spare the use of protein for energy production, so improving nitrogen balance. See Table 18.5 for an example of the method for calculating macronutrient requirements.

The choice of diet depends upon an understanding of how a particular illness affects the normal physiology. For sick patients, highly digestible protein sources with a high biological value, e.g. meat-based ingredients (chicken, fish, liver, egg, milk proteins), may be combined with a highly digestible carbohydrate source, e.g. rice, potato. The fibre intake should be reduced. For the majority of patients meat-based canned, liquid or powdered foods containing adequate amounts of protein, fat and carbohydrate (see above for requirements) would suffice (Table 18.6). Where gastrointestinal function may be compromised, highly digestible liquid enteral feeds designed for dogs and cats should be fed.

With anorectic animals several methods are available to improve food intake. Some patients refuse to eat different foods in strange surroundings and therefore returning an animal to its own environment may increase its food intake. Hand-feeding patients increases nutrient intake. The temperature of the food should be between room and body temperature, and in suitably shaped bowls; wide and shallow for cats. Cats may not eat if food is served in bowls which produce off-odours (e.g. plastic bowls). The use of strong smelling food is advocated where there is impairment of the animal's ability to smell, e.g. cats with upper respiratory tract disease, although such foods may not be suitable for nauseous animals. Dogs often prefer animal protein and fat, and sweet foods. Intravenous diazepam (0.1mg/kg) (dogs and cats) or oral oxazepam (2.5mg/cat) (cats only) may act as appetite stimulants.

Enteral Nutrition

If a patient is unable to eat (e.g. fractured jaw) or remains unwilling to eat, food must be provided by enteral or parenteral means. Enteral nutrition is the provision of a patient's nutritional requirements via a functional gastrointestinal tract. As a general rule, **'If the gut works, use it'**. This method of feeding is contraindicated in patients with gastrointestinal failure, e.g. severe malabsorption, pancreatitis, gastric or intestinal obstruction, uncontrolled vomiting, severe bleeding from the upper gastrointestinal tract or severe inflammatory bowel disease. Several routes are available for enteral nutrition (Tennant and Willoughby, 1993).

- Force feeding is only suitable for short-term use. Liquid foods may be squirted into the mouth through a syringe, whilst canned foods may be administered by placing pre-formed boluses on the back of the tongue. Alternatively, food may be administered through an orogastric tube. Liquids in particular should be administered carefully to reduce the risk of laryngotracheal aspiration. For both methods a cooperative patient is required. If a patient is uncooperative or if nutritional support is intended to be prolonged, other techniques should be considered.

- Clinical history: 8-year-old castrated male DSH.10 day history of respiratory distress, inappetance, depression.
- Physical finding: Dyspnoea, dull lung sounds ventrally on right side. Body condition score 1.5, loss of lean body mass. Pyrexia (39.5°C).
- Diagnostic plan: Thoracic radiography — right sided pleural effusion.
  Thoracocentesis — cloudy, thick exudate containing large numbers of toxic neutrophils.
  Staphylococcus aureus isolated from the fluid.
- Diagnosis: Pyothorax.
- Treatment: Pleural lavage with lactated Ringers solution and systemic antibiotics.

Nutritional assessment

Intensive nutritional support was indicated in this case as a large septic focus was present. This is a nutrient-depleting injury because of its hypermetabolic and hypercatabolic effects. Loss of lean body mass is already evident in this case and the cat is likely to remain inappetant for several days.

Enteral nutritional support is indicated as the gastrointestinal tract is functioning adequately. Given the probable prolonged requirement for nutritional support and the need to anaesthetise the cat to place a chest drain, a gastrostomy tube was placed percutaneously using an endoscope. The cat weighed 3.3kg (optimal weight 4.5kg).

Dietary strategy

Maintenance energy requirement (MER) (at optimal weight) = 98 x $4.5^{0.75}$ = **303**kcal.[1]
Illness energy requirement (IER) = MER x Illness factor = MER x 1 = **303**kcal

Protein requirement estimated at 8g protein/100kcal IER = **24**g protein/day.
Energy yield from protein = 3.5kcal/g.
Thus, energy provided by protein = 24g x 3.5kcal/g = 84kcal/day
Proportion of energy from protein = 84/303 = 28% of IER.

Fat requirement estimated at 50% of IER = 151kcal
Energy yield from fat = 8.5kcal/g
Thus, amount of fat required = 151/8.5 = **17.8**g fat

% IER from **Carbohydrate** = 100 - %Protein energy (28%) - %Fat energy (50%) = 22%
Thus, carbohydrate supplies = (22/100) x 303 kcal = 67 kcal.
Energy yield from carbohydrate = 3.5kcal/g
Thus, amount of carbohydrate required = 67/3.5 = **19**g carbohydrate

1 tin Feline p/d (Hills) liquidised with water to a total volume of 650ml.
- Energy density of the slurry approximately 99kcal/100ml.
- Protein content 10g/100ml.
- Carbohydrate content 2.2g/100ml.
- Fat content 6.6g/100ml.

300ml of the slurry was fed per day, thereby providing the cat with:
- Energy: **297**kcal
- Protein: **30**g - (30 x 3.5)/297 = 35% of IER from protein
- Carbohydrate: **6.6**g - (6.6 x 3.5)/297 = 8% of IER from carbohydrate
- Fat: **19.8**g - (19.8 x 8.5)/297 = 57% of IER from fat

Although this diet provided the cat with more protein and less carbohydrate than had been calculated, the amounts were approximately within recommendations.
The cat was fed three times a day (100ml per feed) over a 5 minute period at each feed. Prior to each feed the tube was aspirated to ensure that it was empty and the tube was also flushed with water at the end of each feed. She was offered food from day 1. The enteral feeding was continued until 75% of her daily requirement was consumed voluntarily.

***Table 18.5:** Example of the method used to determine the macro-nutrient requirements of a cat.*

1 1kcal = 4.184kJ.

Product	Energy density (kcal (kJ) /100g DM)	Protein content (g/100g DM)
a/d (Hill's)	493 (2062)	45.7
Canine p/d (Hill's)	490 (2050)	31.4
Feline p/d (Hill's)	510 (2133)	50
Pedigree® Canine Concentration instant diet (WALTHAM)*	437 (1826)	41
Whiskas® Feline Concentration instant diet (WALTHAM)*	478 (2000)	42
Pedigree® Canine Concentration diet (WALTHAM)	442 (1848)	36.8
Whiskas® Feline Concentration diet (WALTHAM)	451 (1886)	41.7
Reanimyl (Virbac)	500 (2092)	29.5
Clinicare canine (PetAg)	550 (2301)	28
Clinicare feline (PetAg)	511 (2138)	39
Renal care canine (PetAg)	470 (1966)	12
Renal care feline (PetAg)	441 (1845)	24

Table 18.6: *Commercial veterinary diets suitable for enteral nutritional support in the dog and cat.*

* *Instant type powder – add water.*

- Nasal feeding tubes are probably the route of choice for most inappetant or anorectic sick animals. Polyvinyl tubes may be passed through the external nares and oropharynx into the stomach. Nasal feeding tubes can be left in position for several weeks and are usually well tolerated. Commercial liquid diets are used with these tubes
- Pharyngostomy tubes are placed under general anaesthesia, through the lateral aspect of the oropharynx into the oesophagus. The popularity of the pharyngostomy tube has declined in favour of other forms of feeding.
- The use of gastrostomy tubes is becoming increasingly popular with the advent of techniques which allow their placement without the need for a laparotomy. Such tubes may be placed percutaneously with or without an endoscope.

Feeding Methods

When using feeding tubes check the tube is in the correct position at each feed by administering sterile saline and that the stomach has emptied by aspirating through the tube. For feeding, the patient should be in an upright position. Tube feeding may be administered continuously with an enteral pump, or more commonly by intermittent boluses. In critically ill patients continuous infusion is recommended at an initial flow rate of 1ml/kg/hr, increasing gradually over 48 hours until the total daily volume can be given over an 18 hour period. If overfilling of the stomach occurs, then the rate should be reduced. With bolus feeding the required volume of food should be divided into three or four feeds initially. The volume given at each feed should not exceed 50mls/kg body weight nor should more than 1/3 of the total daily volume be given at any one time. The food should be at room temperature, and the animal should be fed over a 5 to 10 minute period to reduce the incidence of vomiting or regurgitation. If either of these occur, stop feeding and clear the mouth of food. After feeding flush the tube with 5 ml of water and cap it.

The volume of food required is calculated as indicated below:

Volume of food (ml/day) = IER (kcal or kJ) ÷ energy density of the food (kcal (kJ)/ml).

Observe the patient for a few minutes after feeding for signs of discomfort or vomiting. It is essential that all feeds are recorded on the patient's case record along with its daily weight and any problems encountered.

Animals with feeding tubes are usually able to eat voluntarily and should be offered food as they respond to treatment. The feeding tube can be removed once the patient voluntarily consumes 75% of its daily caloric intake. Hospitalisation is necessary during the initial stages of nutritional support. However, many patients can be discharged with the feeding tube in place as most owners are able to accept the presence of the tube and to manage it successfully.

Complications of nutritional support include mechanical, gastrointestinal, metabolic or infectious problems. Several mechanical problems may be seen. Tube occlusion is occasionally encountered, with fragments of tablets being the commonest cause. If tablets are to be administered through tubes they must be dissolved first. Other causes of occlusion should be infrequent so long as liquid diets only are used with fine-bore tubes and that liquidised canned diets are sieved prior to use with wide-bore tubes. If occlusion does occur, the tube should be flushed with water or cola, or replaced. Pharyngostomy and occasionally nasal feeding tubes may compromise oropharyngeal function, thereby causing gagging, regurgitation, airway occlusion or aspiration pneumonia. Susceptible patients, particularly brachycephalic dogs and cats, should be monitored regularly for any signs of oropharyngeal discomfort.

Regurgitation of naso-oesophageal tubes is occasionally seen in dogs and more frequently in cats. The use of tubes with weighted ends may help to prevent this.

Gastrointestinal complications include vomiting and bloat due to rapid administration of food or obstruction of the pylorus by the mushroom tip if the tube should migrate into the stomach. Diarrhoea may develop as a result of a low fibre intake, lactose intolerance, too rapid delivery or, most likely, the concomitant administration of drugs. Constipation may occur if the fibre intake is too low.

Metabolic, fluid and electrolyte abnormalities are uncommon in uncomplicated cases where a food formulated specifically for dogs or cats is used. Human liquid diets should not be used. Careful attention to the dietary make-up is necessary where organ dysfunction, such as renal or hepatic failure, is present.

Infectious complications including necrosis and cellulitis at an ostomy site may occur if there is excessive pressure on, or too large an incision in, the skin. With percutaneously placed gastrostomy tubes, discharge from the ostomy site is commonly encountered for up to 7 days after tube placement. This is usually self-limiting but may occasionally develop into a more serious diffuse cellulitis. Cellulitis may also develop as a result of the leakage of gastric contents, if the exit site for gastrostomy tubes are too far ventral in the body wall. Aspiration pneumonia may develop if pharyngostomy, or occasionally nasal feeding tubes compromise oropharyngeal function.

REFERENCES

Bistrian BR, Blackburn GL, Hallowell E and Heddle R (1974). Protein status of general surgical patients. *Journal of the American Medical Association* **230,** 858.

Bistrian BR, Blackburn GL, Vitale J, Cochran D, Naylor J (1976). Prevalence of malnutrition in general medical patients. *Journal of the American Medical Association* **235,** 1567.

Dowe, Curt and Meguid (1989). Trauma. In: *Nutritional Medicine; A Case Management Approach.* Eds GL Blackburn, SJ Bell and JL Mullen. WB Saunders, Philadelphia.

Haider M and Haider SQ (1984). Assessment of protein-calorie malnutrition. *Clinica Chemica Acta* **3,** 1286.

Hill GL, Blackett RL, Pickford I, Burkinshaw L, Young GA, Warren JV, Schorah CJ and Morgan DB (1977). Malnutrition in surgical patients. An unrecognised problem. *Lancet* **i,** 689.

Schlichtig R and Ayres SM (1988). Modes of delivery: Rationale, implementation, and mechanical complications. In: *Nutritional Support of the Critically Ill.* Eds R Schlichtig and SM Ayres. Year Book Medical Publishers, Chicago.

Souba WW (1991). Glutamine: A key substrate for the splanchnic bed. *Annual Reviews in Nutrition* **11,** 285.

Tennant BJ and Willoughby K (1993). The use of enteral nutrition in small animal medicine. *Compendium on Continuing Education* **15,** 1054.

Wilcutts HD (1977). Nutritional assessment of 1,000 surgical patients in an affluent suburban community hospital. *Journal of Parenteral and Enteral Nutrition* **1,** 25.

FURTHER READING

The Waltham Book of Clinical Nutrition of the Dog and Cat (1994). Eds JM Wills and KW Simpson. Pergamon Press, Oxford.

Clinical Nutrition of the Dog and Cat (1993). Simpson JW, Anderson RS and Markwell PJ. Blackwell Scientific Publications, Oxford.

CHAPTER NINETEEN

Urolithiasis – a Nutritional Perspective

David F. Senior

ASSESSMENT OF PATHOLOGICAL STATES

Formation, Dissolution and Prevention of Urolithiasis

Canine and feline urine is usually supersaturated with respect to several mineral components. Crystals spontaneously precipitate when urine is above critical supersaturation as shown in Figure 19.1 (Nancollas, 1976). Even though spontaneous precipitation will not occur in the metastable range, already formed crystalline particles can continue to grow. On the other hand, crystal particles only dissolve when urine is undersaturated with respect to their mineral composition. Thus, for dissolution of uroliths, dietary adjustments and medication must induce formation of undersaturated urine. However, for prevention of urolith formation, when the urinary tract has been freed of all crystalline material, dietary adjustment and medication need only keep urine from achieving critical supersaturation. Naturally, increased urine volume reduces the risk of precipitation of all solutes in urine. Evaluation of urine concentration has been determined on an investigative basis for several mineral types but such calculations are not clinically practical and current recommendations are based on extrapolation from experimental data and previous experience (Senior *et al.*, 1985; Porter, 1963a, b).

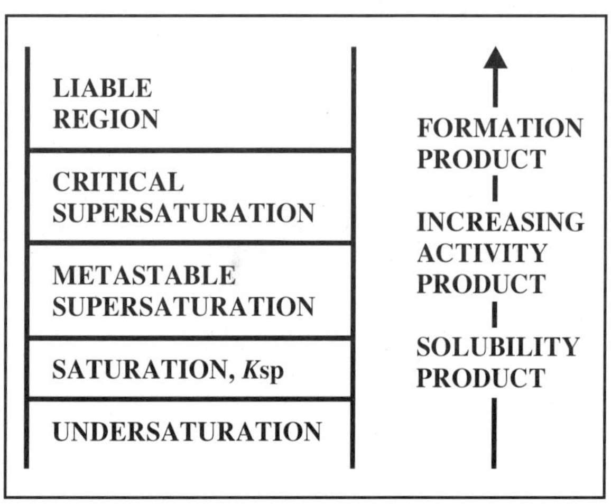

Figure 19.1: *The effect of increasing activity product on solution saturation.*

Accurate assessment of the mineral composition of uroliths is essential because the appropriate dietary and medical strategy for dissolution and prevention varies by mineral type. A strategy for dissolution and prevention of the wrong mineral may predispose formation of uroliths composed of other minerals. The most accurate assessment of mineral composition is direct analysis of a urolith that has been passed spontaneously or recovered by a surgical or non-surgical removal procedure. Quantitative analysis such as crystallographic analysis, infrared spectroscopy, and x-ray diffraction are more accurate than chemical analysis for determination of mineral composition. Crystallographic analysis is capable of determining the composition of most uroliths but infrared spectroscopy or x-ray diffraction are necessary in some instances e.g. to distinguish between urate and xanthine uroliths.

When uroliths are not available for analysis, prediction of urolith composition must be based on epidemiological and clinical evidence such as age, breed, sex, urinalysis findings, anatomical location, plain and contrast radiographic appearance and ultrasonic image.

The composition of uroliths from various surveys is shown in Table 19.1. In dogs, struvite uroliths predominate. While previous surveys indicated that struvite was the most common component of feline uroliths, recent reports in the USA suggest that struvite and calcium oxalate are now equally represented (Osborne *et al.*, 1989, 1994). The relative frequency of cystine uroliths depends on the breed disposition within the survey population. For instance, cystine uroliths are more represented in German surveys because the Dachshund, which is predisposed to cystine urolith formation, is a popular breed (Hesse, 1990). The relative likelihood of each of the major mineral components of dogs based on age, breed and sex can be seen in Table 19.2.

Urinalysis should be performed to determine urine pH, the presence or absence of infection and the mineral composition of crystals. If the urinalysis indicates the presence of urinary tract infection, a bacterial culture and sensitivity test should be performed. Crystals in the urine sediment usually match the mineral composition of the urolith. However, patients with

	Year of Report	Total # Examined	Struvite	Urate	Cystine	Oxalate	Other	Location
DOG	1955[1]	52	42	10	-	-	-	1
	1966[2]	350	211	18	67	54	-	2
	1970[3]	73	62	6	5	0	-	1
	1970[4]	100	53	13	20	14	-	2
	1974[5]	110	49	2	24	35	-	2
	1977[6]	438	307	21	95	12	3	1
	1981[7]	299[a]	151	16	37	4	18	3
	1984[8]	272[a]	187	19	9	27	30	1
	1989[9]	2700[a]	1584	161	49	427	368	1
	1990[10]	1731[a]	951	118	387	87	199	3
	1990[11]	171[a]	79	13	44	28	7	4
CAT	1989[9]	1200[a]	842	67	2	127	162	1
	1990[12]	150[a]	121	5		11	13	1
	1990[13]	491[a]	290	29		138	34	1
	1994[13]	1429[a]	619	115	9	601	85	1

Table 19.1: *Analysis of uroliths from dogs and cats.*

Locations: 1 = United States; 2 = United Kingdom; 3 = Federal Republic of Germany (West Germany); 4 = Spain

References: 1) Brodey, 1955; 2) White, 1966; 3) Finco et al., *1970; 4) Weaver, 1970; 5) Clark, 1974; 6) Brown* et al., *1977; 7) Hicking* et al., *1981; 8) Bovee and Maguire, 1984; 9) Osborne* et al., *1989; 10) Hesse, 1990; 11) Escolar, 1990; 12) Ling* et al., *1990; 13) Osborne* et al., *1994.*

a These surveys used accurate crystallographic, x-ray diffraction or infrared spectroscopy methods of urolith analysis.

Radiographic appearance: cystine: small, often multiple, rounded, mildly radiopaque calcium oxalate: often spiky projections, very radiopaque calcium phosphate: smooth, very radiopaque struvite: smooth, multiple or single, mild to very radiopaque ammonium urate: smooth, often multiple, poorly radiopaque
Urinalysis: crystalluria - same as urolith composition pH: acid: cystine alkaline: struvite variable: calcium oxalate, ammonium urate culture: urease producers - *Staphylococcus, Proteus* induce struvite[1] uroliths urolith analysis (if urolith passed): accurate quantitative crystallographic techniques are required
Serum chemistry: hypercalcaemia - calcium oxalate[2] metabolic acidosis (renal tubular acidosis) - calcium phosphate[2] bile acid pre- and post-prandial elevation - ammonium urate
Age of dog immature animals (not Dalmatian) - usually struvite
Breed Dalmatian: ammonium urate Bulldog, Dachshund, Bassett, Chihuahua, Irish and Yorkshire Terrier (mature age males) - cystine
Sex female dogs: struvite

Table 19.2: *Criteria for determining the most likely mineral composition of uroliths in dogs.*

1 Struvite uroliths can be formed in a sterile environment and uroliths composed of other minerals can become infected by urease-producing organisms

2 Extremely rare.

non-struvite uroliths can develop urinary tract infection with a urease-producing organism so that struvite crystals appear in the urine sediment. Cystine crystalluria is definitive evidence that the patient has a reabsorption defect for cystine. Examination of urine sediment should be made on fresh urine as soon as possible after collection because precipitation can develop in urine left at room temperature or refrigerated for a prolonged period. Such crystal formation may be irrelevant to the mineral composition of uroliths.

Radiographic analysis of the anatomical location and radiodensity of uroliths is helpful because calcium salt and struvite uroliths are the most radiopaque. In male dogs, about 60% of radiopaque uroliths are composed of calcium salts (mostly calcium oxalate), whilst about 20% are pure struvite. In female dogs, around 50% of radiopaque uroliths are composed of struvite, whilst only around 40% are composed of calcium salts. However, in cats, the vast majority of radiopaque uroliths contain calcium salts (mostly calcium oxalate) and only about 5% are composed of struvite (Osborne *et al.*, 1993). Cystine and ammonium urate uroliths tend to be more radiolucent and may require contrast studies for detection. Ultrasonic evaluation allows location of radiolucent uroliths when a contrast study is deemed to be too time consuming or yields equivocal results.

This evaluation should allow a decision concerning appropriate management options which may include surgical removal, urethrohydropropulsion, lithotripsy via cystoscopy, dietary/medical dissolution or vigilant observation. More importantly, the information should allow determination of the mineral composition of uroliths so that appropriate strategies for dissolution and subsequent prevention of reformation of uroliths once they are removed. Surgical removal of multiple tiny uroliths is often required to relieve and prevent urethral obstruction. Complete removal of all urolith particles is often impossible. Such patients should undergo a full dissolution protocol for at least 6 weeks postoperatively before conversion to a prevention protocol. Surgical removal of renoliths by the "clamshell" technique can induce rapid loss of function in the operated kidney so non-dissolvable renoliths may be best left untreated. Renoliths composed of dissolvable minerals tend to dissolve more slowly than uroliths in the bladder.

STRUVITE UROLITHIASIS

Dietary Strategy

Both dissolution and prevention of struvite uroliths can be achieved by a dietary/medical approach in dogs and cats (Abdullahi *et al.*, 1984; Osborne *et al.*, 1990). The struvite molecule is $MgNH_4PO_4.6H_2O$ and increases of magnesium, ammonium and trivalent orthophosphate in urine all increase the driving force for precipitation. In most dogs, struvite uroliths are induced by urinary tract infection; however in some dogs and most cats, struvite uroliths form in the absence of infection. In the infection-induced form, a urease-producing infection, usually *Staphylococcus intermedius* hydrolyses urea to ammonia. Ammonia further hydrolyses to ammonium with the generation of hydroxyl ion according to the reactions:

$$NH_2\text{-}CO\text{-}NH_2 + H_2O \overset{\text{urease}}{\rightleftharpoons} 2NH_3 + CO_2 \quad (1)$$

$$NH_3 + H_2O \rightleftharpoons NH_4^+ + OH^- \quad (2)$$

The subsequent alkalinisation of urine increases the concentration of bivalent and trivalent orthophosphate by shifting the following reactions to the right:

$$H_3PO_4 \rightleftharpoons H_2PO_4^- + H^+ \qquad pK = 2.1 \quad (3)$$

$$H_2PO_4^- \rightleftharpoons HPO_4^{2-} + H^+ \qquad pK = 6.8 \quad (4)$$

$$HPO_4^{2-} \rightleftharpoons PO_4^{3-} + H^+ \qquad pK = 12.7 \quad (5)$$

Current dissolution and prevention strategies in dogs and cats call for control of urinary tract infection, when present, with antimicrobials to reduce urinary excretion of ammonium. In addition, special diets are necessary to reduce urinary excretion of magnesium and phosphate; to reduce urine pH; and to increase urine volume.

Magnesium and Phosphorus

Gastrointestinal absorption of magnesium and phosphorus are affected by the palatability and energy density of the diet. Excessive palatability can result in greater food intake with a tendency toward obesity and higher intake and urinary output of dietary minerals. The energy density of a ration determines the daily intake of magnesium and phosphorus because animals usually eat sufficient food to satisfy their energy requirements. Thus, two diets with the same stated content for magnesium and phosphorus (usually expressed as a percentage of weight on a dry matter basis, i.e. % DMB) but different energy density can result in vastly different daily mineral intake.

Digestibility varies with binding interactions with other ions in the intestinal lumen and the form of mineral in the diet because inorganic salts of magnesium and phosphorus are much more readily absorbed than organic salts as found in poultry, meat, or fish meals (Lewis *et al.*, 1978; Finco *et al.*, 1989). Even though phosphorus may be consumed in both organic and inorganic forms, most phosphorus undergoes renal excretion as salts of orthophosphoric acid distributed according to the dissociation constants and urine pH in reactions 3-5. Although the concentration of orthophosphate salts in urine is important in determining struvite supersaturation in urine, for diets containing recommended levels of phosphorus, the powerful impact of urine acidification on the proportion of orthophosphate that exists in the trivalent form renders urine pH much more significant in affecting struvite supersaturation than the total concentration of urinary orthophosphate (Buffington *et al.*, 1985, 1990).

Urine pH

Urine pH can be reduced by adjusting the composition of the diet. The most common strategies include:

- increased sodium content
- appropriate selection of mineral salts e.g. $MgCl_2$ instead of MgO, $CaCl_2$ instead of $CaCO_3$
- selective feeding of dietary amino acids e.g. lysine, arginine, histidine, methionine and cysteine
- direct addition of acidifying chemicals to the diet. Acidifying agents added to foods by manufacturers include D, L-methionine, ammonium chloride and phosphoric acid.

Urine Volume

Urine volume is dramatically increased in dogs fed a low protein, high sodium diet. This could be caused by thirst, solute diuresis induced by the high sodium content of the diet, and/or reduced medullary hypertonicity. In cats, where the ability to reduce dietary protein is limited, urine volume can be increased by adding water to the diet.

Dissolution in Dogs

Requirements

A proven dissolution strategy in dogs is as follows (Abdullahi *et al.*, 1984):

1) Feed a diet that severely reduces the activity product of struvite in urine.

A commercial diet specifically formulated to induce dissolution of struvite uroliths in dogs is low in magnesium (3.3mg magnesium/100kcal (418kJ) ME) and phosphorus (24mg phosphorus/100kcal (418kJ) ME) and uses a low protein-high sodium chloride combination (1.47g protein/100 kcal (418kJ) ME; 23.3mg sodium/100kcal (418kJ) ME) to increase urine volume. The diet induces formation of acidic urine by selecting amino acid and mineral ingredients that generate hydrogen ions on metabolism. Specific information regarding the formulation of the diet is protected by the manufacturer and is not available.

2) Treat with antimicrobials to control urinary tract infection.

Urine culture and sensitivity is usually not necessary because the sensitivity of urinary staphylococci tend to be predictable. Synthetic penicillins such as ampicillin and amoxicillin are most commonly used. Sulphonamide antimicrobials should be avoided because they can precipitate around the urolith and set up a barrier that prevents or slows further dissolution.

3) Extended treatment

When all urolith material has been eliminated based on radiography or ultrasound, the dissolution protocol should be continued for a further 4 weeks.

Feeding

A dissolution diet should be fed exclusive of all other food. The amount fed should satisfy energy requirements and clean water should be available at all times. The frequency of feeding does not seem to be important.

Evaluation

Prior to commencing a dissolution protocol a thorough physical examination should be performed and a complete blood cell count, serum chemistry panel and urinalysis should be run to evaluate the patient for cardiac, hepatic and renal function. Ideally, blood pressure should be measured. The high sodium dissolution diet can cause decompensation of congestive heart failure and exacerbate hypertension which is quite common in renal failure patients. Severely reduced protein in the diet can induce hypoalbuminaemia and anaemia particularly in patients with hepatic and renal insufficiency. Almost all dogs fed the commercial struvite urolith dissolution diet develop a mild elevation of serum alkaline phosphatase, however, this does not appear to be clinically significant (Abdullahi *et al.*, 1984).

Dogs should be rechecked every 3-4 weeks during dissolution as follows:

1) Radiographs or ultrasound to determine if uroliths are becoming smaller.

If progress is not satisfactory, serum chemistry values and urinalysis results can often help to determine the cause of delayed dissolution. Failure to induce dissolution in the face of appropriate values suggests that the urolith is not composed of struvite.

2) Blood urea nitrogen (should be 0.58 ± 0.4mmol/l); urine specific gravity (should be less than 1.015).

Higher values indicate that the patient is consuming a significant proportion of food other than the prescribed diet.

3) Urine pH (should be less than 6.0); urine sediment (no crystals or bacteria should be apparent).

Inappropriately increased pH indicates either dietary indiscretion or uncontrolled urinary tract infection. Owners should be counselled carefully concerning alternative food sources and persistence in giving the antimicrobial. If the antimicrobial appears to be ineffective, a culture and sensitivity test on urine may be necessary to choose a more appropriate drug.

Prevention in Dogs

Requirements

Because most struvite uroliths in dogs are induced by infection, prevention of recurrence involves prevention of urinary tract infection. A satisfactory prevention strategy is:

1) Feed a low magnesium–low phosphorus diet that induces acid urine.

A commercially available diet for this purpose contains 14.8mg magnesium/100kcal (418kJ) ME and 89mg phosphorus/100kcal (418kJ) ME.

2) Monitor weekly for return of infection caused by urease-producing bacteria.

When the patient is fed an appropriate diet, the pH of urine collected before feeding after an overnight fast should be acidic. Urease-producing infections induce alkaline urine.

Feeding

Foods other than the preventive diet should be avoided. The amount fed should satisfy energy requirements and clean water should be available at all times. On the day prior to regular urine pH measurement, the patient should not be fed after 10:00pm. Collection after an 8–12 hour fast precludes confusion due to the post-prandial alkaline tide.

Evaluation

Routine urinalysis should be performed on a regular basis. Urine pH should be less than 6.5 and there should be no struvite crystals in the urine sediment. A shift toward alkalinity may be due to urinary tract infection with urease-producing bacteria which could set the stage for struvite urolith formation. Formation of alkaline urine requires that patients be checked for infection by urinalysis and bacterial culture of urine. Repeated episodes indicate a predisposition to urinary tract infection and afflicted patients should be worked up for a primary underlying cause that reduces normal host defences. If a predisposing factor cannot be identified or eliminated, patients are best treated with long-term low-dose antimicrobials as prevention for recurrent urinary tract infection. The most frequently used drugs for this purpose are synthetic penicillins and potentiated sulphonamides given once a day at night after the last void.

Feeding a diet that is low in magnesium and phosphorus and induces formation of acidic urine can prevent sterile struvite uroliths but may fail to prevent infection-induced struvite uroliths because strong urease-producing organisms can overcome the effects of such diets. However, feeding diets that induce aciduria is advantageous because they allow easier recognition when urease-producing bacteria induce alkaline urine.

Dissolution in Cats

Requirements

A proven strategy for struvite urolith dissolution is as follows (Osborne *et al.*, 1990):

1) Feed a diet that severely reduces the activity product of struvite in urine.

Commercial diets for this purpose are low in both magnesium and phosphorus and appear to be heavily acidified. As distinct from the situation in dogs, undersaturation with respect to struvite is achieved by extreme acidification rather than by a low protein-high sodium combination because cats cannot tolerate low protein diets as well as dogs.

2) Control urinary tract infection with antimicrobials.

This strategy is usually not required in cats because struvite uroliths are seldom caused by infection. If infection is present, the therapeutic principles are the same as infected struvite uroliths in dogs.

3) Extended dissolution protocol.

When all urolith material has been eliminated based on radiography or ultrasound, the dissolution protocol should be continued for a further 4 weeks.

Feeding

A dissolution diet should be fed exclusive of all other food. The amount fed should satisfy energy requirements and clean water should be available at all times.

Evaluation:

Prior to feeding a struvite urolith dissolution diet, a serum chemistry panel should be performed to evaluate renal function and pre-existing metabolic acidosis. The diet may be detrimental if renal failure and metabolic acidosis are present. During the period of urolith dissolution, radiographs or ultrasound should be performed every 3–4 weeks to assess progress. If uroliths are not getting smaller, the urolith may be composed of another mineral (usually calcium oxalate), the owners may not be strictly adhering to the diet and urease-producing infection may be present. Urinalysis and urine culture should be performed if infection is thought to be present. Cats on a dissolution diet should have a urine pH <6.0.

Prevention in Cats

Requirements

For prevention, commercial diets that reduce struvite saturation in urine should be fed but the reduction in activity product of struvite need not be so low. Many commercial diets that induce aciduria and are somewhat reduced in magnesium and phosphorus currently fit the criteria that would deter struvite precipitation. In the past, ‘off-the-supermarket-shelf’ commercial cat foods usually contained 0.11-0.25% magnesium DMB with an energy density of 4kcal (17kJ) ME/g DMB, thus providing 30-65mg magnesium/100kcal (418kJ) ME. Most recently formulated diets designed to prevent struvite crystalluria tend to contain reduced levels of magnesium: 0.07-0.09% magnesium DMB with an energy density of 4.7-5.5kcal (19.7-23kJ) ME/g DMB, thus providing 15-20 mg magnesium/100kcal (418kJ) ME. The phosphorus content also tends to be reduced to less than 140mg phosphorus/100kcal (418 kJ) ME. Adding acidifiers such as D, L-methionine or ammonium chloride to any diet induces urine acidity (Senior *et al.*, 1986).

Feeding
A dissolution diet should be fed exclusive of all other food. The amount fed should satisfy energy requirements and clean water should be available at all times.

Evaluation
Routine urinalysis on a regular basis should indicate urine pH less than 6.3 even during the post-prandial alkaline tide and there should be no evidence of struvite crystals in the urine sediment.

URATE UROLITHIASIS

Dietary Strategy

Both dissolution and prevention of urate uroliths can be achieved in dogs by a combination of dietary and medical treatment (Bartges *et al.*, 1994). So far there are few data concerning medical management of urate uroliths in dogs with a portosystemic vascular shunt and in cats.

The metabolites of nucleic acid metabolism are excreted as uric acid and allantoin. In most dogs, hepatic uricase converts uric acid to highly soluble allantoin. In Dalmatian dogs, individuals of other breeds and patients with portosystemic vascular shunts, the conversion of uric acid to allantoin is impaired and ammonium urate precipitation in urine leads to urolith formation (Figure 19.2). In many male Dalmatian dogs, urethral outflow obstruction is the first indication of urate urolithiasis. Affected patients must be relieved of obstruction on an emergency basis prior to commencing dietary management.

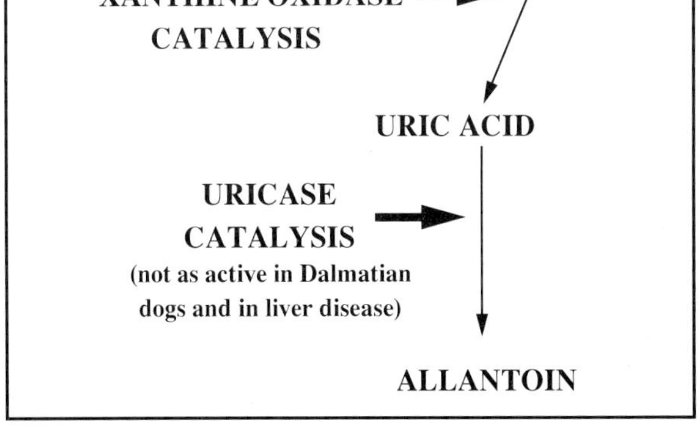

Figure 19.2: *Allantoin production from nucleic acid metabolism is impaired and leads to urate urolith formation.*

Low protein diets reduce daily urate excretion and neutral or slightly alkaline urine reduces renal excretion of ammonium. Additional treatment with allopurinol, a xanthine oxidase inhibitor, to reduce urate excretion further is necessary for dissolution and in many patients to prevent recurrence.

Dissolution in Dogs

Requirements
The following protocol has induced urate urolith dissolution in about 60-70% of Dalmatian dogs:

1) Feed a low protein diet.
Diets with 1.6-2.2g protein/100kcal (418kJ) ME reduce urinary urate excretion. To minimise nucleic acid intake, the protein source should not be from organ meats such as kidneys, liver etc. A home-cooked low protein diet is shown in Table 19.3.

2) Treat with a xanthine oxidase inhibitor.
Allopurinol 15mg/kg PO bid should be given concurrently. The effect of a given dose on urate excretion varies with individual patients so dose adjustments may be necessary.

3) Induce mild urine alkalinisation to reduce renal ammonium excretion.
Potassium citrate given to effect (start at 50-100mg (0.25-0.5mEq)/kg PO bid) has proven popular and is even incorporated into the formulation of one commercial low protein diet.

Feeding
A dissolution diet should be fed exclusive of all other food. The amount fed should satisfy energy requirements and clean water should be available at all times.

Evaluation
Prior to initiation of a dissolution strategy, non-Dalmatian patients should be evaluated for portosystemic vascular anastomosis. Feeding a very low protein diet to such patients may induce anaemia, hypoalbuminaemia, oedema and ascites.

During the dissolution period, patients should be rechecked every 3-4 weeks by radiography and ultrasound to determine progress. Good owner compliance will result in a urine pH greater than 7, a urine specific gravity less than 1.015 and urate crystals will be absent on examination of the urine sediment. Xanthine oxi-

Home-cooked Low Protein Diet for a 20 lb dog
This assumes dog is not athletic and is half the requirement of a similarly active 60 lb dog.

Recipe 1:

Ingredient	For 1 day	For 4 days
Rice	3 oz.	12 oz.
Egg	1	4
Corn oil	2 tblspns	8 tblspns
Dicalcium phosphate	1 tspn	4 tspn
Light salt	1/2 tspn	2 tspn
Centrum Senior Multivit (USA)	1/2 tab.	2 tab.
or Intervet SA37 (UK)	3/4–1 tsp.	3/4–1 tsp.

Recipe 2:

Ingredient	Mod. salt (Na ≈ 0.9mg/kcal)	Low salt (Na ≈ 0.2mg/kcal)
Rice	3 oz.	3 oz.
Skinless chicken	1 oz.	1 oz.
Corn oil	2.5 tblspn	2.5 tblspn
Dicalcium phosphate	1 tspn	1 tspn
Light salt	1/2 tspn	Pinch
Centrum Senior Multivit (USA)	1/2 tab.	2 tab.
or Intervet SA37 (UK)	3/4–1 tsp.	3/4–1 tsp.
Saly Substitute (Leo K or Slow K)		1/2 tspn.

These supply = 680 kcal/day, and contain, on an energy basis, approximately:
8% Protein
46% Carbohydrate
46% Fat

Instructions

Quantities: amounts given are for ***level*** teaspoons/tablespoons and ***uncooked*** weights

Usual Ingredients:
1) **Carbohydrate** e.g. rice has to be thoroughly cooked.
2) **Protein** e.g. meat or egg.
3) **Fat** any vegetable oil is O.K.
4) **Dicalcium phosphate**.
5) **Salt:** iodized.
6) **Vitamin/minerals supplement**.

Cooking Instructions: (similar to those for human food)

All ingredients (except vitamin tablets must be thoroughly cooked. All ingredients (except vitamin tablets) can be casseroled or microwaved together. Rice must be completely cooked. Ideally they should be cooked, in part at least, with meat so that they will absorb flavour. Vitamin tablets are added ***after*** the food has cooled. Enough for 4 days may be cooked at one time, then divided and frozen for subsequent reheating; however, vitamins should be added on the day of feeding. Food may also be divided and given as 2–3 meals per day.

Water should be offered free choice.

Monitoring: Your dog must be checked regularly while on this diet. Though this diet has been formulated to comply with the clinical needs of your dog and where possible to conform with the current recommendations for an ***average*** dog, your dog may not exactly correspond to this average animal. Careful monitoring is essential because your dog is an ***individual***. Albumin, PCV, and electrolytes (e.g. K^+) should be checked.

Treats: If you like to feed treats, keep some of the meat back and feed that as a treat. Do not feed other foods unless specifically directed.

Body Weight: Your dog's weight should be measured and recorded every 2 weeks. This can be achieved using bathroom scales, picking the dog up and subtracting your own weight. The amount of food suggested is for an average dog taking little or no exercise. Some dogs may need up to 40% less or a lot more than we have suggested. If your dog is gaining weight, reduce the amount of carbohydrate in the diet slightly (e.g. if your recipe says 8 oz rice, reduce it to 6 oz.) If your dog is losing weight, increase the amount of carbohydrate slightly (8 oz rice becomes 10 oz).

Prepared by: Dr. Richard Hill MA VetMB PhD MRCVS
(Waltham Visiting Assistant Professor of Clinical Nutrition)
University of Florida, College of Veterinary Medicine

Table 19.3: *A home-cooked low protein diet for a dog.*

dase inhibition with allopurinol predisposes to xanthine in urate urolith formers. Xanthine can precipitate around the outside of existing ammonium urate uroliths and cause formation of new uroliths made entirely of xanthine. Unfortunately, the dose of allopurinol cannot be titrated based on urinary urate estimations. An empirical approach calls for the dose of allopurinol to be increased by 10-25% if urate uroliths recur or ammonium urate crystals persist in the urine sediment and reduced by 25% if xanthine uroliths develop (Bartges *et al.*, 1994). Xanthine and urate cannot be distinguished with routine crystallographic analysis using refractive indices. X-ray diffraction or infrared spectroscopy must be used.

Prevention in Dogs

Prevention of urate urolithiasis involves the same strategies as for dissolution but the dose of allopurinol often can be reduced. However, when a low protein diet is used alone, uroliths recur in about 30% of patients.

CYSTINE UROLITHIASIS

Dietary Strategy

Cystinuria is a metabolic defect where the reabsorption of filtered cystine in the proximal tubule is impaired (Bovee, 1984). Cystine is very insoluble, particularly in acidic urine. Affected animals have the defect for life although the magnitude of cystinuria may vary. Low protein diets can reduce the total daily excretion of cystine. Sodium excretion can enhance cystine excretion in experimental animals so diets should also be restricted in sodium (Norman and Manette, 1990). Low sodium, low protein diets tend to increase urine volume which further decreases the urinary concentration of cystine. Urinary alkalinisation increases cystine solubility; however, this should be achieved by the addition of a non-sodium containing alkaliniser such as potassium citrate or by selecting the mineral composition of the diet to induce alkaluria. Cystinuria tends to occur in several breeds as shown in Table 19.2 and in South American maned wolves and certain strains of North American timber wolves. The condition is only rarely observed in cats where there is no information on dietary and medical management.

Dissolution in Dogs

Requirements

The following protocol has proven effective (Hoppe *et al.*, 1988):

1) Treat with the disulphide exchange drug, tiopronin (Thiola®, Mission Pharmacal Inc.) 15mg/kg PO bid.

D-penicillamine (Cuprimine®, Merck) has been used in the past but it causes anorexia and vomiting in most patients. Gastrointestinal signs are much less frequently seen with tiopronin.

2) Feed a low protein–low sodium alkalinising diet.

Low protein, low sodium diets alkalinised with potassium citrate are commercially available and commonly fed to patients with chronic renal failure. One example contains 9% protein DMB, 0.24% sodium DMB, 4.5kcal (19kJ) ME/g DMB.

3) Alkalinise the urine to pH 7.5 or higher.

To appreciably increase cystine solubility, urine pH should exceed 7.5. Renal failure diets may require additional supplementation with potassium citrate, (50-100 mg (0.25-0.5mEq)/kg PO bid) to achieve this goal.

Feeding

A dissolution diet should be fed exclusive of all other food. The amount fed should satisfy energy requirements and clean water should be available at all times. Tiopronin should be given after or with meals rather than before meals in patients where the drug tends to cause vomition.

Evaluation

During dissolution, patients should be checked every 3-4 weeks to ensure that uroliths are becoming smaller and disappearing. The urine specific gravity should be less than 1.015 and the urine pH should be greater than 7.5. No cystine crystals should be detectable in the urine sediment. The dissolution protocol should be continued for 30 days after a recheck shows no evidence of remaining uroliths.

Prevention in Dogs

Cystine uroliths recur very often and diet alone is seldom sufficient for prevention. For prevention, essentially the same protocol should be continued but the dose of tiopronin can be reduced in some patients. The minimum dose of tiopronin that will prevent cystine urolith formation cannot be predicted. The dose of tiopronin can be progressively reduced then maintained just above the level at which cystine crystalluria appears.

CALCIUM OXALATE

Dietary Strategy

The causes of calcium oxalate urolithiasis remain obscure in dogs and cats. In Miniature Schnauzers, hyperabsorption of calcium and renal calcium "leak" have both been described (Lulich *et al.*, 1991); however, in most patients, such characterisation is seldom performed and treatment is empirical.

Direct animal experimentation and extrapolation from clinical experience in human medicine suggest several dietary strategies (Robertson *et al.*, 1979; Schuette *et al.*, 1980). High protein feeding enhances intestinal calcium absorption and subsequently increases urinary calcium loss. Diets with acidic ash tend to enhance gastrointestinal calcium absorption while alkaline ash diets tend to reduce it. Diets that induce aciduria deplete urinary citrate, a major inhibitor of calcium oxalate crystal growth. In addition, low sodium diets reduce calcium excretion (Kleeman *et al.*, 1964). Based on these findings, an appropriate diet for prevention of calcium oxalate uroliths would be reduced in protein and sodium and would enhance urinary citrate excretion with a urine pH of 7.0-7.5.

At the moment, there is no dietary regimen to dissolve calcium oxalate uroliths, but there is reasonable evidence that they can be successfully prevented.

Prevention in Dogs and Cats

Requirements

The following protocols are suggested for prevention of calcium oxalate uroliths in dogs and cats:

DOGS:

1) Feed a low protein-low sodium alkalinising diet.

Protein levels of 1.6-2.2g protein/100kcal (418kJ) ME have been suggested. An adequately sodium restricted diet would contain 0.10-0.20% sodium DMB in a diet that provides 4.5-5kcal (19-21kJ) ME/g DMB (45-55mg sodium/100kcal (418kJ)ME).

2) Alkalinise the urine to pH 7.0-7.5.

A non-sodium alkaliniser should be used. Potassium citrate 100-200mg (0.25-0.5mEq)/kg PO bid is usually sufficient.

3) Treatment with hydrochlorothiazide 2-4 mg/kg PO bid.

This dose reduces urinary calcium excretion, particularly with concurrent feeding of a low sodium diet. Long-term diuretics cannot be given to cats because they tend to become extremely dehydrated.

4) Add water to the food to reduce urine concentration.

Aim for a urine specific gravity less than 1.015.

CATS:

1) Feed a low protein-low sodium diet.

There is a limit to the degree of protein restriction in cats and the diet should contain no less than 5g protein/100kcal (418kJ) ME and about 70mg sodium/100kcal (418kJ) ME.

2) Alkalinise the urine to pH 7.0-7.5.

A non-sodium alkaliniser such as potassium citrate, to effect, should be used. A starting dose would be 100-200mg (0.25-0.5mEq)/kg PO bid.

3) Add water to the food to reduce urine concentration.

Aim for a urine specific gravity of less than 1.020.

Feeding

A dissolution diet should be fed exclusive of all other food. The amount fed should satisfy energy requirements and clean water should be available at all times.

Evaluation

Routine urinalysis can be performed on a regular basis to ensure that urine specific gravity is less than 1.015 for dogs and less than 1.020 for cats; that urine pH is 7.0-7.5; and that no calcium oxalate crystals are present in the urine sediment.

REFERENCES

Abdullahi S, Osborne CA, Leininger JR, Fletcher TF, Griffith DP (1984). Evaluation of a calculytic diet in female dogs with induced struvite urolithiasis. *American Journal of Veterinary Research* **45,** 1508-1519.

Bartges JW, Osborne CA, Koeler L, Felice LJ, Lulich JP, Bird K, Unger L (1994). An algorithmic approach to canine urate uroliths. *Proc. 12th ACVIM Forum, San Francisco* pp 476-477.

Bovee KC (1984). Genetic and metabolic diseases of the kidney. In: *Canine Nephrology.* Ed KC Bovee. Harwell Publ Co, Media, PA pp 339-354

Bovee KC and Maguire TGT (1984). Qualitative and quantitative analysis of uroliths in dogs: Definitive determination of chemical type. *Journal of American Veterinary Medical Association* **185,** 983-987.

Brodey RS (1955). Canine urolithiasis. A survey and discussion of fifty-two clinical cases. *Journal of American Veterinary Medical Association* **126,** 1-9.

Brown NO, Parks JL and Greene RW (1977). Canine urolithiasis: Retrospective analysis of 438 cases. *Journal of American Veterinary Medical Association* **170,** 414-418.

Buffington CA, Rogers QR and Morris JG (1990). Effect of diet on struvite activity product in feline urine. *American Journal of Veterinary Research* **51**(12), 2025-2030.

Buffington CA, Rogers QR, Morris JG and Cook NE (1985). Feline struvite urolithiasis: Magnesium effect depends on urinary pH. *Feline Practice* **15**(6), 29-33.

Clark WT (1974). The distribution of canine urinary calculi and their reoccurrence following treatment. *Journal of Small Animal Practice* **15,** 437-442.

Escolar E (1990). Structure and composition of canine urinary calculi. *Journal of Veterinary Research* **49,** 327-333.

Finco DR, Barsanti JA, Brown SA (1989). Influence of dietary source of phosphorus on fecal and urinary excretion of phosphorus and other minerals by male cats. *American Journal of Veterinary Research* **50**(2), 263-266.

Finco DR, Rosen E, Johnson KH (1970). Canine urolithiasis: A review of 133 clinical and 23 necropsy cases. *Journal of American Veterinary Medical Association* **157,** 1225-1228.

Hesse A (1990). Canine urolithiasis: Epidemiology and analysis of urinary calculi. *Journal of Small Animal Practice* **31,** 599-604.

Hicking W, Hesse A, Gebhardt (1981). Analytiche untersuchungen an harnsteinen von säugetieren. In: *Harnstein-Symposien Bonn-Wien.* Eds W Vahlensieck and G Gasser. Steinkopff Verlag, Darmstadt.

Hoppe A, Denneberg T and Kagedal B (1988). Treatment of clinically normal and cystinuric dogs with 2-mercaptopropionylglycine. *American Journal of Veterinary Research* **49**(6), 923-928.

Kleeman CR, Bohannan J and Bernstein D (1964). Effect of variation in sodium intake on calcium excretion in normal humans. *Proceedings of the Society for Experimental Biology and Medicine* **115,** 29-32.

Lewis LD, Chow FHC, Taton GF and Hamar DW (1978). Effect of various dietary mineral concentrations on the occurrence of feline urolithiasis. *Journal of American Veterinary Medical Association* **172(5),** 559-563.

Ling GV, Franti CE, Ruby AL and Johnson DL (1990). Epizootiologic evaluation and quantitative analysis of urinary calculi from 150 cats. *Journal of American Veterinary Medical Association* **196**(9): 1459-1462.

Lulich JP, Osborne CA, Nagode LA, Polzin DJ and Parke ML (1991). Evaluation of urine and serum metabolites in Miniature Schnauzers with calcium oxalate urolithiasis. *American Journal of Veterinary Research* **52**(10): 1583-1590.

Nancollas GH (1976). The kinetics of crystal growth and renal stone formation. In: *Urolithiasis Research.* Eds H Fleisch, WG Robertson, LH Smith, *et al.* Plenum Press, New York pp. 5-23.

Norman RW and Manette WA (1990). Dietary restriction of sodium as a means of reducing urinary cystine. *Journal of Urology.* **143,** 1193-1195.

Osborne CA, Lulich JP, Kruger JM, Polzin DJ, Johnston GR and Kroll RA (1990). Medical dissolution of feline struvite urocystoliths. *Journal of American Veterinary Medical Association* **196**(7), 1053-1063.

Osborne CA, Lulich JP, Polzin DJ, Bartges JW, Unger LK, Koeler LA and Bird KA (1993). Canine and feline nephrolithiasis - Causes and cure. *Proc. 11th ACVIM Forum, Washington, DC* pp 370-373.

Osborne CA, Sanna JJ, Unger LK, Clinton CW and Davenport MP (1989): Analyzing the mineral composition of uroliths from dogs, cats, horses, cattle, sheep, goats, and pigs. *Veterinary Medicine* **8,** 750-764.

Osborne CA, Thumchai JP, Lulich JW, Bartges JW, Lund EM, Marsh WE, Koehler LA, Unger LK and Bird KA (1994). Epidemiology of feline urolithiasis. *Proc. 12th ACVIM Forum* pp 482-483.

Porter P (1963a). Physico-chemical factors involved in urate calculus formation. I. Solubility. *Research in Veterinary Science* **4,** 580-591.

Porter P (1963b). Physico-chemical factors involved in urate calculus formation. II. Colloidal flocculation. *Research in Veterinary Science* **4,** 592-607.

Robertson WG, Heyburn PJ and Peacock M (1979). The effect of high animal protein intake on the risk of calcium stone-formation in the urinary tract. *Clinical Science* **57,** 285-288.

Schuette SA, Zemel MB and Linkswiler HM (1980). Studies on the mechanism of protein-induced hypercalciuria in older men and women. *Journal of Nutrition* **110,** 305-315.

Senior DF, Sundstrom DA and Wolfson BB (1986). Testing the effects of ammonium chloride and D, L-methionine on the urinary pH of cats. *Veterinary Medicine* **81,** 88-94.

Senior DF, Thomas WC, Gaskin JM and Finlayson B (1985). Relative merit of various strategies on non-surgical treatment of infection stones in dogs. In: *Urolithiasis and Related Clinical Research.* Eds PO Schwille, LH Smith, WG Robertson, *et al.* New York: Plenum Press pp 589-592.

Weaver AD (1970). Canine urolithiasis. Incidence, chemical composition and outcome of 100 cases. *Journal of Small Animal Practice* **11,** 93-107.

White EG (1966). Symposium on urolithiasis. I. Introduction and incidences. *Journal of Small Animal Practice* **7,** 529-535.

CHAPTER TWENTY

Nutrition Related Orthopaedic Diseases

Åke Hedhammar

INTRODUCTION

The locomotor system requires an adequate nutritional supply to develop properly in the growing animal and thereafter to maintain its optimal function during adult life. Consequently malnutrition interferes with its normal development, function and integrity. The importance of nutrition to the bony structure of the skeleton has long been evident through observation of such classical deficiency syndromes as rickets and scurvy. Research in orthopaedic disease in the dog and cat has been focused on two main areas: firstly the absorption and distribution of calcium (the major component of bone) within the body and the role of vitamin D (both excesses and deficiencies affect optimal skeletal characteristics (Hazewinkel *et al.*, 1991)); and secondly the influence of total food consumption on growth rates (particularly in canine practice (Hedhammar *et al.*, 1974)). Most nutritionally related orthopaedic diseases in both dogs and cats are seen during growth.

Because the locomotor system is an integrated system of bones, joints and muscles, this chapter will consider the effects of nutrition on orthopaedic disease rather than just its effects on bones and skeletal diseases.

COMPOSITION OF BONE AS IT RELATES TO NUTRITION

Bone is composed of water, a cellular component, an organic matrix and a mineral phase. The organic matrix is mostly composed of collagen fibres with a high content of hydroxyproline. The mineral phase is mainly in the form of hydroxyapatite crystals and amorphous calcium phosphate but does contain many other elements in small quantities. The complex chemical and physical composition of bone changes during growth from an immature status at birth to a more stable but never steady state in adults. In humans much is known about changes in bone composition that occur later in life, particularly on the influence of nutrition on osteoporosis in elderly women. Although little is known about such changes in elderly dogs and cats, the clinical evidence does not indicate that nutrition is of similar importance.

In adults almost all total body calcium (99%) and most body phosphorus (80%) is built into the skeleton. The proportion of calcium to phosphorus by weight is about 2:1 within the skeleton (and hence in bone meal) whereas it is 1.3:1 in the body as a whole. The large amounts and relative proportions of calcium and phosphorus that need to be laid down in the skeleton during growth indicate large and balanced needs for these constituents in the diet of growing animals. It is no coincidence that milk from most mammals, including dogs and cats, is rich in calcium and phosphorus and in the same proportions as occur in the body of their suckling young. Needs are greatest when growth is most rapid and when lactation is at its peak.

Other minerals that are not major constituents of bone are also essential for normal skeletal development. A deficiency of iodine will result in a lack of growth (cretinism) as well as goitre. Whilst a low bioavailability of dietary zinc has been implicated in a number of conditions in dogs (most prominently the zinc responsive dermatoses, see Chapters 2, 3 and 14) it also retards growth. This has been seen in puppies of fast-growing breeds like Great Danes that were inappropriately fed high calcium diets.

Bone also consists of small amounts of minerals such as copper, magnesium, manganese, silicon and vanadium. The requirements for these are easily met under most practical conditions. Theoretically both high calcium diets and those with excessive amounts of zinc may interfere with bioavailability of copper and magnesium. However, bone disorders due to deficiency of copper or magnesium have not been described.

Many microelements seen in bone are simply stored there and not intrinsically beneficial.

Vitamins are another group of nutrients that are essential for development and integrity of the entire skeleton. A deficiency of vitamin A, hypovitaminosis A, results in retarded bone growth. This has been produced experimentally in both cats and dogs but is rarely seen in clinical practice. Dogs are able to convert carotenoids, precursors of vitamin A, into the vitamin itself and are therefore not dependent on a dietary supply. Cats are unable to convert carotenoids to vitamin A and rely on a dietary supply. However, as cats are usually fed diets rich in animal fats, they are rarely vitamin A deficient. Hypervitaminosis A, caused by prolonged excessive intake of vitamin A, is seen occasionally in dogs and cats. It is commonest in adult cats fed an unbalanced diet such as one composed exclusively of liver or certain fish. The characteristic clinical signs are lameness and pain on neck palpation. The animal is also lethargic and apprehensive. Radiographs reveal multiple exostoses, most noticeable on the cervical and thoracic vertebrae, on the forelimbs around articular surfaces and attachment of ligaments and tendons. In growing animals the long bones are shortened due to disturbance of epiphyseal growth.

Vitamin D metabolites stimulate calcium and phosphorus absorption from the gut and increase bone cell activity, endochondral ossification and calcium excretion. After being absorbed from the intestine, vitamin D must first be hydroxylated in the liver to 25-OH vitamin D and then further hydroxylated in the kidney to 24,25-OH_2 vitamin D and 1,2-OH_2 vitamin D. It is these metabolites, functioning more or less as hormones, that regulate calcium homeostasis within the body. Classical rickets may be seen in growing puppies that are ingesting insufficient vitamin D and/or are unable to synthesise vitamin D by UV irradiation. The condition known as 'vitamin D resistant rickets' is not caused by a deficiency of vitamin D in the diet but by faulty hydroxylation of vitamin D to its active metabolites. This occurs most commonly because of inborn errors in an individual's metabolism.

Water-soluble vitamins like thiamin (B_1) and riboflavin (B_2) are needed for the development and integrity of the locomotor system of dogs and cats. Thiamin deficiency results from exclusive feeding of diets that are either rich in thiaminase (such as certain raw white fish) or in which all thiamin has been completely destroyed by processing.

Vitamin C (ascorbic acid) is needed for the synthesis of collagen. Humans and guinea pigs require vitamin C in their diet but most mammals including dogs and cats are able to synthesise their own supply. The need for vitamin C in the diet of cats and dogs has never been proved but there are repeated claims that vitamin C supplements are beneficial.

In addition, protein and small amounts of lipids are needed to form bone's organic matrix.

GROWTH RATE – RETARDED, OPTIMAL OR MAXIMAL

Normal growth depends on, and is regulated by several hormones and the supply of adequate nutrition. The maximum rate of growth achievable is genetically determined but total amount of energy normally regulates whether this rate of growth will be attained. When the diet is deficient in nutrients, there will be specific effects associated with each deficiency. In addition, almost all deficiencies will depress appetite and hence reduce total food intake and retard growth. Reduced intake of a balanced diet reduces rate of growth but does not interfere with either body composition or final size unless the restriction is severe and prolonged. Reduced intake of an unbalanced diet actually prevents the more serious consequences of a greater intake of such a diet. In Sir Edward Mellanby's classical studies on vitamin D, only puppies with the genetic potential to grow rapidly (large breeds and mongrels expected to attain large final size) developed rickets, and puppies that for various reasons ate less of a vitamin D deficient diet developed less severe changes than those eating more.

Of clinical importance is the fact that a decreased growth rate resulting from reduced intake, either by unavailability or poor appetite, will be compensated for by an increase when intake is increased. A period of rapid growth then occurs during which the demand for a balanced diet is critical.

The association of specific deficiencies with stunted growth led to the belief that maximal rate of growth indicated optimal nutrition. As more is learnt about each specific nutrient this belief is now in question (see below).

Dwarfism

Growth may be retarded by malnutrition from dietary deficiencies or intestinal parasitism; by abnormal endocrine regulation; by genetic disorders of bone and cartilage; by congenital disorders of cell metabolism; and by congenital or acquired major organ failure. It is difficult to differentiate clinically between various reasons for retarded growth.

Pituitary dwarfism has been described in German Shepherd Dogs and Carelian Bear-Dogs. Juvenile diabetes mellitus with growth retardation has been described in Golden Retrievers and the Keeshond. Genetic disorders of bone and cartilage expressed in several forms of osteochondrodysplasia have been described in various breeds. Some of these occur together with other abnormalities i.e. with anaemia in Alaskan Malamutes and with ocular defects in Labradors and Samoyeds. Others result solely in dwarfism i.e. in Beagles, Cocker Spaniels, English Pointers, Great Pyreneans, Irish Setters, Newfoundlands, Norwegian Elkhound, Poodles and Scottish Terriers. Congenital and inherited disorders of cell metabolism, like lysosomal and glycogen storage diseases, have been described in many breeds of dogs as well as in cats.

The most common metabolic causes of retarded growth are probably liver diseases like portosystemic shunt and kidney diseases such as progressive nephropathies. Achondroplasia due to decreased zinc absorption has been reported in Alaskan Malamutes. Individuals affected by congenital heart failure or chronic progressive lung diseases often fail to attain normal size.

As retarded growth can result from a variety of causes, it is mandatory to take a complete clinical history and perform a clinical examination, including clinical biochemistry and other diagnostic aids. This will help to define and differentiate the functional and morphological background of each clinical case.

Normal Growth – Disturbed Growth

To define normal growth characteristics is almost as difficult as to define optimal rate of growth. With the diversity of breed and breed characteristics in dogs it is hard to know what a puppy of a certain breed should look like at different stages of growth.

To allow for longitudinal growth the metaphyseal region of bones must be broadened. At faster rates of growth, broadening is more pronounced. But to what extent does the external appearance lead to the suspicion of faulty development? During periods of rapid growth all puppies of giant breeds have, to some extent, cartilaginous cores at their most active metaphyses which are retained in an irregular fashion. When this is exaggerated it may lead to permanently retained cartilage and deviation of the bone axis. Puppies do not have straight front legs when viewed from the side; their tendency to angulate at their carpal joint varies a great deal but is most pronounced at 2–4 months of age.

It is rare in modern practice to see orthopaedic diseases caused by nutritional deficiencies. Knowledge of requirements and availability of balanced diets has made it extremely rare to see clinical cases of rickets (the classical orthopaedic condition of growing dogs before their great need for calcium and vitamin D was appreciated). Cases of nutritional secondary hyperparathyroidism (NSH) are still seen occasionally in cats fed on an all-meat diet which is too low in calcium and too high in phosphorus.

Although it is rare to see orthopaedic diseases caused solely by nutrition, many prevalent clinical conditions are affected by nutritional factors. Nutrition affects the occurrence, severity and outcome of orthopaedic conditions and will influence the operation of inheritance and environmental factors. Excessive intake of food or specific nutrients is as detrimental to optimal development as deficiencies.

As yet there has been little investigation into the role of nutrition as a determinant rather than the cause of orthopaedic disease. As with other determinants, like hereditability, it would be worthwhile quantifying its effects on various conditions.

CONGENITAL, DEVELOPMENTAL AND DEGENERATIVE ORTHOPAEDIC DISEASES

Diseases affecting the locomotor system can be divided into congenital, developmental, degenerative and traumatic (Table 20.1).

Congenital orthopaedic diseases may be obvious at birth or during the neonatal period but some will not present with overt clinical signs until much later in life. Developmental orthopaedic diseases are commonly seen during the most rapid period of growth. The exact period varies with breed and is affected by both inheritance and nutrition. Degenerative orthopaedic diseases are most commonly associated with old age but occur when detrimental effects interfere with development and function. These detrimental factors may be obvious, e.g. trauma, but may also be determined by inheritance and nutrition.

Optimal bone /skeletal conformation and function result from an interaction between inheritance, nutrition and other environmental factors such as training.

INTERACTIONS BETWEEN ORTHOPAEDIC DISEASES, NUTRITION AND GENETICS

Congenital or developmental orthopaedic diseases commonly have a proven or strongly indicated hereditability. Any breed predisposition and/or a family pattern of occurrence is strongly indicative of a genetic component. A few diseases are inherited by

CONGENITAL
Dwarfism:
cretinic
chondrodysplasia
hypophyseal
Osteopetrosis
DEVELOPMENTAL
Osteochondrosis
Fragmented coronoid process
Ununited anconeal process
Metaphyseal osteopathy
Enostosis
Wobbler syndrome
Hip dysplasia
Calcinosis circumscripta
Legge Perthes
Patellar luxation
DEGENERATIVE
Secondary arthrosis
Anterior cruciate ligament rupture
Osteosarcoma
TRAUMATIC
Fractures
Luxations/Distorsions

Table 20.1: *Classification of diseases affecting the locomotor system.*

Condition	Inheritance		Nutritional Factors	
Rickets	+	breed predisposition	+++	vitamin D deficiency
Retained cartilage	+	breed predisposition	++	overfeeding / calcium excess?
Metaphyseal osteopathy	+	breed predisposition	+	overfeeding / calcium excess?
Wobbler syndrome	+	breed predisposition	+	overfeeding / calcium excess?
Enostosis	+	breed predisposition	+	overfeeding / calcium excess
Osteochondrosis	++	hereditability estimate	++	overfeeding / calcium excess
Fragmented coronoid process	++	hereditability estimate	+	overfeeding / calcium excess?
Ununited anconeal process	+++	simple recessive	+	overfeeding
Hip dysplasia	++	hereditability estimate	+	overfeeding
Anterior cruciate ligament rupture	+	breed predisposition	+	overfeeding

Table 20.2: *Interactions between inheritance and nutrition in nutrition related orthopaedic diseases.*
Relative importance graded from (+) to (+++).

simple recessive inheritance and some have a polygenic inheritance with hereditability estimates published for defined populations. Congenital orthopaedic disease can sometimes be affected by nutrition but it is the developmental orthopaedic diseases that are mostly influenced by nutrition. Both congenital and degenerative diseases may be influenced in their course and severity by nutritional factors.

The interaction between the effects of inheritance and nutrition on orthopaedic diseases in dogs is shown in Table 20.2; the relative importance of each factor has been graded subjectively as either (+), (++) or (+++).

Interactions between Nutrition and Other Environmental Factors

An animal that is overweight, even though it may be eating a balanced diet, is predisposed to develop both developmental orthopaedic diseases during growth and degenerative orthopaedic disorders throughout life. The progress and outcome of degenerative orthopaedic disease is adversely affected by obesity. Whilst there are no published studies proving adverse effects of obesity on the incidence of ruptured cruciate ligament or on the success rate of surgical correction, there is a strong clinical impression that dogs and cats that are overweight sustain this injury more commonly and are less successful candidates for surgical correction.

Malassimilation of food will affect the supply of various nutrients though this may be difficult to quantify. Pancreatic insufficiency, for example, interferes with availability of the fat-soluble vitamins A, D and E. Severe damage to the intestinal mucosa caused by endoparasites interferes with total caloric uptake as well as with absorption of specific nutrients.

Developmental orthopaedic diseases are often influenced by nutrition. Lack of specific nutrients during periods of rapid growth and development cause specific changes — rickets in growing puppies being a classic example. An excess of specific nutrients also causes most damage if it occurs during a period of rapid growth; hypervitaminosis A in kittens is a typical example.

In dogs and cats nutritional secondary hyperparathyroidism (NSH) is manifested to a greater extent during the period of growth. Puppies or kittens fed diets almost exclusively made from meat and meat by-products will get too little calcium and too much phosphorus. Lowered concentrations of plasma calcium stimulates release of parathyroid hormone. If dietary calcium is not available parathyroid hormone causes calcium to be resorbed from bone to restore plasma calcium concentration. 'Juvenile osteodystrophy' will result if such feeding practices are not corrected. It is rare to see NSH in adult animals unless heavily unbalanced diets are fed for very long periods. In the old dog and cat renal secondary hyperparathyroidism (RSH) may be seen more frequently. RSH is not alleviated by dietary correction. In both NSH and RSH the most pronounced changes are seen when they occur in conjunction with congenital renal failure which is manifested early in life, i.e. progressive nephropathy. This may be seen quite commonly in some breeds.

Developmental orthopaedic diseases with a strong genetic background (see Table 20.2) may be influenced unfavourably by deficiency or excess of specific nutrients. However, the energy supply from total food consumption has the most important impact on these conditions.

PREDISPOSITIONS TO ORTHOPAEDIC DISEASES

Species

Cats are not as prone to developmental orthopaedic problems as dogs because they grow less rapidly. Rickets has not been described in cats nor have true osteochondrotic lesions, metaphyseal osteopathy nor wobbler syndrome. Developmental orthopaedic diseases seen in cats are most commonly associated with genetic disorders like mucopolysaccharidosis in Siamese cats, or with heavily unbalanced diets causing NSH, hyper- or hypovitaminosis A. Developmental orthopaedic diseases seen in dogs are almost exclusively manifested in large and giant sized breeds.

Age

Depending on whether the cause is mainly congenital, developmental or degenerative, different nutrition related orthopaedic diseases become manifest at different ages (See Table 20.3).

Breed

Developmental orthopaedic diseases have variable prevalence and manifestation in different breeds. This depends partly on adult size but constitutional and hereditary predispositions seem to operate as well.

Period	Disease	Caused by
Gestation	Congenital defects	maternal influences nutritional deficiencies /excess i.e. iodine-goitre
Birth	Developmental defects	lack of nutrition factors affecting lactation malnutrition inappropriate milk substitute
Weaning		inappropriate weaning diet or regimen
New Home		inappropriate feeding: diet amount
12+ Weeks	Nutritional secondary hyperparathyroidism	calcium deficiency / phosphorus excess
	Rickets	vitamin D deficiency
	Hypervitaminosis D	vitamin D excess
	Hypovitaminosis A	vitamin A deficiency
	Hypervitaminosis A	vitamin A excess
	Hypovitaminosis E	vitamin E deficiency / unsaturated fat excess
	Chastek's paralysis	thiamin deficiency / thiaminase excess
Period	**Disease**	**Affected by**
12+ Weeks	Osteochondrosis:	overfeeding / calcium excess?
	epiphyseal	overfeeding / calcium excess?
	metaphyseal	overfeeding / calcium excess?
	retained cartilage	overfeeding / calcium excess?
	Fragmented coronoid process	overfeeding / calcium excess?
	Ununited anconeal process	overfeeding
	Hip dysplasia	overfeeding
	Metaphyseal osteopathy	overfeeding / calcium excess?
	Enostosis	overfeeding / calcium excess?
	Wobbler syndrome	overfeeding / calcium excess?
12+ Months	Degenerative diseases:	
	secondary arthrosis	overweight
	anterior cruciate ligament rupture	overweight
	degenerative myelopathy	overweight
	Osteosarcoma	malnutrition

***Table 20.3:** Age disposition to nutrition related orthopaedic diseases.*

Reported breed predispositions may or may not be universal (see Table 20.4).

Sex

It has been documented that prevalence and severity of developmental orthopaedic diseases is higher in males. However, hip dysplasia in some breeds is a notable exception.

SYMPTOMS OF NUTRITION RELATED ORTHOPAEDIC DISEASES (TABLE 20.5)

Clinical signs of nutrition related orthopaedic diseases usually relate to rate of growth and /or normal growth characteristics:

- Retarded or stunted growth is almost a hallmark of deficiency, whether of total energy, protein or specific nutrients.
- Exaggerated growth characteristics with broadened metaphyseal regions of long bones, bulging of costochondral junctions and deviation of angulation of long bones is not only seen grossly with rickets but also as a manifestation of a wide variety of abnormal skeletal developments.
- Lameness in nutrition related orthopaedic diseases most commonly involves more than one leg.
- Pain on palpation of metaphyseal regions is seen in metaphyseal osteopathy. Pain on palpation of diaphyses is seen in enostosis (panosteitis).
- Pain on manipulation of joints is seen in osteochondritis dissecans, fragmented coronoid process, ununited aconeal process and hip dysplasia.

Predisposition	Cat	Dog	Breed
Cretinism	?	birth	
Hypochondroplasia	?	weaning	Alaskan Malamute
Rickets	-	weaning	larger sized
Nutritional secondary hyperparathyroidism		young-adult	
Hypovitaminosis A	young	young	
Hypervitaminosis A		adult	
Osteochondrosis: shoulder elbow knee hock	-	4 months	larger sized Rottweiler
Retained cartilage	-	4-8 months	larger sized
Fragmented coronoid process	-	4 months	Bernese, Mountain Rottweiler, Newfoundland
Ununited anconeal process	-	6 months	German Shepherd Dog, St Bernard
Metaphyseal osteopathy	-	3-8 months	Great Dane, Boxer
Hip dysplasia	?	6 weeks	
Calcinosis circumscripta	-	4 months	German Shepherd Dog
Enostosis	-	6 months	German Shepherd Dog
Wobbler syndrome	-		Great Dane, Dobermann Pinscher, Saluki, Borzoi

Table 20.4: *Age and breed predisposition in nutrition related orthopaedic diseases.*

DIAGNOSTIC FEATURES OF NUTRITION RELATED ORTHOPAEDIC DISEASES

Haematology and Clinical Biochemistry

Haematological examinations are of limited value in diagnosis of nutrition related orthopaedic diseases other than to differentiate from polyarthritis and canine leucocyte adhesion defect (CLAD). Serum calcium initially is low in secondary hyperparathyroidism but compensatory mechanisms in both NSH and RSH make interpretation difficult later in the course of the diseases.

Clinical biochemistry during growth must be interpreted with great caution. Serum calcium, phosphorus and alkaline phosphatase all decrease to some extent with age. Adult reference values cannot be used until growth ceases completely. The age at which animals stop growing varies with breed: by 6 months in toy breeds but at well over 12 months in giant breeds.

Serum alkaline phosphatase has been shown to be affected by the level of nutrition; dogs fed a restricted amount of a high calcium diet had a higher serum alkaline phosphatase than dogs fed the same diet ad libitum.

Radiology

Radiographic appearance often helps to diagnose nutrition related orthopaedic diseases. However diagnosis solely by radiology is difficult at a young age, early in the course of low grade disease and with combined aetiologies. Newer imaging techniques may prove to be helpful in diagnosis of certain skeletal diseases.

Importance of a Thorough Dietary History

In orthopaedic conditions seen in very young animals a dietary history should include information on the maternal diet. Although fetal growth and lactation are protected from deficiencies in maternal diet, an inadequate diet may reduce the amount of milk produced. Theoretically toxic substances and amounts of nutrients in the maternal diet may interfere with normal development. For example, sledge dogs on accidental high intake of lead have given birth to stunted pups.

If milk substitutes are given instead of maternal milk or as supplements, their ingredients and chemical composition should be evaluated critically.

The type of weaning diet and the amount fed is the next critical stage for evaluation. As soon as a significant part of a young animal's diet is no longer supplied by maternal milk then all nutrient requirements should be accounted for by the weaning diet, whether this is commercially prepared or homemade, together with snacks or supplements. As diets of puppies and kittens are frequently changed, these changes in composition and amount should be documented along with any extended periods of diarrhoea or other signs of malassimilation.

Evaluation of a Dietary History

The composition of the diet and the total amount fed (i.e. ordinary diet, snacks and supplements) should be evaluated to see whether it supplies a complete and balanced diet for that animal at that particular stage of life (see Chapters 2 to 7). Information on exercise regimens should be considered and allowances made for individual and environmental variation. The final estimation of adequacy must, of necessity, often be a crude one.

THERAPY

If a dietary history indicates an unbalanced diet and /or too high or too low an intake, a change in feeding regimen and /or choice of food should be instigated. It may be necessary to modify the diet rather than instigate a drastic change if the client is reluctant to abandon the original diet. Successful therapy will then depend on the ability to calculate the formulation of the modified diet to provide a complete and balanced diet (see Chapter 2) and to estimate the appropriate amount to be fed.

Changing to an alternative complete and balanced diet with a validated claim of adequacy requires the compliance of both client and patient, and precludes the feeding of supplemental food sources. Rough guidelines

Symptom		Differential Diagnosis
Conformity	Bulging / Broadening of metaphyseal regions	metaphyseal osteopathy / rickets
	Deviation of bone axis	retained cartilage / rickets
Function	Weakness	storage diseases /nutritional myopathy
	Limping	nutritional secondary hyperparathyroidism / enostosis / osteochondrosis
Pain	On manipulation	osteochondroses
	On palpation	enostosis / metaphyseal osteopathy

Table 20.5: *Symptoms related to disease affecting developing bone in general (one or more legs).*

1) Evaluate CLINICALLY the possibility that the condition is either caused or affected by nutrition by comparing with diseases known to be caused or affected by nutrition. (Tables 20.2 and 20.3) epidemiology (age, sex, breed) clinical history clinical signs radiology clinical biochemistry
2) Evaluate NUTRITIONALLY the possibility that nutrition plays a role by obtaining a complete dietary history: dietary composition by analysis or by declaration amount fed by estimation or by approximation and compare it to known needs: nutritional balance of diet relative to stage of life (see Chapters 3 and 5) amount fed relative to body weight stage of life (see Chapters 3 and 5)
IF A CONDITION APPEARS TO BE NUTRITIONALLY RELATED 3) Correct dietary composition: by change of diet or by supplementation / deduction from diet fed
4) Change the amount fed most commonly by a reduction of total food intake

Table 20.6: *Step by step approach to orthopaedic disease suspected of being nutrition related.*

on how much to feed during growth is given for commercial diets, but it should be emphasised how difficult it is to give accurate advice under variable circumstances.

Overcorrection

It is never justified to 'overcorrect' a diet for any nutrient. A complete and balanced diet is the most suitable diet as long as the patient's ability to handle nutrients is normal. Short-term effects of 'overcorrection' are difficult to monitor and may well create new problems.

Therapeutic Measures

Whilst it is beyond the scope of this chapter to give advice on therapeutic measures, it is, however, important to put nutritional therapeutics in perspective. It is important to decide whether nutritional changes alone are sufficient or whether they should be considered as an integrated part of a number of measures. Feeding adequate amounts of a complete and balanced diet is likely to suffice in those orthopaedic diseases which are caused by nutritional inadequacy (like rickets, NSH, hyper- and hypovitaminosis A) but have not been complicated by fractures, bowing and permanent deviations of bone axes.

Because of unknown aetiology little can be done for metaphyseal osteopathy and enostosis besides assuring a balanced diet in restricted amounts. In most cases of osteochondroses, fragmented coronoid process and ununited anconeal process surgery is recommended. Early detection and correction being mandatory for a successful outcome.

Nutrition is crucial in patients undergoing radiotherapy and /or chemotherapy. Nutrition in the case of osteosarcoma is determined mostly by the side effects of the therapy.

Optimal nutrition for various types of osteoarthritic changes still has to be determined, although many compounds including nutrients have been claimed to alleviate symptoms. Until that has been done NSAID and other medications and methods to alleviate pain should be the prime consideration.

Reduced food intake of a balanced diet is always justified in developmental orthopaedic diseases and degenerative conditions; the objective is to avoid or to reduce overweight.

Prevention is the Key

As with most diseases, prevention of nutrition related orthopaedic diseases is more rewarding than treatment. Nutritional secondary hyperparathyroidism, rickets, hypo- and hypervitaminoses A and steatitis are all caused by faulty nutrition and are therefore totally prevented by feeding a complete and balanced diet in optimal amounts. It is equally important to realise that genetic disorders that mimic nutrition related orthopaedic problems are neither prevented nor cured by nutrition. Congenital and developmental diseases like achondroplasia, mucopolysaccharidosis and calcinosis circumscripta will remain regardless of diets. At best diet can be used to partly affected their clinical course.

How Much is Too Much?

In developmental diseases with multiple or unknown aetiology, like enostoses, hip dysplasia, osteochondroses and metaphyseal osteopathy, reduced intake of a complete and balanced diet affects the clinical course to such an extent that it is worth mentioning as a preventive measure.

Thanks to fairly extensive knowledge, precise recommendation can be given about dietary composition for both dogs and cats under various circumstances (see Chapters 3 to 7). The amount of food to be given is much more difficult to define for individual feeding. Breed differences and individual variation in genetic make-up, together with environmental factors such as exercise and ambient temperature, have a major impact on the amount of food consumed. It seems however that the amount of food, as it affects skeletal development, is of paramount importance only for large and giant sized breeds in which the genetic capacity for maximal rate of growth seems exaggerated.

Having advocated optimal rate of growth in these breeds rather than maximal, we are still left with the difficulty of defining optimal growth rate to our clients and advising how it should be achieved. Growth charts, even when subdivided by breed and sex, together with recommended energy intake for stage of growth and projected final size, may still only be regarded as guidelines. Palpable body fat is not sufficiently specific to define optimal nutrition during growth. A lean pup may consume at a rate that would appear to be greater than that compatible with optimal skeletal characteristics.

Comparing an individual with litter-mates and other dogs of the same breed and age as outlined in published growth charts (Kirk and Bistner, 1985) and comparing caloric intake to published guidelines is advisable (see Chapter 5). If the dietary composition is right, it is safe to recommend that the amount to be fed during the most rapid growth phase in large and giant breeds should be too little rather than too much. At worst such a feeding practice could only marginally affect final size as the period of growth will be extended. At best it would allow for less serious manifestations of nutrition related orthopaedic disease.

REFERENCES/SUGGESTED READING

Chambers JN (1993). Lameness. In: *Small Animal Medical Diagnosis, 2nd edition.* Eds MD Lorenz and LM Cornelius. Lippincott, Philadelphia.

Groendalen J and Hedhammar Å (1982). Nutrition of the rapidly growing dog with special reference to skeletal disease. In: *Nutrition and Behaviour in Dogs and Cats.* Ed RS Anderson. Pergamon Press, Oxford.

Hazewinkel HAW, Van den Brom WE, Van't Klooster ATH *et al.* (1991). Calcium metabolism in Great Dane dogs fed diets with various calcium and phosphorus levels. *Journal of Nutrition* **112,** S99.

Hazewinkel HAW (1994). Skeletal Disease. In: *The Waltham Book of Clinical Nutrition of the Dog and Cat.* Eds JM Wills and KW Simpson. Pergamon Press, Oxford pp 395-423.

Hedhammar Å, Wu F, Krook L *et al.* (1974) Overnutrition and skeletal disease: an experimental study in growing Great Dane dogs. *Cornell Veterinarian* **64**(Suppl.), 1.

Kirk RW and Bistner S (1985). Normal physiological data. In: *Handbook of Veterinary Procedures and Emergency Treatment, 4th edition.* WB Saunders, Philadelphia.

Lorenz MD (1993). Retarded growth. In: *Small Animal Medical Diagnosis, 2nd edition.* Eds MD Lorenz and LM Cornelius. Lippincott, Philadelphia.

Nap RC, Hazewinkel HAW, Voorhout G *et al.* (1991). Growth and skeletal development in Great Dane pups fed different levels of protein intake. *Journal of Nutrition* **121,** S107.

Toombs JP and Widmer WR (1993). Bone, joint, and periskeletal swelling or enlargement. In: *Small Animal Medical Diagnosis, 2nd edition.* Eds MD Lorenz and LM Cornelius. Lippincott, Philadelphia.

PART IV

Small Pets and Exotics

CHAPTER TWENTY-ONE

Small Pets – Food Types, Nutrient Requirements and Nutritional Disorders

Graham Tobin

INTRODUCTION

This chapter describes the main foods that are commonly used for small pets such as rats, mice, gerbils, rabbits, guinea pigs and hamsters, the nutrient requirements of these species, and the most common disorders arising from malnutrition.

CHARACTERISTICS OF COMMERCIALLY PREPARED FEEDS AND SUPPLEMENTS

Commercially prepared feeds may be complete feeds, complementary feeds or feed supplements. Complete feeds should provide all the nutrients required by an animal in the correct quantities. Sometimes feeds marketed as complete may not meet this objective, either because the manufacturer is unaware of the amounts of nutrients required, or does not adequately allow for the losses that occur in manufacture and storage or for financial reasons does not add adequate amounts of some of the more expensive ingredients such as vitamins.

Complementary feeds are a mixture of feedstuffs that contain ingredients that provide high levels of certain nutrients, for example protein, minerals and vitamins, that may be deficient in the balance of the diet. Such feeds are most likely to be used in conjunction with home-prepared feeds based on simple easily obtainable ingredients, for example hamster seed mixes.

Feed supplements are usually concentrated sources of trace minerals and vitamins and are usually used to supplement complete diets where there may be doubt as to the nutritional adequacy. The supplements may be powders that are to be dissolved in drinking water or oil-based. The main forms of these diet types are described below.

Pelleted Feeds

Pelleted feeds are cylinders of compressed feed ingredients usually about 9–15 mm in diameter for rats, mice and hamsters and 3–4 mm for rabbits and guinea pigs.

The use of pelleted feed allows the introduction of ingredients on the basis of their nutritional qualities rather than visual appeal. It also permits easy incorporation of dusty mineral and vitamin premixes with often unpleasant texture and taste. Such minerals and vitamins may also be toxic if ingested in excess and blending them in the feed will ensure even distribution and ingestion in appropriate amounts.

Pelleting usually ensures the intake of a balanced diet since the grinding, blending and compression means that the animal is unable to select out favoured ingredients, though identifiable traces of the ingredients can usually be detected in the pellet. However animals such as the rat may waste much feed if the pellet contains a high level of an unpalatable ingredient.

Pellet hardness is very important. A diet that is too hard may prevent the intake of an adequate amount of food and lead to poor growth and often hair loss. The rat is more sensitive to pellet hardness than the mouse. A diet that is too soft may be good for growth but lead to high wastage. A good generalisation is that the pellet should be capable of being snapped between the thumb and first finger without undue force and pain to the digits.

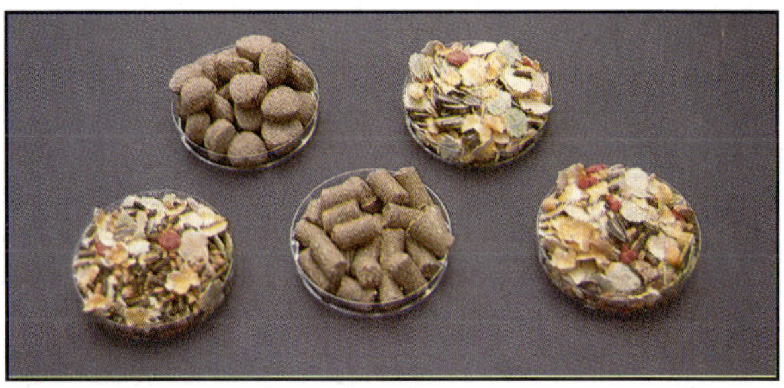

Figure 21.1: Rat, mouse and hamster diets. Front left: rat and mouse coarse mix. Clockwise: extruded rat and mouse diet, hamster mix, 'high grade' hamster mix, pelleted rat and mouse diet.

Extruded (Expanded) Feeds

Extruded feed typically has a lower density than the equivalent conventional pellet, and is porous and biscuit-like. A greater variety of shapes is possible with extruded diet, e.g. cylinders, rings, star shapes, and these may affect food intake. Extruded diet can be produced with a much higher fat content than a conventional pelleted diet, though this is more relevant to the feeding of dogs and cats.

A high operating temperature during manufacture and a drying stage results in a low microbiological count in the product and with good storage conditions very long shelf lives can be obtained. The process is more damaging to vitamins than conventional pelleting but digestibility and palatability is improved. Wastage by animals is reported as being less than with conventional pellets.

Extruded diets have the same advantages as pelleted diets in terms of providing a blend of ingredients from which the animal cannot select favoured items, thereby providing a balanced diet.

Currently, apart from being extensively used for dogs and cats, extruded diets are fed primarily to rats, mice and hamsters used in research, but there is no reason why the benefits of such diets cannot be spread more widely. Rabbits and guinea pigs are not fed extruded diets.

Coarse Mixes

Coarse mixes are blends mainly of whole ingredients. The mixes may be supplemented with molasses and vegetable oil to aid palatability and reduce dust levels. Typical ingredients include cereals, oilseeds, dried vegetables such as peas and beans and pieces of dried forage. The cereals, oilseeds and vegetables may be intact whole seeds or have received some form of processing. The main forms of processing may be 'cold', such as coarse grinding, cracking, crushing and rolling, or 'hot', such as flaking, micronising or popping. The cold processes allow the endosperm to be made easily available to the animal's digestive system. The 'hot' processes increase the digestibility of the material.

Coarse mixes may also include conventional pellets. These pellets may be a convenient way of introducing individual ingredients such as lucerne or may contain blends of ingredients that contribute nutrients that otherwise would be in short supply. Such pellets may be used to carry trace elements and vitamins and boost the protein level of the mix. However many manufacturers imply that pellets are a second rate ingredient, which nutritionally may be nonsense.

Coarse mixes look more attractive than simple pelleted product, and this has caused them to become probably the main form of food for small pets. The more bland looking pelleted feeds, despite their ability to delivered a balanced range of nutrients, have come to be regarded as 'second rate' since visual appeal to the owner is unfortunately often more important than a nutritional declaration. Coarse mixes also provide variability in the diet of the animal. However it is more difficult to ensure a balanced intake of nutrients with such feeds, since some items may be preferentially selected by the animal and bland pelleted diets may be better in achieving a healthy long life.

Powders

The use of diets and feeds whose adequacy in providing minerals, particularly trace minerals, and vitamins is doubtful, has led to the development of powdered supplements, usually to be added to the drinking water. These supplements are often called conditioning powders and provide, in the correct dosage, the animal's requirement for minerals and vitamins. The ingredients are in water-soluble or water-dispersible forms. A good well balanced diet will not require additional supplements.

Liquid Feeds

Liquid feeds for healthy small pets are unusual, however some manufacturers provide oil-based supplements that are to be added to the dry feed to provide the fat-soluble vitamins. It is relatively easy to produce hypervitaminosis of the fat-soluble vitamins. Great care needs to be taken in supplementing with fat-soluble vitamins, and the manufacturers' instructions must be followed precisely.

Treats

Treat sticks are available commercially and are often known as honey treats. These are usually mixtures of seeds, nuts and dried fruits, and sometimes other ingredients, including minerals and vitamins, set in a honey or caramelised base around a stick. As well as providing nutrients, the sticks provide an opportunity for gnawing.

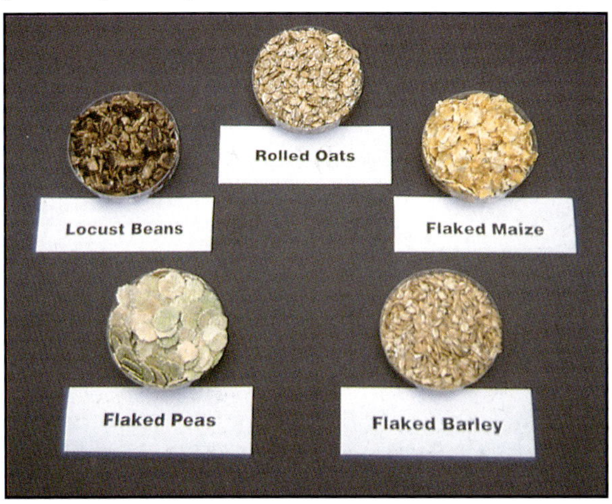

***Figure 21.2:** Some common coarse mix ingredients.*

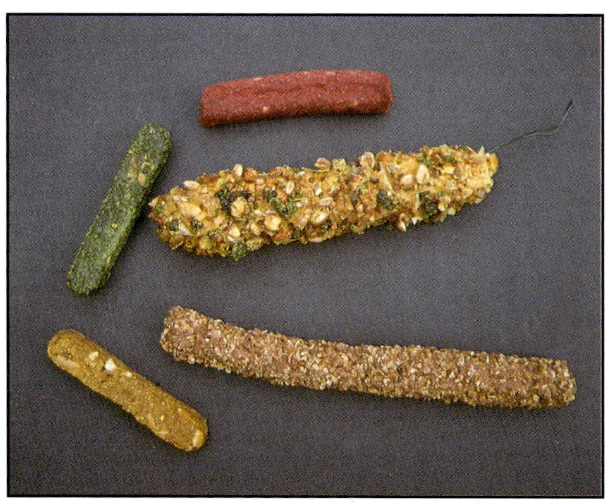

***Figure 21.3:** Treats for rabbits and hamsters.*

CHARACTERISTICS OF INGREDIENTS FOR COMMERCIAL AND HOME-PREPARED FOODS

Diets for small pets can be made up by the owner from ingredients available from agricultural merchants, pet shops, and food retailers. The use of home-produced foods should be treated with caution unless the owner has a good grasp of the animal's nutritional requirements and is able to formulate diets to meet the requirement. Diet formulation and nutritional knowledge are skills that are not easily attained, and there is much to be lost by the approach of trial and error.

Many of the materials below are used in commercially prepared feeds and the comments apply equally to those feeds.

Cereals

The main cereals that are used for diets are barley, maize, oats and wheat. They are good sources of energy, with modest levels of protein, typically 8–12%. The main amino acid deficiency is that of lysine, and they are not unduly rich in methionine and cystine. With the exception of oats, they are low in fibre. Cereals are deficient in calcium, and although phosphate levels are about twice those of calcium much is in the form of phytates and about half is unavailable. The phytates also make several of the other minerals unavailable, for example calcium, magnesium and zinc. The cereals are deficient in vitamin D and, with the exception of maize, vitamin A and its provitamins. They are good sources of vitamin E and B_1 (thiamin).

Whole cereals may be difficult for some animals to eat, so they are often processed. However whole maize, because of its relatively large size, can be handled by many rodents. Crushed, rolled, flaked, micronised, and popped forms of cereals are usually available. Heat treatment increases the digestibility of the cereals.

Processed cereal products for human consumption can also be used, but are a relatively expensive option.

Vegetables

The main vegetables that are used in small animal diets are roots, tubers, 'leafy vegetables' and legume seeds such as peas and beans. Roots, tubers and leafy vegetables are usually fed in their 'as harvested' state whilst peas and beans are in the dried form.

Roots

Roots such as carrots, fodder beet, mangolds, parsnips, sugar beet, swedes and turnips have a high moisture content (75–95%), and a low protein, starch and fibre content. Most of the dry matter is in the form of sugars. Carrots have rich supplies of carotenes, and these provitamin A compounds are also found in parsnips. Generally the roots are poor sources of vitamins.

Tubers

The primary tuber is potato. It has a higher dry matter content than the roots, though it still has a low fibre and protein content. Instead of sugars, the main carbohydrate is starch.

About half the crude protein (N x 6.25) content is in the form of non-protein nitrogenous compounds, of which probably the main one is solanidine. Solanidine is a toxic alkaloid that is found in the free form or as a glyco-alkaloid in the form of chaconine and solanine. The concentration of these alkaloids may be increased in potatoes that have been exposed to light. These alkaloids can cause severe gastrointestinal disturbances.

Cooking the potatoes substantially decreases their toxicity, and this is the form in which they are usually eaten. Cooking also improves the digestibility of the starch and also of what little protein there is. Green potatoes, caused by the production of chlorophyll, should never be fed, and nor should the young potato shoots, which are rich in alkaloids.

Potatoes are poor sources of minerals and of most vitamins. They do contain small quantities of vitamin C, though this is decreased in storage and by about 50% during cooking.

Leafy Vegetables

Several leafy vegetables can be fed to small pets. They include items such as Brussels sprouts, cabbage, celery, endive, kale, lettuce, spring greens, and spinach. In the fresh form they have a high moisture content (90–95%), and a low content of protein and fibre. The carbohydrate is a mixture of sugars, which predominate, and starch. Because of their role in photosynthesis, leafy vegetables contain quite high levels of minerals and vitamins (on a dry matter basis) that are involved in the process, namely carotene, vitamin K, vitamin C, calcium, iron and magnesium. They also contain moderate amounts of vitamin B_2 (riboflavin) and folate and large amounts of potassium.

The brassicas, which include Brussels sprouts, cabbage, cauliflowers and kale, contain glucosinolate goitrogens in the leaves (and especially their seeds) that decrease the uptake of iodine by the thyroid gland. Whilst it is very unlikely that small amounts of brassica leaves would cause a problem, many experts suggest that they should not be used.

Legume Seeds

The main legume seeds used in home-prepared feeds are field beans and peas. These are usually incorporated in the dry form, either as intact seeds or in flaked form. They are quite rich in protein (over 20%), with a high level of lysine, though they are deficient in methionine and cystine. Their amino acid pattern complements that of the cereals, and a blend of the two can produce a good protein source. Legume seeds are rich in fibre, but low in oil. The seeds are poor sources of calcium but are high in phosphorus; they contain little or no sodium, chloride or manganese. They contain modest levels of most of the B vitamins but little or no carotene, or the fat-soluble vitamins.

Legume seeds often have antinutritional factors such as tannins in the seed coat, phytohaemagglutinins, and trypsin inhibitors. Plant breeders have now produced varieties in which the level of such factors is low, and most of the new varieties grown in Europe contain little or no antinutritional activity. Steam treatment will inactivate most of the antinutritional factors, and flaking of peas and beans involves the application of steam. Nevertheless the inclusion of these ingredients should be restricted.

Many of the beans of the genus *Phaseolus*, including kidney beans, navy beans and butter beans, are toxic to rodents when fed raw, and should never be used.

Other Seeds

Locust beans seem to be a popular ingredient in the UK both for home and commercial coarse mixes. There are two materials commonly referred to as locust beans: the Mediterranean carob bean (*Ceratomia siliqua*) and the African locust bean (*Parkia filicoidea*). The carob tree is grown for its fleshy pods, which with its enclosed seeds is ground and used as an animal feed. The main material used in pet foods is the African locust bean, which is supplied as the whole dark brown seed. Both materials are very sweet but the carob bean, although highly palatable, contains tannic acid which reduces digestibility. The African locust bean contains modest levels of protein (c. 14%) and oil (c. 8%) but is a poor source of vitamins.

Fruits

Many fruits can be used in small quantities in home-prepared diets. Generally their most significant contribution to the diet, other than variety, is vitamin C. They also contain high levels of fibre and can make a minor contribution to the intake of carotene and the B vitamins. They contain little protein or fat, but do have modest levels of available carbohydrate mainly in the form of sugars. Fruits also contain high levels of organic acids whose concentrations fall during the ripening process. Some care must be taken that these acids do not irritate the membranes of the mouth of the feeding animal.

Oilseeds

Several oilseeds are used whole in diets, mainly groundnut (peanut), and sunflower and sesame seeds. Several other extracted oilseeds, such as soya bean and linseed, are used as ingredients in complete feeds but are not usually sold for inclusion in home-prepared diets. The intact seeds have modest levels of protein (15-25% protein and high levels of fat (20-50%). The protein in the seeds is of good quality being readily digested but the protein is usually low in lysine, methionine and cystine. Sunflowers have a large amount of fibre, but this is primarily in the husk, which animals usually discard. The seeds have a low calcium content but a high phosphorus level. The intact seed contains modest levels of vitamin E, but little or no other fat-soluble vitamins; they also contain modest levels of the B vitamins.

Care needs to be taken in the use of peanuts: they must always be of best quality. Poor quality and mouldy peanuts may contain aflatoxins.

Herbage

One of the most common herbages commercially available for inclusion in home-prepared diets is lucerne (alfalfa); this is usually supplied in dried, chopped form or in pellets. It is a good ingredient for diets for herbivores such as rabbits and guinea pigs. It has a modest content of protein and is rich in fibre and many minerals, including calcium (though it is low in phosphorus). It contains high levels of carotene (provitamin A) and vitamin E.

Hay is also used both as a bedding and a feed supplement in diets for herbivores. It can be produced from a range of grass types and from legumes such as lucerne. Its quality can be highly variable, and only good sweet smelling hay should be used. Good quality hay has a modest level of protein, 8-12% in grasses and 14-22% in legumes, and a high level of fibre, 25-35%. It is a good source of carotene.

Home-prepared diets can also use freshly gathered grass, clover and edible plant leaves. They contain a variable level of protein, which is usually higher in fresh immature material, and fibre; the protein level is inversely related to the fibre level. The mineral content is variable and depends on environmental and soil conditions. Fresh herbage contains high levels of carotene, and is usually a good source of vitamin E and B vitamins. Some experts suggest that fresh material should only be introduced in small quantities. Some plants may contain toxic materials and care must be taken in their selection for use.

Animal Matter

A variety of animal products can be used in home-prepared diets, even for some herbivores. They include meats, fish, fat, eggs, cheese and live animals such as meal worms. Generally such material is rich in protein, which is of very good quality with an amino acid profile that matches the animal's requirement. The amount of fat will vary with the product. Meats are usually rich in iron and phosphorus but are poor in calcium; they are good sources of B vitamins but contain little fat-soluble vitamins. Fish contains only small amounts of vitamins and minerals, though fish oils are rich sources of the fat-soluble vitamins. Many species of fish contain thiaminase which destroys thiamin, and any fish used should be cooked to remove any thiaminase that might be present. Eggs are good sources of calcium, iron, vita-

	Rats, Mice, Gerbils, Hamsters	Guinea Pigs, Rabbits
Energy Sources	**Cereals** (Whole, crushed, flaked, extruded, micronised, ground) *barley, maize, oats, wheat* **Kitchen Scraps** *cooked potatoes and vegetables, corn flakes, crisps, crackers* **Oils and Fats** *maize oil, soya oil, vegetable oils, tallow* **Molasses** (Liquid, dried)	**Cereals** (Whole, crushed, flaked, extruded, micronised, ground) *barley, maize, oats, wheat* **Oils and Fats** *maize oil, soya oil, vegetable oils, tallow* **Molasses** (Liquid, dried)
Protein Sources	**Vegetable Proteins** (Whole, crushed, flaked, micronised, ground) *linseed meal, maize gluten meal, wheatfeed, soyabean meal, peas, peanuts, field beans, locust beans, oilseeds* **Animal Proteins** (ground) *Fish meal, meat meals, meat and bone meals* **Kitchen Scraps**[1] *raw and cooked meat, boned cooked fish* **Synthetic Amino Acids** *lysine, methionine*	**Vegetable Proteins** (Whole, crushed, flaked, micronised, ground) *linseed meal, maize gluten meal, wheatfeed, soyabean meal, peas, field beans, locust beans, oilseeds* **Animal Proteins** (ground) *Fish meal, meat meals, meat and bone meals* **Synthetic Amino Acids** *lysine, methionine*
Fibre Sources	Not usually specifically required.	**Cereal Products** (ground) *oatfeed, wheatfeed, wheat bran* Vegetable Fibre *grass meal, hay, lucerne, sugar beet pulp* Root Crops *carrots, swedes, turnips, fodder and sugar beet*
Vitamin Sources	**Natural Raw Materials** *brewer's yeast (B vitamins), grass meal, lucerne (provitamin A), wheat germ, whey powder (B-vitamins), raw vegetables and fruits* **Pure Vitamins**	**Natural Raw Materials** *brewer's yeast (B vitamins), grass meal, lucerne (provitamin A), wheat germ, whey powder (B vitamins), raw vegetables and fruits* **Pure Vitamins**
Mineral Sources	**Natural Raw Materials** limestone flour (Ca), dicalcium phosphate (Ca, P), calcined magnesite (Mg), magnesium oxide (Mg), salt (Na, Cl), vegetables and fruit Mineral Salts *Trace elements*	**Natural Raw Materials** limestone flour (Ca), dicalcium phosphate (Ca, P), calcined magnesite (Mg), magnesium oxide (Mg), salt (Na, Cl), vegetables and fruit Mineral Salts *Trace elements*

	Rats, Mice, Gerbils, Hamsters	Guinea Pigs, Rabbits
Fresh Forage	Not usually supplied to rats and mice, though access is unlikely to be deleterious. Hamsters should be given fresh fruits and vegetables. These can be taken from the list opposite.	**Vegetables**[2] *carrot leaves, cauliflower and cauliflower leaves, celery, chicory, Chinese cabbage, corn-on-the-cob, endive, kale, lettuce leaves, parsley, spinach, spring greens, string beans* **Fruits**[3] *apples, melons, pears, strawberries, tomatoes* **Wild plants** *wide variety of grasses and plants, including bindweed, chickweed, clover, coltsfoot, dandelions, groundsel, lucerne, plantains, poppies, sainfoin, shepherd's purse, sorrel, vetches and wild radish*

Table 21.1: *Typical ingredients used in small pet diets.*

1 *Not usually given to gerbils.*
2 *Individual vegetables should be given in small quantities, since some may cause digestive disturbances when fed at high levels.*
3 *Many fruits are acidic and may irritate the lining of the mouth. The quantities should be limited and the fruit cut into small pieces. The material should be removed if problems arise.*

min A and B vitamins, and cheese is a good source of calcium, vitamin A and riboflavin.

Great care must be taken to remove uneaten material before food spoilage occurs.

Potential Contaminants

When using freshly gathered materials, great care must be taken to ensure that such materials are clean and disease-free. For example, a disease such as coccidiosis may be spread to pet rabbits if grass is collected from areas where wild rabbits graze. Materials gathered from the road side may be contaminated with vehicle exhausts and may be fouled by dogs. Care must also be taken to ensure that materials have not been recently treated with pesticides and herbicides. To minimise the introduction of contaminants, fresh materials should be washed in a mild disinfectant like Savlon (ICI), rinsed and then dried.

Many wild plants are toxic to animals, so only plants that can be identified and are known to be safe should be used.

INGREDIENTS USED IN SMALL PET DIETS

Table 21.1 provides examples of typical ingredients used in diets for small pets. The pets have been divided into two broad groups, those that require a high fibre diet and those that do not. Materials used in pelleted diet are finely ground whilst those used in coarse mixes are whole or crushed. Items listed as being a source of a particular dietary component will inevitably contribute other components, but are categorised on the basis of their main contribution.

Plants to Avoid

Many weeds, for example belladonna, buttercups, celandine, docks, dogbane, foxglove, hemlock and nightshade, may be poisonous or produce adverse effects and should be avoided. A small amount of dried buttercups in hay should not pose a problem. As a 'rule of thumb', plants raised from bulbs should be avoided. Pets should not be fed any plants that cannot be recognised as non-poisonous. Some vegetables such as cabbage, dandelions, head lettuce, and potato tops should not be fed in large quantities because they can cause flatulence and diarrhoea.

Food Composition Tables

Information on the nutrient levels of feed ingredients can be obtained from many sources. It is important to recognise that these are typical figures and may not accurately reflect the composition of the ingredient in use. They may be averages of only a few analyses. A list of some good sources of information is given below.

Useful Reference Sources

Several of the National Research Council (NRC) publications on the nutrient requirements of domestic animals contain nutrient composition tables for ingredients used in their diets. Tables are included in the publications for dogs, cats, mink and foxes, and rabbits.

The National Academy of Sciences, Washington D.C., publishes two compilations of feed ingredients:

- Publication 1684, *United States-Canadian Tables of Feed Composition.*
- Publication 1919, *Atlas of Nutritional Data on United States and Canadian Feeds.*

UK Tables of Feed Composition and Nutritive Value for Ruminants compiled by the Ministry of Agriculture, Fisheries and Food Standing Committee on Tables of Feed Composition and published in 1986 by Chalcombe Publications, Marlow, Bucks provides data that are equally useful for a range of small pets.

Many commercial companies provide data on the nutritional content of feed ingredients. Roche Products Ltd (Welwyn Garden City, Herts, UK) produced an excellent compilation called Vitec, Animal Nutrition and Vitamin News that over three volumes provided much valuable data on food composition and Novus (Cirencester, Glos., UK) produces a book of raw material tables entitled 'Raw Material Compendium'.

McCance and Widdowson's The Composition of Foods edited by B. Holland, A.A. Welch, I.D. Unwin, D.H. Buss, A.A. Paul and D.A.T. Southgate and published in 1994 in its 5th Edition by The Royal Society of Chemistry provides data on human foods that might be used for pets.

Data on Nutritional Requirements

Availability and Reliability of Data

For purposes of simplicity and brevity the values given in the sections below are estimates made by the author on the basis of published data. There has been no attempt to justify scientifically these estimates, for this is outside the scope of a chapter of this size. The values given are the levels that should be present when the diet is fed to the animal, and which are unlikely to result in nutritional deficiency. In judging whether a specific diet is adequate, allowance will have to be made for losses in any manufacture and storage.

Variation in Dietary Ingredients

One of the difficult areas in feeding small pets is whether to have variation in the ingredients in the diet or whether to feed a fixed-formula diet. Both approaches have advantages and a sensible approach needs to be taken.

Advantages of Diet Variation

Novelty. Many owners consider the feeding of their pets with human emotions. Thus just as they wish for variety and novelty in their own diet, most owners consider that such factors are important for healthy contented pets. Even 'treats' with different colours and flavours are now available for small pets.

Stimulation. In restricted conditions, with little other stimulation in the cage, a constantly changing range of dietary ingredients may do much to alleviate boredom, particularly if it involves some foraging activity.

Balanced diet. A diet composed of a wide range of ingredients taken from the main feed categories, i.e.

	Weight (g)	10	15	20	25	30	35	40	45
	$W^{0.75}$	0.032	0.043	0.053	0.063	0.072	0.081	0.089	0.097
Stage	kcal/$W^{0.75}$ [1]								
Maintenance	110	3.5	4.7	5.9	6.9	7.9	8.9	9.8	10.7
Growth	145	4.6	6.2	7.7	9.1	10.5	11.7	13.0	14.2
Gestation	145	4.6	6.2	7.7	9.1	10.5	11.7	13.0	14.2
Lactation	440	14.0	18.8	23.6	27.6	31.6	35.6	39.2	42.8

Table 21.2: *Estimated daily metabolisable energy requirements (kcal) for mice at different stages of development.*

	Weight (g)	50	100	150	200	300	400	600	800
	$W^{0.75}$	0.106	0.178	0.241	0.299	0.405	0.503	0.682	0.846
Stage	kcal/$W^{0.75}$ [1]								
Maintenance	110	11.6	19.6	26.5	32.9	44.6	55.3	75.0	93.0
Growth	145	15.3	25.8	34.9	43.4	58.8	72.9	98.9	122.7
Gestation	145	15.3	25.8	34.9	43.4	58.8	72.9	98.9	122.7
Lactation	440	46.4	78.4	106.0	131.6	178.4	221.2	300.0	372.0

Table 21.3: *Estimated daily metabolisable energy requirements (kcal) for rats at different stages of development.*

[1] *1kcal = 4.184kJ.*

cereals, oilseeds, vegetables, fruits, etc., is less likely to result in a nutritional deficiency than a diet based on a few ingredients of similar type. However it is important that particular favoured items are restricted in availability to ensure that there is no preferential ingestion of one or a few items at the expense of a balanced diet.

Disadvantages of Diet Variation

Gastrointestinal disturbances. Substantial sudden changes in dietary ingredients often lead to gastrointestinal disturbances until the digestive system adjusts to the new pattern of nutrients. Any changes should be phased in over one or two weeks. Where a mixture of ingredients are fed, it is usually possible to change one item from each of the categories each day.

Inappetance. A sudden change of diet in some species, particularly the rabbit, may lead to inappetance, and the animal may starve itself to death rather than eat a new diet.

Overeating and obesity. One of the advantages of diet variation was stated to be novelty. Unfortunately novelty may lead to overeating - the animal eating for pleasure rather than energy. Whilst this may give a contented animal, it will also give a fat, even obese animal, whose life expectancy is severely decreased. With this in mind, the animal given a well designed but bland conventional pelleted diet may be better off in the long term. Certainly it is good practice to avoid giving the animal treats and tit bits.

RATS AND MICE

Because of their widespread use in research, the nutrient requirements of rats and mice are well defined. Nutrient requirements for rats and mice have been published by Clarke *et al.* (1977) and the NRC (1978).

Nutrient Requirements

Energy

Based on published data, the daily metabolisable energy requirements of rats and mice are set at:

maintenance energy requirement = 110kcal (462kJ) per $kg^{0.75}$

growth energy requirement = 145kcal (609kJ) per $kg^{0.75}$

gestation energy requirement = 145kcal (609kJ) per $kg^{0.75}$

lactation energy requirements = 440kcal (1840kJ) per $kg^{0.75}$

Estimates of energy requirements of mice and rats at different body weights can be seen in Tables 21.2 and 21.3, respectively.

Uncertainty in the estimates of the energy needs of rodents is of little practical importance since they are usually able to adjust their food intake to meet their energy requirements. Because rat and mouse diets typically have a high metabolisable energy density, unlike rabbit and guinea pig diets, these rodents are usually able to meet most of their increased energy requirements in pregnancy and lactation by increased food intake provided that the diet is of high quality and unrestricted in supply. It is not unusual for pregnant or lactating rats to increase food intake 3-4-fold. Modest deficits will be made up by utilising body energy stores, and the animal may reduce its level of activity to conserve energy.

Nutrients

A summary of the nutrient requirements of rats and mice is given in Appendix 1. The data are extrapolated from published tables of nutrient requirements and the author's own experience.

Protein. In practice, breeding diets that contain about 17-20% protein seem satisfactory. Many nutritionists seem reluctant to consider using low protein diets for maintenance, nevertheless there seems to be good evidence for using maintenance diets containing 13-14% good quality protein from soon after weaning at 4 weeks of age.

Fats and fatty acids. The main function of fat in the diet is to provide essential fatty acids, primarily linoleic (18:2) acid. NRC (1978) recommend a level of linoleic acid of about 0.6% of the diet for male and 0.3% for female rats and mice. Maize oil contains about 50% linoleic acid, so that its inclusion in the diet at about 1.2% should meet the requirement. In practice most diets contain more than 3% fat and essential fatty acid deficiency is rare.

Fat also improves palatability and increases the energy density of the diet since it contains about twice the metabolisable energy (9kcal/g) (38kJ/g) as available carbohydrate (4kcal/g) (16.8kJ/g) or protein (4kcal/g) (16.8kJ). If it is difficult for animals to get sufficient energy from low fat diets during pregnancy and lactation, a high fat diet may be beneficial. However high fat diets should be avoided for maintenance since they will cause obesity.

Minerals. There is quite good agreement between Clarke *et al.* (1977) and the NRC (1978) on the requirements of rats and mice for minerals. There are however few data on variation in mineral requirements with age or stage of development, and a single requirement seems to be used throughout life.

Phytates in the diet may limit the availability of some minerals, particularly calcium, phosphorus and zinc. However the levels recommended by Clarke *et al.* (1977) and NRC (1978) will accommodate the presence of typical levels of phytate.

Vitamins. Rats and mice require a dietary source of the fat-soluble vitamins A, D, E, and K. Rats and mice are coprophagic and in theory they may obtain at least some of their requirement for B vitamins by the ingestion of faeces. Because of uncertainty of the effectiveness of coprophagy in meeting all the animals requirements, particularly those on mesh-bottomed cages, it is probably safer for diets to include a vitamin supplement containing B vitamins.

Special Needs

Rats and mice are robust animals and have no special nutritional needs beyond a well balanced nutritionally-sound diet.

Food Types

Rats and mice are omnivorous, and will eat virtually anything that is edible. They will even eat other rats and mice if they detect that they are weakened or injured and can be killed.

The main types of commercial diets for rats and mice are pelleted, though some coarse mixes are available (see Figure 21.1). The omnivorous nature of rats and mice means that all human foods as well as the standard feed ingredients may be used to supply nutrients (see Table 21.1).

The diet needs sources of energy, such as cereals and cereal products, protein, and of minerals and vitamins. There is some evidence that rats and mice can select from a variety of ingredients to produce a reasonably balanced diet. A sensible approach to feeding would be to include elements from each group.

Assessment of Feeding

Most Probable Nutritional Disorders

Obesity. Giving rats and mice unrestricted access to highly palatable foods, and feeding foods as treats is likely to lead to obesity. Obesity in rodents has been shown to be associated with the development of tumours and reduced life span. The welfare of the animal will be better served by feeding a bland purpose-designed pelleted diet.

Further improvements in life expectancy and tumour profile can be achieved by restricting the intake of food to about 60–80% of the typical voluntary intake.

Nephritis. It is common to feed rats and mice excessive amounts of protein, particularly during the maintenance phase. Whilst animals are generally well able to degrade surplus protein, to detoxify the metabolites produced and excrete them, over a period of time this process can lead to kidney damage (referred to as chronic nephritis, nephropathy and several other synonyms). This disease can be recognised as early as 3–6 months of age, progressively developing in severity with increasing proteinuria, and it can lead to death in old animals.

Feeding diets containing 17–20% for breeding and 13–14% for maintenance will minimise the risk of nephritis. There are additional benefits from feeding a low protein diet, since there are observations that high protein intake, particularly in early adult life, can lead to increased risk of neoplasms.

Nephrocalcinosis. Inappropriate dietary levels of calcium, phosphorus and magnesium can lead to nephrocalcinosis, a severe renal disease particularly affecting female rats and mice. The disease is very common and a major cause of premature death.

The disease is typified by deposition of crystals of calcium phosphate in the renal pelvis, the peripheral parts of the renal papillae and tubules. Nephrocalcinosis may be observed in animals within a few weeks of life. There is a strain difference in susceptibility of animals to the disease.

The disease has been extensively studied in animals used in research. It is associated with high levels of dietary calcium and with a calcium:phosphorus ratio of less than unity.

Typically one sees Ca at 1% and P at 0.8% of the diet or more, whilst the NRC requirements are 0.5% for Ca and 0.4% for P. There seems no reason why the concentrations of these elements in maintenance diets cannot more closely approach the NRC values. The main note of caution is that since there is often variation between expected and actual levels of dietary nutrients, as one decreases the absolute values of calcium and phosphorus there is an increasing risk of inadvertently getting an adverse Ca:P ratio.

Dietary magnesium has been found to protect against diet-induced nephrocalcinosis, the protective effect being optimal, with reasonable ranges of calcium and phosphorus, at a level of about 0.20–0.25% of the diet. Any factor that affects the uptake of calcium and phosphorus will affect the incidence of nephrocalcinosis, for example vitamin D concentration and phytates, as will factors that affect the solubility of calcium salts in the kidney such as acidity of the urine (acid urine usually results in decreased nephrocalcinosis).

Vitamin and mineral deficiencies. Vitamin and mineral deficiencies in rats and mice remain a possibility but are unusual with diets from reputable commercial manufacturers. There are several summaries of the symptoms of deficiency, for example NRC (1978) and Rogers (1979).

GERBILS

The natural diet of the gerbil is based on grains and seeds, and when they are available fresh vegetables and roots. The gerbil obtains most of its water requirement from the metabolism of its diet, though drinking water should be made available when only a dry diet is available. Little is known about the precise nutrient requirements of the gerbil, though what is known is covered by the NRC (1978).

Nutrient Requirements

There are few data on the effect of stage of development or age on nutrient requirements.

Energy

In the absence of any other data, the energy requirements of the gerbil can be assumed to be similar to the rat and mouse. The weight of the Mongolian gerbil varies from about 5g at birth to about 50–60g in the adult. Thus the energy requirement can be estimated by combining data from Tables 21.2 and 21.3 that cover mice and rats.

Nutrients

Protein. The protein requirement for growing gerbils is about 17%, which is similar to that for rats and mice.

Fats and fatty acids. The fat and essential fatty acid requirements of the gerbil have not been determined. However gerbils grow better on a 12% fat diet than a natural raw material diet containing about 3–5% fat. Gerbils have a passion for sunflower seeds (30% oil) and gorging may cause a grossly lipaemic serum.

Minerals. No special mineral requirements have been noted and the levels recommended for rats and mice are adequate.

Vitamins. No special vitamin requirements have been noted and the levels recommended for rats and mice are adequate.

Special Needs

No special nutritional requirements have been noted.

Food Types

Gerbils can be fed the same food types as reported for rats and mice. Since the gerbil is largely vegetarian, it is not usual to feed it meat or meat products.

Whilst the juvenile and adult gerbil will perform well on standard rat and mouse pellets, pre-weaning animals may have a high mortality on such diets. The pelleted diet should be supplemented with chopped green vegetables and fruit, and a seed mix that contains only a few sunflower seeds. It is not clear whether the supplement is needed because the pups cannot find or chew the pellets, or because they need an intake of moisture.

Seed mixes are commonly fed, but they should contain few sunflower seeds since the gerbil will select these at the expense of other types. The seed mix should be supplemented with chopped green foods, roots and fruit.

'Honey' treats are also available for gerbils.

Assessment of Feeding

Most Probable Nutritional Disorders

With the exception of lipaemia following ingestion of excessive quantities of sunflower seeds, few nutritional disorders have been described in the gerbil. Like many other rodents their teeth grow continuously and malocclusion may occur unless the diet contains materials that the animal can gnaw on, or unless pieces of wood are added to the animal's environment. It is likely that they suffer from the same problems as rats and mice.

RABBITS

There are several sources of information on nutrient requirements of rabbits at various stages of development, reflecting the widespread use of rabbits for research and commercial meat and wool production. Those published by the NRC (1977) are for rabbits used primarily for research, whilst those of Lebas (1980) and Schlolaut (1982) are for rabbits used for commercial production.

	Weight (kg)	1.0	1.5	2.0	2.5	3.0	3.5	4.0	4.5	5.0
	$W^{0.75}$	1.00	1.36	1.68	1.99	2.28	2.56	2.83	3.09	3.34
Stage	kcal/$W^{0.75}$ [1]									
Maintenance	100	100	136	168	199	228	256	283	309	334
Growth	200	200	272	336	398	456	512	566	618	668
Range	±10	±10	±13	±17	±20	±23	±25	±29	±31	±33
Early gestation	135	135	183	227	268	308	345	382	417	451
Late gestation	200	200	271	336	398	456	512	566	618	669
Lactation	300	300	408	504	597	684	768	849	927	1002

Table 21.4: *Estimated daily metabolisable energy requirements (kcal) for rabbits at different stages of development.*

[1] *1kcal = 4.184kJ.*

Nutrient Requirements

Energy

From published data, an estimate can be made of the energy requirements of rabbits at various stages of development:

maintenance requirements are
100 kcal (418.4kJ).$W^{0.75}$ per day

growth requirements are
190-210 kcal (798-882kJ).$W^{0.75}$ per day.

Requirements at the onset of gestation are maintenance requirement plus one-third, increasing to twice maintenance at the end of gestation. This would give a figure of 135kcal(567kJ).$W^{0.75}$ per day rising to 200kcal (840kJ).$W^{0.75}$ per day.

Requirements for lactation are 300kcal (1260kJ).$W^{0.75}$ per day.

Calculated estimates for the energy requirements of the rabbit using the assumptions above are given in Table 21.4 .

Uncertainty in the estimates for the energy needs for rabbits is not of practical importance since they eat for energy, and will adjust food intake to compensate for the energy concentration of the diet, except where the required food intake exceeds gut capacity. However with a typical diet containing about 2.5kcal ME/g, it is extremely unlikely that the rabbit can eat sufficient food during lactation to meet all its energy requirements, and it is probable that part of the requirement must be met by catabolism of body tissues.

Nutrients

A summary of the nutrient requirements of rabbits is given in Appendix 1. The data are extrapolated from published tables of nutrient requirements and the author's own experience.

Protein. In the absence of further information, it is assumed that the protein requirement as a proportion of available energy is similar over the range of phases of development from the lactating doe to the growing rabbit. Thus about 15-18% protein in the diet will be adequate, providing that protein is of good quality. Where rapid growth is not required, and that will be true for most non-breeding pet rabbits, a lower protein level of 12-13% is beneficial, reducing the likelihood of nephritis and of tumours.

Fats and fatty acids. A fat level of 2% is adequate for the rabbit, and appears to supply adequate amounts of essential fatty acids. The tendency of rabbits to become overweight suggests that dietary fat levels should be kept within the range 2-5%.

Minerals. There is reasonable agreement between authorities on the mineral requirements of rabbits. Nevertheless there is a lack of accurate data on the requirement for minerals at different stages of development and generally similar levels are used throughout.

A substantial proportion of zinc in the diet may be made unavailable by the presence of phytates. A total of 50mg/kg diet should be adequate to overcome this effect.

Vitamins. There seems to be little evidence to determine whether the rabbit requires different levels of dietary vitamins at different stages of development. It is generally accepted that rabbits achieve adequate amounts of the B vitamins to meet their requirements from coprophagy (see below), though some supplementation with B vitamins is usually advisable.

Whilst green material in the diet will contain ß-carotene, a precursor of vitamin A, its level will decline in dried and treated material such as hay and lucerne. Up to 80% of the carotene may be lost in slow sun-drying of forages and there may be losses of about 50% over 6 months of storage of grass meal. Rabbits have been reported as suffering from vitamin A deficiency (xerophthalmia, neural disorders).

Rabbits are also known to be particularly sensitive to vitamin E deficiency, developing muscular dystrophy and myocardial damage; coccidiosis is reported to increase the requirement for vitamin E.

Whilst one would expect coprophagy to meet the rabbit's requirements for vitamin K, there has been evidence of deficiencies adversely affecting reproductive performance. Consequently rabbit diets should at least be fortified with vitamin A, E and K; Clarke *et al.* (1977) recommend 7000IU vitamin A/kg diet, 40mg vitamin E/kg diet, and 2mg of vitamin K/kg diet.

Despite the possibility of coprophagy, many commercial diets will also be fortified with the other vitamins as well to ensure adequacy.

Coprophagy. In addition to the usual hard faecal pellets, the rabbit produces soft 'green' faecal pellets, usually in the morning, that it removes from its anus and ingests. This process is described as coprophagy or pseudo-rumination.

The coprophagous pellets contain about twice the protein of standard faecal pellets, 25-30% of the dry matter, and about half the fibre. The coprophagous pellets also contain large quantities of the B vitamins, which are synthesised in the large intestine. The ingestion of these pellets is thought to supply adequate amounts of the B vitamins and make supplementary B vitamins unnecessary. However, as described above, several manufacturers of rabbit diet do add such vitamins so that reliance on coprophagy is not necessary.

Special Needs

Fibre. Low levels of fibre in the diet give rise to gastrointestinal disturbances, often manifested by diarrhoea. There is some debate as to the minimum amount of fibre necessary. It seems wiser to veer on the safe side and recommend that diets should contain no less than 14% crude fibre to ensure absence of diet-induced enteritis. Ideally one ought to use dietary fibre (a better measure of indigestible fibre) as a measure of adequacy. Unfortunately there are no published data on recommended levels of dietary fibre, though diet-induced enteritis and diarrhoea have been rarely observed in diets containing 30-40% dietary fibre.

If there is doubt about the adequacy of the diet to provide sufficient fibre, hay can be used to supplement the diet. However hay may contain dust and fungal spores that have an adverse affect on the rabbit's health; if hay must be used it should be fresh and of high quality.

ß-Carotene. It is generally assumed that the function of ß-carotene in the rabbit's diet is as precursor of vitamin A; however there is good evidence that ß-carotene has an ability to improve the breeding performance of rabbits even when the level of vitamin A is adequate. The mechanism is unclear, but justifies the recommendation that rabbit diets contain at least 30mg ß-carotene/kg diet, even with adequate dietary vitamin A.

Vitamin E. The rabbit seems to be particularly sensitive to muscular dystrophy induced by vitamin E deficiency. Vitamin E in diet and ingredients may decline by 5-20% per month during storage. As an anti-oxidant, its rate of loss can be accelerated by the presence of oxidisable materials. It seems prudent to ensure that dietary levels of vitamin E are well above the requirement of about 40-50 mg/kg. Diets should always be supplemented with vitamin E, since few diet ingredients contain adequate amounts. Vegetable oils are rich sources of vitamin E; however cod liver oil should not be given since this increases the rate of destruction of vitamin E. The effect of increasing oil content of the diet on vitamin E requirements should be noted: for every 1% oil in the diet, an additional 5mg of vitamin E are needed.

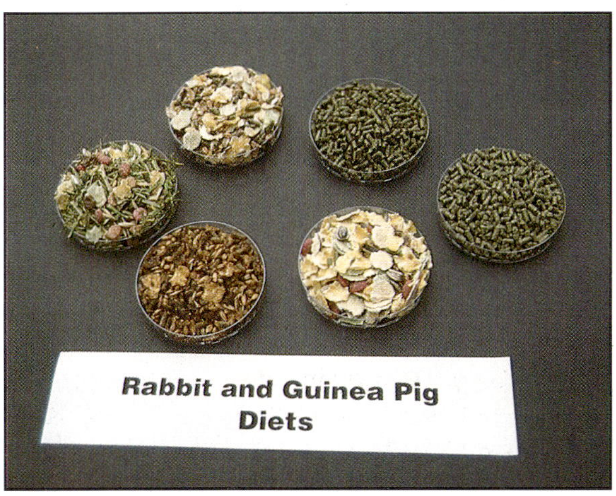

Figure 21.4: *Rabbit and guinea pig diets. Read clockwise from 'brown' diet. Molassed coarse mix for rabbits, coarse mix with lucerne, rabbit coarse mix with pellets, rabbit pellets (dark green), guinea pig pellets (green), guinea pig coarse mix (note sunflower seeds).*

Calcium. The rabbit is unusual in that it appears not to regulate calcium uptake from the gastrointestinal tract. Thus plasma calcium levels reflect dietary levels, and any surplus calcium must be excreted in the urine. Dietary calcium concentrations must closely reflect requirements, being neither excessively high (see below) or even marginally deficient.

Food Types

The main types of commercial diets for rabbits are pelleted or coarse mixes, with the emphasis on the latter. Many of the coarse mixes are finely sprayed with molasses to aid palatability and minimise dust levels (see Figure 21.4).

Some rabbit diets may contain a coccidiostat.

Assessment of Feeding

Most Probable Nutritional Disorders

Obesity. Most pet rabbits are confined with little opportunity to take significant exercise. Given ad libitum access to good food they will gain weight rapidly and may become very fat. There is a lot of evidence that overfed animals develop tumours and have a reduced life span. Because the rabbit is so good at utilising fibre in the diet, it is not possible to restrict body weight gain by feeding high fibre diets, as one can with other many species of pet. The only solution is the physical restriction of feed, either by supplying daily an amount of feed about 70-80% of voluntary intake, or alternatively by providing no food at all on one day of the week.

Diarrhoea/Enteritis. The gastrointestinal tract of the rabbit seems very susceptible to disturbance. Low levels of fibre (see above), sudden changes of diet and feed contaminated with pathogenic bacteria, protozoans and moulds may be significant dietary causes of diarrhoea and enteritis. However there are many other possible causes of gastrointestinal disturbances that should not be excluded, and these are reviewed by Flecknell (1991).

Colon impaction ('the blows'). Rabbits fed on clover in the summer months have been reported to have hard dry caecal contents, with faecal matter some-

	Weight (kg)	0.3	0.4	0.5	0.6	0.7	0.8	0.9	1.0
	$W^{0.75}$	0.405	0.503	0.595	0.682	0.765	0.846	0.924	1.000
Stage	kcal/$W^{0.75}$ [1]								
Maintenance	110	45	55	65	75	84	93	102	110
Growth	145	59	73	86	99	111	123	134	145
Gestation	145	59	73	86	99	111	123	134	145
Lactation	165	68	83	98	113	126	140	153	165

Table 21.5: *Estimated daily metabolisable energy requirements (kcal) for guinea pigs at different stages of development.*

[1] *1kcal = 4.184kJ.*

times adhering to the walls of the large intestine. The blockage of the gut often leads to the formation of gas that sometimes extends the stomach leading to congestion of the lungs because of mechanical pressure.

Inappetance. Rabbits will occasionally refuse to eat food, and may even starve themselves to death. The most likely causes of inappetance are a sudden change of diet and stress, including that of transportation. Thus the early days after the purchase of a pet rabbit may be difficult. If possible any change of diet should be phased in gradually. Where inappetance occurs, moist hay, changed very frequently to prevent spoilage, may tempt a rabbit to begin eating again.

Alopecia. Rabbits may show excessive grooming and fur chewing (barbering), often with extensive hair loss. This is often the result of the presence of inadequate amounts of fibre in the diet, which can be corrected by feeding a diet with increased fibre levels or the provision of hay. The accumulation of a hairball in the stomach may lead to inappetance and diarrhoea that results from secondary disturbances of the digestive tract.

Urolithiasis. The presence of urinary stones and gravels, primarily composed of calcium salts, is not uncommon in rabbits. It seems that the condition is largely related to high levels of dietary calcium, and the lack of a regulatory mechanism that controls uptake of calcium from the gut. Any excess absorbed dietary calcium must be excreted in the urine. To minimise the risk of urolithiasis, a low level of dietary calcium should be used: where practicable about 0.5% for maintenance and 0.8% for growth and breeding.

Deposition of calcium salts is enhanced because the urine of the rabbit is usually alkaline, which reduces the solubility of mineral salts. Unfortunately, diets containing large amounts of grass and lucerne will also have high levels of potassium, which contributes to the base excess and thus the alkalinity of the urine.

To minimise the deposition of calcium in soft tissues, dietary vitamin D should be less than 1000IU/kg diet.

GUINEA PIGS

The main source of information on the nutrient requirements of guinea pigs or cavies is the NRC (1978) publication on the nutrient requirements of laboratory animals. Precise requirements are not available for many of the nutrients. There are no data showing variation of requirements with age.

Clarke *et al.* (1977) have published estimates of the amounts of minerals and vitamins with which diets for guinea pigs should be supplemented.

It should be noted that the guinea pig has a relatively long gestation period resulting in newborn animals that are advanced and able to eat semi-solid and solid food.

Requirements

Energy

There are few determinations of the energy requirements of the guinea pig at different stages of development. Apart from the energy for lactation, the values are assumed to be similar to rats and mice:

maintenance energy requirement = 110kcal (462kJ) per $kg^{0.75}$

growth energy requirement = 145kcal (609kJ) per $kg^{0.75}$

gestation energy requirement = 145kcal (609kJ) per $kg^{0.75}$

lactation energy requirements = 165kcal (690kJ) per $kg^{0.75}$

The milk energy of the guinea pig at peak lactation is about one third that reported for the rat, and a lower lactation energy requirement of 165kcal (690kJ) per $kg^{0.75}$ is more appropriate.

Estimates of energy requirements at different body weights can be seen in the table above.

With high fibre diets, the guinea pig may have difficulty in eating sufficient bulk to meet its energy requirements.

Nutrients

Appendix 1 provides estimates of the nutritional requirements of the guinea pig based on published data and the author's own experience.

Protein. For growing animals, dietary protein levels of 18-20% seem to produce satisfactory growth. It is probable that at maintenance lower levels of protein, about 12%, would be adequate.

During the unusually extended gestation, the fetal mass often reaches the weight of the guinea pig's non-pregnant weight. This can create problems in excreting waste nitrogenous materials, so that increasing the protein level is not recommended.

Fats and fatty acids. Like the rabbit, the guinea pig tolerates fat levels much higher than the 3-5% typically included in diets, and up to about 7-15% oil improved growth rate, after which it declined.

The essential fatty acid requirement was met by 0.3% linolenic acid. Thus the guinea pig's requirement for essential fatty acids will be met by the inclusion of 1% maize oil, which contributes about 0.5% linoleic acid.

Minerals. There has been no attempt to define requirements for different phases of growth and development, so that the values given are for growing and breeding guinea pigs.

Clarke *et al.* (1977) suggest that the requirement for minerals by the guinea pig seems little different from that of mice and rats.

Vitamins. Recommended vitamin levels for guinea pigs are summarised in Appendix 1. There are no modifications to these levels for different stages of development.

The guinea pig can utilise some ß-carotene derived from grass meal or lucerne in the diet, but inefficiently. Furthermore the amount of ß-carotene in such materials is highly variable and declines with treatments such as drying and with storage (see above). Thus it is important to ensure supplementation of the diet with vitamin A to achieve about 10-20IU/g of total vitamin A, which will be adequate and allow for some losses in manufacture of the diet and in storage.

The guinea pig has an unusually low requirement for vitamin D, and it is difficult to produce rickets with a diet deficient in vitamin D providing that the calcium to phosphorus ratio is within the normal range.

Many of the B vitamins can be supplied by coprophagy, but it is usual in commercial diets to add vitamin supplements to achieve the levels seen above. The guinea pig, particularly when young, is reported to have an unusually high requirement for folate.

The guinea pig has a requirement for vitamin C (ascorbic acid) that is unusual. It is discussed below.

Special Needs

Fibre. Like the rabbit, the guinea pig has a requirement for substantial levels of fibre. Commercial diets usually contain 7-18% crude fibre, and even at these levels it is usual to supply hay. Low levels of fibre may produce gastrointestinal disturbances such as caecal impaction and excessive grooming with the formation of hairballs in the gut. NRC (1978) recommend a level of crude fibre of no less than 10%.

Vitamin C. The guinea pig shares with humans and primates a distinct requirement for vitamin C. NRC (1978) state a minimum requirement of 200mg/kg. Other estimates set the vitamin C requirement for growth at 75-150mg/kg. The stress of pregnancy may increase the requirement.

Vitamin C is highly labile and much is destroyed in manufacturing processes and in storage. With this in mind, Clarke *et al.* (1977) suggest that diets should be supplemented with 1500mg/kg diet.

Many commercial diets for pet guinea pigs contain added vitamin C at levels little more than the NRC recommended requirement of 200mg/kg. Diets for research animals are supplemented with vitamin C at about 7-15 times this level, and even then have shelf lives restricted to about 3 months. Roche recommend an initial minimum level of 400mg/kg for dry meals or mixes and 1400mg/kg for pelleted products at time of manufacture. We would regard these as marginal levels for products with a shelf life of 3 months.

The diet of the guinea pig may be supplemented with fruit or leafy vegetables known to contain high levels of vitamin C. Such materials should be fresh and replaced in the cage regularly. The use of such materials should be approached with caution: the materials should be thoroughly washed to reduce bacterial contamination and sudden changes in the materials used should be avoided otherwise there may be digestive disturbances.

Vitamin C, obtainable at most pharmacists in powder or tablet form, may also be added to the drinking water at a concentration of 1g/litre, and may be a more reliable way of supplementation. However vitamin C is unstable in water and fresh solutions must be made up daily. To minimise losses, ideally the bottles should be amber or made light-proof with glass, stainless steel or Pyrex spouts, since many metals will increase the rate of destruction of vitamin C.

Recently a new form of vitamin C activity has appeared from Roche called, appropriately, Stay-C. This is reported to be very stable, losing only a few percent of its activity during processing and storage.

Food Types

The main types of commercial diets for guinea pigs are pelleted or coarse mixes, with the emphasis on the latter (see Figure 21.4). Whilst some manufacturers provide diets specifically for guinea pigs, others produce diets said to be suitable for both rabbits and guinea pigs, though requiring supplementary sources of vitamin C when used for the latter.

Care must be taken if rabbit pellets are used as the basis for the diet since it is thought that coccidiostats, present in some rabbit diets, may cause liver and kidney damage in guinea pigs.

The foods that can form the basis of a diet for guinea pigs can be divided into five broad groups, cereals, root crops, fruits, green materials and hay.

Assessment of Feeding

Most Probable Nutritional Disorders

Many of the common nutritional problems of guinea pigs have been discussed by Navia and Hunt (1976) and Wagner (1976).

Caecal impaction. As in the rabbit, an inadequate intake of fibre in the guinea pig may cause caecal impaction and death; an adequate supply of hay is likely to prevent the condition. Other causes of caecal impaction may be the presence of a hairball, caused by fur chewing (again thought to be caused by a shortage of fibre) and the ingestion of wood shavings or chips used as bedding. Ingestion of wood chips may occur in conditions of vitamin C deficiency.

Constipation may be treated with oral administration of 0.5-1.0 ml of paraffin per day, but for no more than 2 days.

Inappetance. The guinea pig does not like sudden changes of diet, and where this occurs inappetance may occur as a consequence. The condition may be so severe that death results from starvation. Any changes in diet should be phased in gradually. Moist hay, changed frequently to prevent spoilage, may encourage the guinea pig to eat again.

Alopecia. Fur chewing, or barbering, may occur in guinea pigs. The main cause is thought to be an inadequate supply of fibre, which can be corrected by the provision of good quality hay. Where barbering occurs, it is important to be conscious of the risk of the formation of hairballs that might lead to caecal impaction and inappetance.

True alopecia commonly occurs in many guinea pigs in late pregnancy, in the absence of any clear nutritional causation.

Scurvy. Of all the possible nutritional disorders of guinea pigs, scurvy - the deficiency of vitamin C - is the best known. It is probably the most common vitamin-related disorder in guinea pigs used in research.

The main symptoms are severe weakness of the hind limbs, gingivitis, and fluffy hair, accompanied by petechial haemorrhages on the serous surfaces and subcutaneously, with larger haemorrhages in the muscles and joints. Bone growth will also be impaired. The animal will show signs of difficulty in walking, a steady loss of body weight and will finally die. On post mortem, severe enlargement of the costochondrial junctions of the ribs will be seen, together with a depletion of body fat. The inability of the guinea pig to store ascorbic acid means that the appearance of a deficiency may be swift — the first stages are seen after 11-14 days of feeding a diet devoid of vitamin C, with death at 18-26 days.

Scurvy is quite common in pet guinea pigs, the major causes being:

- inadequate vitamin C supplementation of the diet
- the use of diet beyond its expiry date
- poor storage of diet, leading to a greater rate of loss of vitamin C than predicted by the manufacturer
- destruction of vitamin C during processing of diet or supplements.

Soft tissue calcification. The guinea pig is reported to be particularly sensitive to a nutritional disorder called soft tissue calcification (STC) and a probably related condition called wrist stiffness syndrome (WS). The main symptoms are poor growth, muscular stiffness particularly in the forelegs, abnormal posture, bone defects, and calcification of the soft tissues. The condition may be fatal. STC-WS is thought to be caused by an imbalance of calcium, phosphorus, and magnesium, occurring when the diet contains a high level of phosphorus in relation to the cation level. It is known that increasing phosphorus increases the requirement for magnesium, and many of the symptoms of STC-WS are similar to those of magnesium deficiency. An acid-base disturbance may also be involved since the guinea pig uses cations rather than ammonia to neutralise acids excreted by the kidney. Thus an 'acid' diet will further deplete cation levels. STC-WS will be unlikely if the recommendations for the dietary levels of phosphorus and calcium, magnesium and potassium set out above are followed.

Deposition of calcium in soft tissues may occur with high levels of vitamin D. Since vitamin D is relatively stable there seems little point in levels exceeding about 2000IU/kg.

Ketosis or pregnancy toxaemia. Ketosis is reported to occur sporadically in guinea pigs in late pregnancy, and it appears to be similar to ketosis in cattle. The condition may be linked to the prolonged gestation period which places great demands on the supply of glucose for the fetuses. During this phase the mother may find it difficult to increase the intake of a high fibre diet to meet its energy intake.

The overt signs of the condition usually commence within 7-10 days of parturition, and include sudden reduction in activity, a ruffled coat, and cessation of eating and drinking. Within 2 days the animal refuses to move, even when startled, and becomes prostrate and dyspnoeic. Skeletal muscle spasms may be observed. Unless treated the cond-ition will lead to death within 2-5 days of onset. The condition can be confirmed by measurements of plasma glucose levels. There is little information on the treatment of the condition, but unlike the ruminant, glucose could be administered orally. There is some suggestion that inadequate supply of vitamin C may be implicated, so oral supplementation with vitamin C may be beneficial.

The precipitating factors of the pregnancy ketosis seem to be similar to those in cattle and include excess body fat before and during early gestation, and an inadequate energy intake in late gestation. Stress in late gestation such as a change of housing or diet may initiate the condition. It is generally agreed that the best means of prevention is to prevent obesity.

Nephritis. A high proportion of aged guinea pigs are reported to die of chronic renal disease. Nephritis is commonly associated with excessive intake of dietary protein, and thus may reflect the usual practice of feeding what amounts to a breeding diet with 18-20% protein throughout life. It is probably better practice to feed a maintenance diet with a protein level of about 12-14% within a few weeks of weaning.

'Slobbers'. The teeth of the guinea pig continue to erupt throughout life balancing the normal wear. Any interference with wear may lead to malocclusion that may become sufficiently severe to prevent prehension and swallowing. The animal may be unable to drink efficiently and swallow its saliva. The saliva drains from the mouth — hence the term 'slobbers'. The usual signs are continual wetness around the mouth, on the chin and the ventral surfaces on the neck. Subsequent symptoms may appear that reflect decreased food and water intake and losses of electrolytes in the saliva. Death may occur within 6 days of the signs of 'slobbers'.

The condition should be prevented by feeding a diet that requires gnawing. Excessive dietary fluoride, usually introduced through dietary minerals such as dicalcium phosphate, has also been associated with 'slobbers'.

HAMSTERS

There are few data on the nutritional requirements of the hamsters, and particularly of strains other than the Golden or Syrian hamster. Most recommended nutrient values are based on diets that give adequate performance.

There is some disagreement whether in practice the hamster requires a diet specifically formulated to meet its requirements or whether a standard rodent diet will be adequate. However the main reviews of nutrient standards (Clarke *et al.*, 1977; NRC, 1978) take the view that standard rodent diets can be used. Reviewing the nutrient levels in hamster diets, there seems no reason why good rat and mice diets would not be adequate.

Requirements

There are no data showing a change in nutrient requirement with age or stage of development, though it would not be unreasonable to assume that the requirement for protein and vitamins declines during the maintenance stage. The hamster is unusual in that the female is heavier than the male.

Energy

There are no details of the energy requirements of the hamster. It is accepted practice (Clarke *et al.*, 1977) to use the guidelines for rats and mice for the hamster. On that basis the following assumptions for the daily energy requirement have been made:

maintenance energy requirement = 110kcal (462kJ) per $kg^{0.75}$

growth energy requirement = 145kcal (609kJ) per $kg^{0.75}$

gestation energy requirement = 145kcal (609kJ) per $kg^{0.75}$

lactation energy requirements = 330kcal (1386kJ) per $kg^{0.75}$

	Weight (g)	50	60	70	80	90	100	110	120	130	140	150
	$W^{0.75}$	0.106	0.121	0.136	0.150	0.164	0.178	0.191	0.204	0.216	0.229	0.241
Stage	kcal/W(kg)$^{0.75}$ [1]											
Maintenance	110	11.6	13.3	15.0	16.5	18.1	19.6	21.0	22.4	23.8	25.2	26.5
Growth	145	15.3	17.6	19.7	21.8	23.8	25.8	27.7	29.6	31.4	33.2	34.9
Gestation	145	15.3	17.6	19.7	21.8	23.8	25.8	27.7	29.6	31.4	33.2	34.9
Lactation	310	34.8	39.9	45.0	49.5	54.3	58.8	63.0	67.2	71.4	75.6	79.5

Table 21.6: *Estimated daily metabolisable energy requirements (kcal) for Syrian hamsters at different stages of development.*

* *1kcal = 4.184kJ.*

Estimates of energy requirements at different body weights can be seen in the table below (estimates for smaller strains of hamster such as the Djungarian and Chinese can be obtained from the data for mice).

Nutrients

Data presented in Appendix 1 are based on the recommended nutrient allowances proposed by the NRC (1978) and the nutrients in Epperley diet No 2. This is a diet reported to outperform most commercial diets against which it was tested.

Protein. Diets suitable for breeding contain 18-22% protein, but hamsters will thrive on protein levels as low as 14-17%. Whilst there are no data on requirements for maintenance, there seems to be little doubt that levels of 13-14% protein, as for mice and rats, would be acceptable.

Fats and fatty acids. A fat level of 5% is said to be optimal for the hamster. At fat levels of 7% and 9% growth rate was not improved, but mortality increased significantly. The cause of the mortality is not clear, but it may be linked with the hamster's unusually high plasma cholesterol level and tendency to produce gall stones. The adverse effect of these moderate fat levels is unusual considering the hamster's like of sunflower seeds (30% fat), sesame seeds (50% fat) and peanuts (49% fat).

Hamsters suffer from deficiency of essential fatty acids but the requirement for linoleic acid has not been defined. However, a diet containing the typical level of fat, 3-5%, is likely to contain adequate linoleic acid.

Minerals. Mineral levels that are suitable for rats and mice seem to be satisfactory for the hamster.

Vitamins. Hamsters will thrive on vitamin mixtures designed for rats and mice.

The NRC (1978) level of 3mg vitamin E per kg of diet for the hamster seems unusually low, and is not supported by the evidence. A safer estimate would be 60-80 mg/kg for diets containing 3-5% fat.

There is some doubt on the need for vitamin C. The fact that they perform adequately on standard rodent diets without additional vitamin C would seem to suggest that under normal conditions vitamin C is unnecessary. However some commercial diets do have vitamin C incorporated.

Special Needs

Carbohydrates. The hamster is unusual in that it has a high mortality rate on diets rich (>60%) in simple sugars such as glucose, lactose, fructose and sucrose. It performs much better when the carbohydrate source is starch.

Vitamin C. The hamster may require small amounts of vitamin C, but the evidence is not strong.

Food Types

The hamster is omnivorous. The main types of commercial complete diets for hamsters are pelleted and coarse mixes, with the latter predominating. Some diets are described as complementary, formulated to be fed in conjunction with the seeds preferred by the hamster.

The hamster mix, commonly found in pet shops, can be made up at home from a mixture of cereals, seeds, and fresh vegetables. To provide supplementary minerals and vitamins, good quality guinea pig pellets can be added. Rabbit pellets should be avoided since they may contain a coccidiostat that might be damaging to the hamster.

To encourage gnawing and prevent overgrowth of teeth, a hard low protein dog biscuit or whole cereal seeds, particularly maize, can be provided. There is a need to limit access to sunflower seeds.

Assessment of Feeding

Most Probable Nutritional Disorders

Tooth malocclusion. One of the most common nutritional problems of the hamster is malocclusion caused by the absence of wear on continuously growing teeth. The problem can be prevented by ensuring that the diet contains items that are hard and require gnawing. Extruded diets might be more suitable for hamsters than either conventional pelleted diets or coarse mixes.

REFERENCES

Clarke HE, Coates ME, Eva JK, Ford DJ, Milner CK, O'Donoghue PN, Scott PP and Ward RJ (1977). Dietary standards for laboratory animals: report of the Laboratory Animals Centre Diets Advisory Committee. *Laboratory Animals* **11,** 1.

Flecknell PA (1991). Rabbits. In: *Manual of Exotic Pets.* Eds PH Beynon and JE Cooper. BSAVA, Cheltenham.

Lebas F (1980). Les recherches sur l'alimentation du lapin: évolution au cours des 20 dernières années et perspectives d'avenir. *II Congr. Mund. Cunic, Barcelona.*

National Research Council (1977). *Nutrient Requirements of Rabbits. 2nd Revised Edition.* National Academy of Sciences, Washington, D.C.

National Research Council (1978). *Nutrient Requirements of Laboratory Animals. 3rd Revised Edition.* National Academy of Sciences, Washington, D.C.

Navia JM and Hunt CE (1976). Nutrition, nutritional diseases, and nutrition research applications. In: *The Biology of the Guinea Pig.* Eds JE Wagner and

PJ Manning. Academic Press, New York.
Rogers AE (1979). Nutrition. In: *The Laboratory Rat. Volume 1, Biology and Diseases.* Eds HJ Baker, JR Lindsey and SH Weisbroth. Academic Press, New York.
Schlolaut W (1982). *The Nutrition of the Rabbit.* Roche Information Service Animal Nutrition Department, Basel, Switzerland.
Wagner JE (1976). Miscellaneous disease conditions of guinea pigs. In: *The Biology of the Guinea Pig.* Eds JE Wagner and PJ Manning. Academic Press, New York.

CHAPTER TWENTY-TWO

Small Pets and Exotics – Feeding Methods and Techniques

Martin P.C. Lawton

INTRODUCTION

An increasing number of small and exotic animals are now being kept as pets. The requirements for feeding these animals are varied and often differ even for members of the same family. Cooper (1990) stated that there are few reliable data on the nutritional requirements of most exotic animals, other than laboratory kept species. It is all too common for these type of animals to be presented to the practising veterinary surgeon with clinical problems which are associated with incorrect diet, either food type or nutrient content. A basic knowledge of the requirements of the more commonly kept exotics is essential to prevent disease or nutritional problems.

This chapter will only cover the basic feeding methods and techniques for the commonly kept taxa, including rodents (guinea pigs, hamsters, gerbils, rats, mice), lagomorphs, some members of the reptilian orders of Chelonia and Squamata (snakes and lizards) together with the commonly presented bird groups (passerines, psittacines and raptors).

FEEDING HEALTHY ANIMALS

Rodents and Lagomorphs

The majority of rodents are herbivores, granivores, fruigivores and insectivores in their natural environment. The digestion of cellulose plant walls requires the help of microorganisms which are found in abundance within the gastrointestinal tract of all rodents and lagomorphs. Storage is a natural instinct which is carried to extremes in the hamster, which with their distendable pouches are able to carry food items around and then store them in their nest. Guinea pigs and lagomorphs are grazers and in their natural environment will be eating grass and small plants. Neither tend to store food due to their ability to ferment their food and thus produce large amounts of heat (which is of additional benefit in the colder months).

All rodents and lagomorphs practice coprophagy (Ford, 1987), where a moist, mucoid lined pellet (a caecotroph) is eaten direct from the anus to allow a second passage through the intestinal tract. This allows the maximum amount of nutrient to be obtained from the food as well as the recovery of the intestinal flora and vitamin B group that was manufactured by the intestinal bacteria. This practice makes both rodents and lagomorphs highly efficient in their digestive processes.

The guinea pig is unique among the rodents in that it is unable to synthesise adequate amounts of vitamin C, thus supplementation is required when feeding them. Although the majority of commercial guinea pig food is already supplemented, it is important that this food is fresh due to the rapid deterioration of the vitamin C. All food should be used within 6 months of manufacture. Failure to provide adequate amounts of vitamin C will result in scurvy. In cases of stress (such as infection with *Trixacarus caviae*), the addition of vitamin C may be advantageous in helping the guinea pig to cope and recover (Harvey and Lawton, 1993).

The dietary requirements of rodents and lagomorphs have been well investigated due to the use of these animals as research models. There are many diets which are specially formulated to provide all the nutrients, vitamins and minerals that are required for various life stages and for reproduction. However, commercially produced diets come as pellets which are often not aesthetically pleasing to the pet owner and thus not accepted as the sole food for these pets. If commercially prepared pellets are not to be used, a balanced and varied diet should be fed together with a soluble vitamin C supplement. In the case of guinea pigs the addition of a soluble vitamin C to the water is advised.

Frequency of feeding is often *ad libitum*, however this can lead to obesity. Commercially produced pellets are often produced to be fed *ad libitum* as the energy density is lower. Where a high energy diet of seeds is given, it is best to restrict feeding to twice daily periods with a measured amount of food. The amount of food is based on regular weighing of the animal to prevent either weight loss or gain.

The major problem with the food that is offered to these animals when they are kept as pets, is often one of overindulgence so that they are either being overfed or they are on a food which is too high in energy, both resulting in obesity. Fatty liver syndrome may occur. Obesity is also a contributory factor to pregnancy toxaemia in guinea pigs. It is a good husbandry technique regularly to weigh all rodents and lagomorphs to try and prevent them from becoming obese (see Table 22.1), an adult animal should maintain its weight and not be expected to increase or decrease this. The feeding of high energy food in preference to other foods should be avoided. The concentrates in the diet commonly purchased from pet shops should be restricted to being offered once a day, so that roughage is then eaten the rest of the day.

The amount of food eaten is difficult to control for some rodents due to the storage behaviour. If the feeding times are restricted then the rodent will still remove food to its nest and feast at its leisure later. Most of the rodents (except guinea pigs) are nocturnal and therefore if perishable food items are to be fed it is better to offer them in the late evening. The nest of rodents who store food should also be regularly 'raided' to remove food and try and prevent the eating of food that has deteriorated.

Artificial foods should not be offered and sweets should be avoided as these can cause caries or problems with impaction of pouches in hamsters.

Food is usually offered in bowls although there is always the risk that these may become contaminated or knocked over. Especially when youngsters are involved, the bowl should be designed and weighted to try to prevent it from being knocked over or the contents becoming contaminated. Coccidiosis is particularly a problem in rabbits and is usually spread by the ingestion of contaminated food. Hoppers, a better method of offering concentrates, are unfortunately seldom used for pets.

Water Requirements

Water should always be readily available for all rodents and lagomorphs. In order to prevent contamination, open bowls should be avoided. Dripper bottles are the most frequently used. These can be of glass or plastic and often have an aluminium nozzle. The better bottles are available with a stainless steel tip for the nozzle to prevent the rodent or rabbit from chewing through, also reducing the chance of aluminium toxicity. Nozzles should not leak or this may result in wet bedding and hypothermia or drowning of smaller rodents or litters of pups.

The water should be changed daily at least to ensure freshness. There are two main problems with these water bottles, the first is breakage and the second is the growth of algae. It is advisable to always have a second bottle, so that if a breakage occurs then a spare is readily available. A spare bottle also allows for regular washing without depriving the animal of water in the mean time. If the bottles are washed on a regular basis the problem with algae and contamination is substantially reduced. Washing in a dish washer on a regular basis is a good way of preventing contamination and reducing the problem of algae growth. The use of water bottles allows a reliable method of monitoring the amount of water that is drunk each day. An increase in water consumption may indicate the possibility of renal or hepatic dysfunction.

Reptiles

The Class Reptilia has approximately 6500 species. A description of preferred food types for the more commonly kept species is given by Scott (1992).

All reptiles are ectotherms and as such are dependent on external temperatures and on behavioural means to regulate their body temperature. It is essential that the reptile is kept at a temperature that allows it to keep its own core body temperature at its optimum for digestion (the enzymes do not function so well below or above this). The external temperature which allows the reptile to achieve this optimum is referred to as the preferred body temperature (PBT)

Species	Weight range	Comments
Chinchilla	400-500g	Females are larger than males
Chipmunks	72-120g	
Gerbils	50-60g	Males are larger than females
Guinea pigs	750-1000g	
Hamsters	85-140g 40-60g	Golden hamster (males usually bigger) Russian hamster
Mice	20-40g	
Rabbits	500-1000g 1-2.5kg 3-7kg	Dwarf types Dutch type Lop ears to Flemmish giants
Rats	400-800g	Males are larger than females

Table 22.1: *Guidelines for average adult body weights.*

(See Table 22.2). The most common reason why a reptile is either not eating or failing to digest its food properly is failure to maintain the reptile within its PBT. Bellairs (1970) showed that a python kept at 28°C and fed a rabbit required 5 days for digestion, while at an environmental temperature of 18°C, digestion took 15 days. It is important always to ascertain that the captive reptile is being kept at its correct PBT.

Chelonia

For the Chelonia, the general rule is that land tortoises are herbivorous or omnivores while terrapins are mainly carnivores and scavengers. Turtles are mainly herbivores (Frye, 1986) but are rarely kept as pets. The main problem with tortoises is trying to offer in captivity food items which are similar to those that would be eaten in their natural environment. Foods such as lettuce, cucumber, tomato, apple and banana are often fed in the UK, although these are not well balanced and require supplementation in order to prevent deficiencies.

Some owners will overindulge their pets and feed abnormal food which would not be eaten in the wild, such as bread, cat food, doughnuts, cheese or milk. Although in small amounts these are unlikely to cause major problems, the tortoise may become 'addicted' to these abnormal foods and will not eat other items (Lawton, 1989). These abnormal diets may lead to obesity and fatty liver syndrome which could even result in the death of the tortoise.

It is quite normal for Chelonia to undergo hibernation when the ambient temperature and daylight lengths decrease. A tortoise, prior to hibernation will stop eating in response to the reduced metabolism and inability of digestive enzymes to work properly. A *Testudo* spp. will often go without food for about 4 weeks, as this is the length of time required for the gastrointestinal tract to be empty prior to hibernation.

Juveniles that are being fed too much or a high protein diet will be growing rapidly which will predispose them to problems such as 'lumpy shell'. Although this is a nutritional secondary osteodystrophy, the same diet has not always been found to cause the deformity, this being dependent on growth rate. Ideally hatchlings should only be fed once a day and on a balanced diet, including watercress, spinach, lettuce, cucumber, tomato and a small amount of fruits. Vitamin and mineral supplements are required.

Terrapins in the wild are scavengers and although they will eat a variety of foods, they are mainly carnivores. The intestines of terrapins are different to the land tortoise in that the small intestines are enlarged and the colon is reduced as fermentation is not required. The diet will partly depend upon the size of the terrapin. Small terrapins may only eat small insects, small shellfish, and amphibian eggs and larvae or the odd mouthful of a carcase that they happen across.

Common Name	Scientific Name	PBT range (°C)
American box tortoise	*Terrapene carolina*	24–29
Boa constrictor	*Constrictor constrictor*	26–34
Corn snake	*Elaphe guttata guttata*	25–30
Garter snake	*Thamnophis sirtalis*	20–35
Green (common) iguana	*Iguana iguana*	26–30
Hermann's tortoise	*Testudo hermanni*	22–28
Hinged back tortoise	*Kinixys belliana*	25–27
Indian python	*Python molurus*	25–30
King snake	*Lampropeltis getulus*	23–30
Leopard gecko	*Eublepharis macularius*	25–30
Leopard tortoise	*Geochelone pardalis*	25–26
Rat snake	*Elaphe obsoleta*	25–30
Red eared terrapin	*Trachemys scripta elegans*	24–30
Royal python	*Python regius*	25–30
Slow worm	*Anguis fragilis*	15–22
Spur thigh (Greek) tortoise	*Testudo graeca*	22–30
Waterdragon	*Physignathus lesueuri*	24–30

Table 22.2: *Some preferred body temperatures of commonly encountered species.*

Medium to larger terrapins will be eating amphibians and fish although the odd small rodent may also be eaten if caught. It is all too common for the pet terrapin, apart from being kept below its PBT, to be fed on dried food which are deficient in minerals and vitamins. Small shellfish and fish (that can be fed whole) should mainly be offered in captivity.

Chelonian water requirements. The supply of water for aquatic or semi-aquatic species is taken for granted, although it is important that the filtration system is efficient in order to maintain adequate hygiene and eliminate the waste products or overgrowth of bacteria. For terrestrial species, most of the water requirements are obtained from the food (of which up to 70% may be water). The production of uric acid in terrestrial species, as the main excretory product, is water sparing thus reducing the overall requirement of fluid intake when compared to mammals. Regular 'baths' up to the marginal shields are advised in order to allow the tortoise the opportunity to take in water. This is more important as hibernation is approaching. During hibernation the bladder acts as a storage organ for water, which is recycled by being reabsorbed in the cloaca (proctodaeum). After awakening from hibernation all tortoises will be severely dehydrated and it is important that they are regularly bathed in tepid water to rehydrate and stimulate the tortoise to defecate and urinate.

Snakes

Of the large order Squamata, the sub-order Serpenta, which includes all the snakes, are the simplest group to feed without a risk of problems, other than obesity or thiamin deficiency in fish-eating snakes. Snakes eat their prey whole and therefore are usually eating a balanced diet. The majority of snakes are carnivores, although the genus *Dasypeltis* are egg-eaters. The prey items include rodents, birds, fish, amphibians, lizards or even other snakes (the genus *Lampropeltis* are snake-eaters - ophiophagous). Except for the reptile-eaters, it is relatively easy to provide a naturally similar food item to the snake kept in captivity.

Snakes that eat fish should not be entirely fed on previously frozen whitebait to the exclusion of all other fish, as this has a high thiaminase activity which could lead to thiamin deficiency. Heavily furred rodents should be avoided or this can result in constipation. Potential problems may occur when 'pieces' of a prey item are fed, especially if it is from an oversized prey item compared to that which the snake would be able to eat whole. Pieces of large fish, especially, should be avoided or bones may stick in the gastrointestinal tract.

The frequency of feeding depends upon the body weight and the surface area of the prey eaten. Small garter snakes and hatchling boas will need to be fed on a daily basis. An African rock python that may be feeding on gazelles, may only need to eat twice a year. As a 'rule of thumb', the snake, when adult, should be fed frequently enough not to put on or lose weight. Even the best feeding snake may normally go off its food at certain times of the year. When it is coming up for a slough, the eyes will go opaque and the snake will refuse food until after it has shed. In certain seasons it is also normal for a snake not to eat and in some instances this may be for several months. Keeping good records will help to identify the patterns associated with shedding or seasonal anorexia. Regular weighing is also advised in order to prevent obesity or excessive weight loss.

Live* versus *dead food for snakes. The problem with feeding snakes is not therefore one of unsuitable diets, provided the correct choice of prey is being offered, but more one of whether the snake is willing to eat dead prey (thawed or freshly killed) or will only eat live prey. Although it is natural in the wild for snakes to seek out and kill live prey, it is not desirable in captivity and for both legal and welfare reasons should be avoided (Cooper, 1987). An important consideration is the potential damage that, with rodents in particular, could be inflicted on the snake by the live prey (Rosskopf and Woerpel, 1981). To prevent any risk of bite or scratch injuries to the pet snake, it is far safer to offer only dead items. The issue of 'cruelty' when considering feeding of live prey to snakes is difficult. If the snake has previously eaten dead prey then this author considers there to be no reason why that snake should be offered any live prey, and that to do so could be considered an act of cruelty and may risk prosecution for causing unnecessary suffering or cruelly terrifying under the Cruelty to Animals Act, 1911. If the snake refuses to eat any dead prey, and it can be shown that every measure has been taken to 'wean' the snake onto dead prey but despite this the snake would only eat live prey, then a case could be made for the feeding of live prey, provided that the prey is not unnecessarily terrified or stressed by being left in the vivarium, in the presence of its predator, longer than would be necessary for the snake to strike and kill that prey. The snake is a very proficient killing machine, either killing its prey by constriction or poisoning (all poisonous snakes are covered by the Dangerous Animals Act, 1986 and therefore the owner/ keeper must be licensed). Providing the snake is hungry and used to feeding on live prey, it will seek out and kill very quickly without causing cruelty. There are, however, very few animals that can not be trained to accept dead prey.

Water requirements of snakes. Water should always be provided for snakes, although it is more important for bathing to assist ecdysis (sloughing) than for drinking, unless there are metabolic or protozoan diseases. The normal water requirements are usually provided from the food and from the ability to conserve water by the production of urates and faeces with a relatively low water content.

Lizards

The second sub-order of Squamata of major importance is Sauria . This sub-order contains a large range of lizards which eat all the varieties of food available. There are insectivores, carnivores, herbivores, fruigivores and omnivores. It is not unusual for a species even to change its feeding requirements during its life. The waterdragon (*Physignathus* spp.) is almost entirely insectivorous as a juvenile but omnivorous as an adult (Lawton, 1991). The substitute diets that are offered to captive lizards are often unsuitable as a balanced diet. The insectivores are mainly fed on mealworms, silk moth larvae, crickets or locusts. All these insects are very high in phosphorus and low in calcium. The sprinkling of a supplement on to these insects is not sufficient to prevent deficiencies. The insects must be fed on a diet which includes an appropriate supplement (such as Nutrobal; Vetark) so that the intestinal tract has the supplement. Any supplement on the exoskeleton may be lost as the insect moves around or is caught and eaten by thc lizard.

The feeding of live insects to lizards is less contentious then feeding rodents to snakes. The concept of causing cruelty to invertebrates is one that seems to be dismissed all too easily. The risk to the lizard is substantially less than when feeding rodents to snakes, and it is only in exceptional circumstances that the lizard is at risk. Insectivorous species chew their food before swallowing (Frye, 1986) (see Figure 22.1). Debilitated or recently anaesthetised lizards should not be fed live insects or these may cause damage within the stomach, especially if they are force fed to the lizard, and not chewed sufficiently.

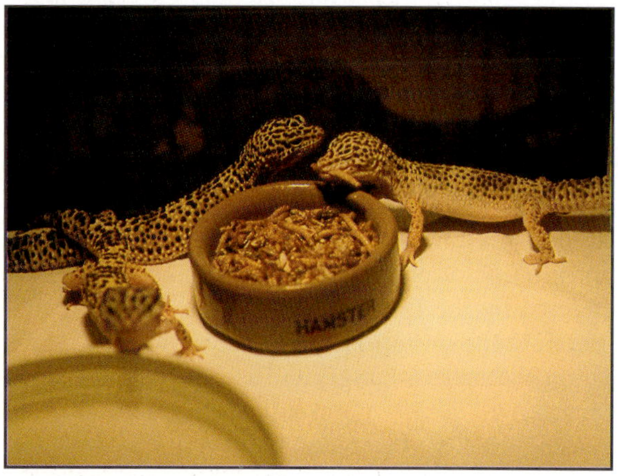

Figure 22.1: *Leopard geckos (*Eublepharis macularius*) eating live mealworms.*

Fruit and vegetables may result in osteodystrophy, unless a supplement is also used. Monitor lizards, which are often fed on eggs, may develop a biotin deficiency due to the avidin content.

Water requirements. It is important that all lizards have access to fresh water. Herbivores and fruigivores will drink little compared to insectivores. Some lizards, such as chameleons (*Chamaeleo* spp.), will not drink from containers but only from droplets of water on plants. To successfully keep these species it is important to mist the tank several times per day either manually or automatically (Cunningham and Gili, 1992; Scott, 1992). Most lizards should be sprayed with water as this reduces the risk of retained bands of skin around digits and the necrosis distal to these that is all too often seen when there are humidity problems.

Birds

Passerines

Passerines are mainly frugivorous or insectivorous in the wild. Due to their soft beaks, the type of seeds that are eaten are the smaller types. In the wild they would eat a variety of seeds and fruits and not just one type. The diet in captivity should try and mimic this, with as wide a variety of fruits and seeds as is possible. The inclusion of grit is important so that the gizzard can work effectively and grind the seed and vegetable matter in order to aid digestion.

Water requirements. Fresh water is important. The use of open bowls or containers is to be avoided in order to prevent contamination. Gravity water bottles can be used for the small passerines. If an open container is used then it should not be under a perch, but ideally slightly higher than the perch in order to try and reduce faecal contamination. The same applies for food containers.

Psittacines

Malnutrition is far too often the cause of disease in parrots (Lawton, 1988). In their natural environment, they would eat a varied diet including fruit, insects and seeds, indeed, Long (1984) observed that some species would eat seeds of up to 52 species in 15 families of plants and six orders of insects. Despite this, the average captive parrot is predominantly fed a seed diet, the bulk of which are sunflower seeds (Lawton, 1988). Sunflower seeds are very low in calcium and vitamin A, but they are high in fats and oils and can lead to obesity as well as deficiencies. Psittacines that are on a solely seed diet, such as sunflower seeds, may become addicted to those seeds and it can therefore be difficult sometimes to change their diets. This may require patience and the use of peeled sunflower seeds mixed in with fruit and other vegetables in order to make it harder for them to pick out the seeds that they prefer and thus have to eat other types of food.

Obesity is an all too common problem in captive psittacines partly due to the diet they are fed and partly due to the boredom factor where they will eat and eat as they have very little else to do. There are many tricks that can be employed to try and reduce the risk of obesity as well as trying to alleviate the boredom. A varied diet should always be the aim. The use of large glass marbles (too big to be eaten) in the food bowls together with chopped pieces of food will make the parrot work for its food, as well as reducing the amount of food that is placed in the container. Budgerigars will often become obese by overindulging on millet sprays. These should be restricted. Obesity in budgerigars will predispose them to the development of lipomata or xanthomata where the skin becomes thickened and yellow. Dietary control will also be able to reduce the size of these tumours so that surgery may not be required.

It is debatable whether psittacines require grit in their diet to the same extent that the passerines do. When grit is provided it is best to avoid the commercial preparations that have additional material such as oyster shell and additional minerals, as it is possible to overdo these especially as the grinding in the gizzard may increase the available concentrations. If grit is to be provided it should be just sand particles, but ideally not too small or this could lead to impaction (Harrison, 1986).

It is common when breeding parrots to rear them by hand. Hand rearing has the advantage in that it also creates a tame, bonded, youngster which is well sought after as a pet. Human baby foods such as Millupa, are often used to hand rear these youngsters. They will readily accept hand feeding when they are ill and thus it is easier to medicate them that way. The advantage of using a proprietary baby food is that it already has vitamins and minerals and is well balanced. When these foods are prepared using a microwave, it is important that the food is equally heated throughout and that there are no hot spots. Severe burns are reported to occur following a single feed if greater than 120°C or several feeds of 115°F (Flammer and Clubb, 1994). Crop necrosis associated with microwaved foods is an all too common occurrence in hand reared birds.

Water requirements. As for passerines, water and food bowls should not be placed where they are likely to be contaminated by faeces or urates. All water containers should be cleaned on a regular basis. The addition of supplements or antibiotics to water sources should be avoided (except in the flock situation) as any change in the taste, colour or smell of the water may result in a reduced intake which could be harmful especially in the sick bird.

Raptors and Stigiformes

This group of birds are carnivores eating a wide variety of rodents, lagomorphs or birds. Some species will also eat insects and earthworms. They will not be able to digest the whole of the prey and therefore will produce casts which are comprised of feathers/hair and nails or beaks in a solid mass which is regurgitated, usually on a daily basis. When feeding these birds it is important that they are not fed pieces of meat or this will lead to nutritional osteodystrophy. The standard types of food offered to birds of prey in captivity include mice, rats, rabbits, chicks or pigeons. Most food types are purchased in bulk and stored in the freezer, being thawed prior to being fed.

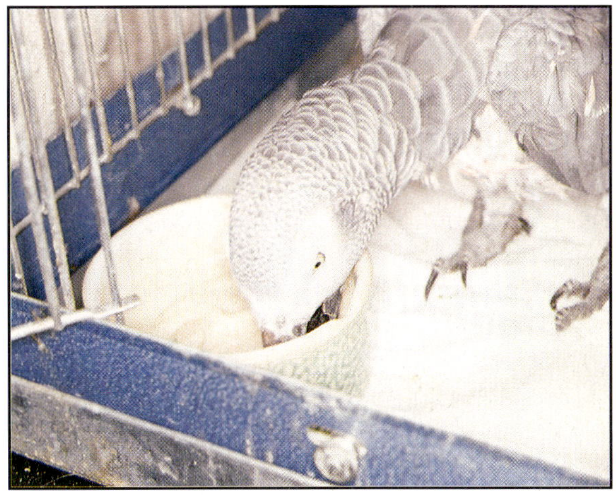

Figure 22.2: *African grey parrot* (Psittacus erithacus) *eating Millupa with added medication.*

Water requirements. It is often the case that water is not constantly provided for raptors or Stigiformes. Enderson (1986) suggested that many species of raptors will survive indefinitely without access to drinking water. When they are healthy and eating well they will obtain their full water requirements from their food. Even when offered water, the majority of raptors will not drink. However, it is important that an uninterrupted access to water should be allowed, especially at times of illness where their requirements may have changed such as when there is diarrhoea or anorexia.

SPECIAL TECHNIQUES FOR FEEDING

Rodents and Lagomorphs

Most rodents and lagomorphs which are unwilling to eat due to ill health may be tempted to eat mashed foods or Millupa vegetable foods. Syringe feeding of rodents and lagomorphs is very easy as they will lap most wet foods that are placed on the tongue.

In small rodents, a firm grip of the scruff and down the back will allow the head and neck to be straightened and the rodent immobilised. A tube is then introduced through the diastema and passed down the oesophagus and into the stomach. There are purpose made gavage tubes for rodents which fit onto syringes and have a ball on the distal end of the tube to prevent this going down the trachea (see Figure 22.3).

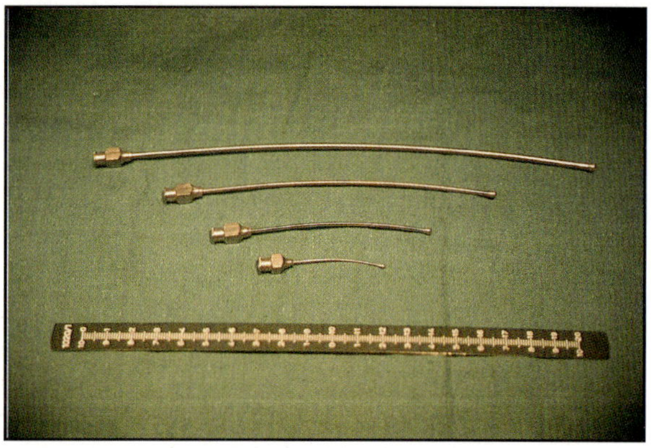

Figure 22.3: *A selection of metal feeding canulae; the smallest are mouse and rat gavage tubes, the larger are bird crop tubes.*

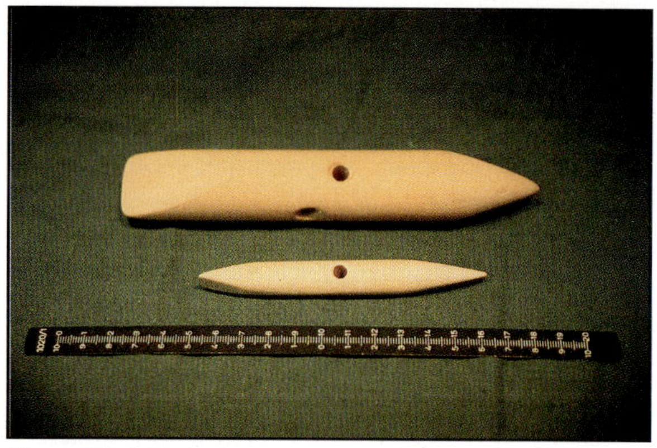

Figure 22.4: *Typical guinea pig (smaller) and rabbit (larger) mouth gags; the hole in the middle is for passing a soft plastic/rubber tube.*

For stomach tubing of guinea pigs and rabbits it is best to use a gag to prevent their biting through the tube. The best type of a gag is a rounded wooden oblong with a hole through the middle (see Figure 22.4). The rabbit or guinea pig should be firmly held around the shoulders, the gag should then be introduced through the diastema and placed behind the incisors, the tube then passed through the hole in the middle of the gag and down the oesophagus.

Reptiles

All reptiles can be tube fed. In Chelonia and Sauria (lizards) it is possible to use a stomach tube, however, in snakes it is usually oesophageal tubing, unless a very long tube is used. Due to the large oesophagus and the trachea being protected by the glottis, it is a safe and easy technique. In all reptilian species, the glottis is easily seen as it is usually found at the base of the tongue and therefore can be avoided. Provided a large tube is passed against the dorsal aspect of the pharynx, there is usually little chance of the tube going down the trachea. The most difficult part about tube feeding a reptile is the handling, restraint and opening of the mouth.

Chelonia

Chelonia may keep their head behind their front limbs and within the shell. In this case it is possible to bring the head out of the shell with patience and possibly the use of whelping forceps. Some terrapins must be handled with care, as they could inflict a painful bite. It may be necessary to sedate some of the more aggressive species, such as snapping turtles. Once the head is restrained, the mouth should be opened with gentle pressure, and the tube inserted. An estimate of the length of tube required may be obtained by measuring the plastron from the gular shields to the junction between the abdominal and femoral shields. With the neck fully extended, this will allow a sufficient length of tube to enter the stomach. Where long-term tube feeding occurs, there is a risk of bruising to the sides of the mandible and the neck. In these cases it is possible to prevent this by the placement of a pharyngostomy tube, similar to that used in mammals. The technique is very similar.

Force feeding pieces of food is possible without the use of a tube. In tortoises, especially if they are sight damaged, this may have to be undertaken on a long-term basis. The food should be cut into small cubes. Once the mouth is open the first piece of food is introduced, then as the tortoise is chewing, the second and subsequent pieces can then be inserted easily, one at a time, until the tortoise has had enough (although it is usually the owner that tires of this first).

Snakes

Snakes are the easiest of all reptiles to tube feed. This technique should never, however, be attempted by one person unaided as there is a possibility that should the snake be supported just by the head, the neck could be dislocated resulting in the death of the snake. The snake's body should be supported by two hands of an assistant, while the head is grasped just behind the mandible and quadrate bones. It is the responsibility of the person supporting the snake to keep the neck straight and the snake reasonably still. The end of the tube is then introduced into the mouth via the labial notch, and down the oesophagus. Once the fluid has been given, the tube should be removed from the oesophagus and the fluid/ food massaged as far down the oesophagus as possible. The snake should be handled for as short a time as possible to reduce the possibility of the snake regurgitating all that has been administered.

Snakes may be force fed with a whole prey item. However, it is important that any dehydration or underlying metabolic or infectious problem has been treated before it is decided to force feed an anorexic snake, especially if there has been long term anorexia. Whether it is a bird or a rodent that is being used, the principle is the same. The prey should be introduced into the snake's mouth head first, so that the fur or feathers do not bunch up and cause an

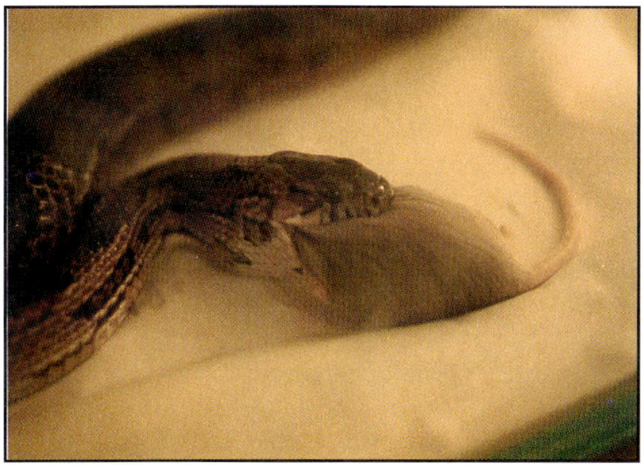

***Figure 22.5:** Corn snake (*Elaphe guttata*) eating a mouse; note that the mouse is being eaten head first.*

obstruction (see Figure 22.5). Once part of the prey is in the mouth, push gently on the head and mandibles to cause the snake to bite on to the prey; this is important as it stimulates the snake to salivate and thus lubricates the mouth and the oesophagus. Alternatively egg white or K-Y jelly may also be smeared onto the prey. The food item is then slowly manipulated into the mouth and eventually down the oesophagus. Most snakes have backward pointing teeth which help to retain the prey within the mouth and prevent the snake from actively spitting it out. Forceps may aid the movement into the pharynx and down the oesophagus, but care has to be undertaken to prevent damage. The food is worked as far down the oesophagus as is possible. The snake is then placed back into its vivaria and left alone. In some cases the snake will regurgitate the food.

Lizards

Although lizards can be hand fed, due to their teeth they are technically more difficult, therefore usually tube or syringe feeding is undertaken. For the long term feeding of lizards with osteodystrophic problems and having soft jaws, the use of baby foods administered via a syringe directly into the mouth is often sufficient, until such time as the jaw hardens and the lizard can chew and bite off pieces of food. The majority of owners are easily shown how to do this procedure.

Where it is necessary to stomach tube lizards, this author uses metal feeding tubes as some species of lizards, such as iguanas, have teeth that are capable of chewing through plastic tubes (see Figure 22.3). Gentle restraint of the lizard is required, usually around the shoulders. The tip of the tube is then gently introduced through the lips and teeth into the mouth and straight down the oesophagus. The length of the tube that should be introduced can be estimated by measuring from the mouth to the site of the stomach, being near the end of the rib cage.

Cage Birds and Raptors

Birds can be easily tube fed by the introduction of a tube into the pharynx and down the oesophagus and into the crop (in those species with this organ) or into the thoracic oesophagus. The choice of tube depends on the species of the birds and in particular the ability of its beak to cut through plastic tubes. Sometimes a soft tube can be used if a reliable gag is also available. Often a metal crop tube is advised. These are usually curved and have a large ball end to prevent them from going down the trachea. Tubing can be performed single handed on small birds, but with the larger parrots and raptors it is advisable to have one person restraining the bird and a second person passing the tube (see Figures 22.6 and 22.7).

Hand reared baby psittacines are usually fed by the use of a spoon. In intensive rearing situations, the technique of 'power feeding' is employed, where a syringe (or dosing gun) is used to fill the crop rapidly. Although this has the advantage that a large number of birds may be fed in a short period of time, there are a number of disadvantages. It is possible to damage the crop or cause some regurgitation and subsequent inhalation will result in pneumonia. Birds that are 'power fed', do not have the human contact time that is required to establish imprinting that is provided in true hand reared birds destined for pets.

If a large amount of food is being fed to hatchlings or they are next fed before the crop is allowed to

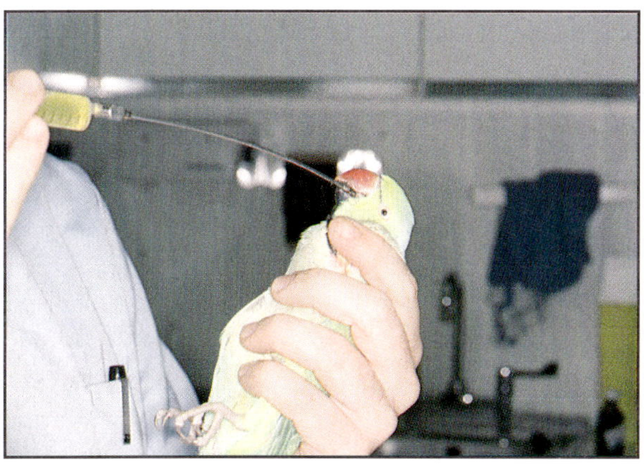

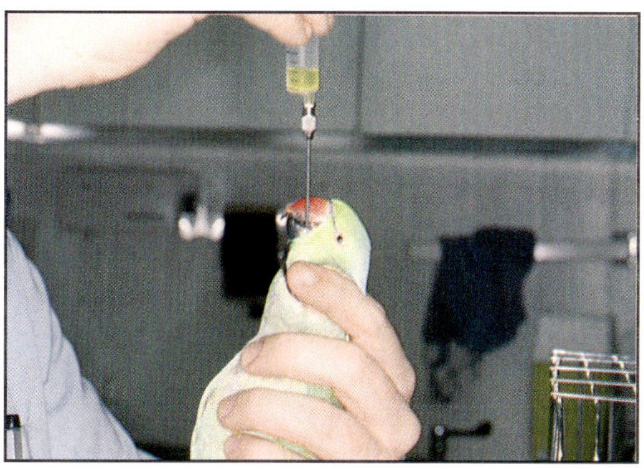

***Figures 22.6 and 22.7:** Ring necked parakeet (*Psittacula krameri*) being crop tubed.*

empty, this may lead to an enlargement or sagging of the crop. The use of a 'crop bra' is recommended in such cases in order to support the crop and prevent further sagging and stretching as well as improving crop emptying (Quesenberry and Hillyer, 1994). This 'bra' can be fashioned from a bandage tied around the neck and supporting and elevating the crop.

REFERENCES

Bellairs Ad'A (1970). *The Life of Reptiles.* Weidenfeld and Nicolson, London.

Cooper ME (1987). *An Introduction to Animal Law.* Academic Press, London.

Cooper JE (1990). Feeding exotic and pocket pets. *Journal of Small Animal Practice* **31,** 482-488.

Cunningham AA and Gili C (1992). Management in Captivity. In: *Manual of Reptiles.* Eds PH Beynon, MPC Lawton and JE Cooper. BSAVA, Cheltenham.

Enderson J (1986). Husbandry and captive breeding of birds of prey. In: *Zoo and Wild Animal Medicine, 2nd edition.* Ed ME Fowler. WB Saunders, Philadelphia.

Flammer K and Clubb SL (1994). In: *Avian Medicine: Principles and Application.* Eds BW Ritchie, GJ Harrison and LR Harrison. Wingers, Lake Worth, FL.

Ford DJ (1987). Nutrition and feeding. In: *The UFAW Handbook on the Care and Management of Laboratory Animals, 6th edition.* Ed TB Poole. Longman Scientific and Technical, Harlow.

Frye FL (1986). Feeding and nutritional diseases. In: *Zoo and Wild Animal Medicine, 2nd edition.* Ed ME Fowler. WB Saunders, Philadelphia.

Harrison GJ (1986). Feeding Psittacine and Passerine birds. In: *Zoo and Wild Animal Medicine, 2nd edition.* Ed ME Fowler. WB Saunders, Philadelphia.

Harvey RG and Lawton MPC (1993). Alopecia and pruritus in small mammals. In: *Manual of Small Animal Dermatology.* Eds PH Locke, RG Harvey and IS Mason. BSAVA, Cheltenham.

Lawton MPC (1988). Nutritional disease. In: *Manual of Parrots, Budgerigars, and other Psittacine Birds.* Ed CJ Price. BSAVA, Cheltenham.

Lawton MPC (1989). Health problems associated with feeding. *Testudo* **3**(1), 75.

Lawton MPC (1991). Lizards and snakes. In: *Manual of Exotic Pets.* Eds PH Beynon and JE Cooper. BSAVA, Cheltenham.

Long JL (1984). The diets of three species of parrots in the South of Western Australia. *Australian Wildlife Research* **11,** 357-371.

Quesenberry KE and Hillyer EV (1994). Supportive care and emergency therapy. In: *Avian Medicine: Principles and Application.* Eds BW Ritchie, GJ Harrison and LR Harrison. Wingers, Lake Worth, FL.

Rosskopf WJ and Woerpel RW (1981). Rat bite injury in a pet snake. *Modern Veterinary Practice* **62,** 871.

Scott PW (1992) Nutritional disease. In: *Manual of Reptiles.* Eds PH Beynon, MPC Lawton and JE Cooper. BSAVA, Cheltenham.

CHAPTER TWENTY-THREE

Nutrition of Captive and Free-Living Wild Animals

James K. Kirkwood

INTRODUCTION

The range of species of wild animals that may be encountered in veterinary practice is wide. It includes the many species kept as companion animals or for educational or conservation reasons, and the growing numbers of sick and injured wild animals taken from the wild for treatment and rehabilitation. Bearing in mind that despite the many thousands of man-years that have been devoted to the study of human nutrition there is still much debate about nutrient requirements of our species, it is not surprising that knowledge of the requirements of most other taxa is as yet very scant. However, as in other aspects of wildlife husbandry and medicine where species-specific data are often not available, patterns of variation between those species which have been studied often provide a valuable basis for predicting the requirements of those that have not.

Nutritional diseases are not uncommon in captive wild animals and in some cases these have been the major bottlenecks in the process of establishing self-sustaining populations in captivity. For example, prior to the discovery that New World primates required dietary vitamin D_3, captive marmosets (Callitrichidae) often failed to thrive (Hunt *et al.*, 1967; Crandall, 1964). Some nutritional diseases remain quite prevalent among wild animals kept as pets or those taken from the wild for treatment and rehabilitation. This is largely a result of ignorance about their requirements. Although a considerable amount of information on aspects of wildlife nutrition is available in the scientific literature (e.g. see reviews by Robbins, 1983; Scott, 1986; Ullrey & Allen, 1986), relatively little is readily available in a form accessible to lay rehabilitators and exotic pet-owners.

The aim of this chapter is to provide some guidelines for the nutrition of captive wild animals. The emphasis here is on energy requirements since these provide a basis for estimating food requirements and in many cases, where the diet composition is well defined (as for example with carnivores that eat whole small rodents or birds), data on specific nutrient requirements may be less often of relevance in practice.

ENERGY AND FOOD REQUIREMENTS

Wild animals maintained in captivity are, in many cases, fed ad *libitum* and, as long as the animals remain healthy and are provided with a suitable diet, knowledge of the quantity of energy and food required each day may not be essential. *Ad libitum* feeding is generally a suitable system because most animals are able to judge their requirements better than their keepers. However, there are many situations in the care or management of captive or free-living wild animals when a knowledge of daily food requirements is very helpful. Without this, degrees of inappetance cannot be assessed and there is no basis for calculating force feeding or parenteral feeding regimens for anorexic or sick animals, or for controlling obesity (Kirkwood, 1991a).

Many species show seasonal variations in appetite and periods of partial or complete anorexia may be a normal aspect of the animal's biology. For example, marked reductions in appetite occur during winter in some species of mammals, there is a marked reduction in appetite at the end of the period of rapid weight gain in some young altricial birds (those that are reared by their parents in nests), and snakes refuse food at time of ecdysis (shedding).

Obtaining Estimates of Energy Requirements for Maintenance

Basal metabolic rate (BMR) or metabolic rate at conditions close to basal have been measured in over 365 (about 5% of) species of birds, at least 685 (about 17% of) species of mammals (Kirkwood and Bennett, 1992), but in smaller numbers of reptiles and amphibians. Food or energy requirements for captive or free-living existence have been measured in considerably fewer species. For most of the 20,000 or so species of terrestrial vertebrates, no data are available on daily energy or food requirements at any stage of their life cycles. Estimates therefore have to be based on findings in other species.

There are several approaches to estimating ME requirements for maintenance (MER, kcal/day), the requirements to sustain energy balance under captive conditions, and these are listed below. The estimates derived should be regarded as first approximations and it is often necessary to refine these after further monitoring intake, body weight and condition.

1) From measurements in the same or in closely related species. Where available in the literature, measurements of ME or food intake from conspecifics or closely related species of similar size are a good basis for estimating requirements. The estimation of food requirements from data on energy requirements and *vice versa* is relatively straightforward (see below).

2) From data on basal metabolic rate. MER is typically about 1.5 to 2 times BMR (e.g. Clarke *et al.*, 1977; Robbins, 1983; Ullrey and Allen, 1986; Blaxter, 1989) and can be estimated this way if BMR data are available.

3) From allometric equations relating MER or BMR to body weight. Data on ME or food intake under existence, or similar, conditions, are available for relatively few species. These intakes have been found to increase with increasing body weight between species in a fairly consistent way. Plotting intake against body weight using logarithmic scales, typically produces a scatter of points about a straight line whose slope is usually within the range 0.5–0.8 and often 0.67–0.75. These relationships can be summarised by allometric equations (see Table 23.1) which provide a basis for predicting MER. The calculation is straightforward and takes only a few seconds using a calculator with an exponent function (see Box 23.1 later). Alternatively, allometric equations (Table 23.1) can be used to predict BMR and MER can be estimated at 1.5–2 times these values (see above).

Whilst predictions from allometric equations can be very helpful, it is important not to lose sight of their limitations. These have been discussed in detail else-

	Taxonomic group	Equation	Source
BMR	Reptiles (30°C)	$6.7\ W^{0.77}$	Bennett and Dawson, 1976
	Reptiles (20°C)	$2.5\ W^{0.80}$	Bennett and Dawson, 1976
	Birds	$80\ W^{0.67}$	Bennett and Harvey, 1987
	Eutherian mammals	$70\ W^{0.75}$	Kleiber, 1961
	Marsupial mammals	$48\ W^{0.74}$	Dawson and Hulbert, 1970
	Echidnas	$34\ W^{0.75}$	Dawson *et al.*, 1979
	Primates	$58\ W^{0.78}$	Ross, 1989
	Artiodactyla	$73\ W^{0.80}$	Hayssen and Lacy, 1985
MER	Snakes	$6.4\ W^{0.75}$	Kirkwood and Gili, 1994
	Passerine birds (30°C)	$115\ W^{0.62}$	Kendeigh, 1970
	Non-passerines (30°C)	$99\ W^{0.75}$	Kendeigh, 1970
	Birds (0°C)	$167\ W^{0.53}$	Kendeigh, 1970
	Birds of prey	$109\ W^{0.68}$	Kirkwood, 1981
	Falconidae	$118\ W^{0.78}$	Kirkwood and Bennett, 1992
	Accipitridae	$110\ W^{0.65}$	Kirkwood and Bennett, 1992
	Eutherian mammals	$145\ W^{0.75}$	Evans and Miller, 1968
	Eutherian mammals	$140\ W^{0.75}$	Robbins, 1983
	Rodents	$85\ W^{0.54}$	Grodzinski and Wunder, 1975
	Insectivora	$67\ W^{0.43}$	Grodzinski and Wunder, 1975
	Primates	$97\ W^{0.75}$	Kirkwood and Underwood, 1984
	Prosimians	$63–136\ W^{0.75}$	Pollock, 1986
ADMR	Lizards	$12.9\ W^{0.80}$	Nagy, 1982
	Birds	$204\ W^{0.61}$	Walsberg, 1983
	Birds	$220\ W^{0.61}$	Bennett and Harvey, 1987
	Mammals	$192\ W^{0.66}$	Garland, 1983

Table 23.1: *Allometric equations describing basal metabolic rate (BMR), maintenance energy requirements (MER), and free-living average daily (ADMR) metabolic rates (kcal/day) for a variety of taxonomic groups in relation to body weight (W, kg).*

1kcal = 4.184kJ.

Bodyweight (kg)	MER (kcal/day)[1]		
	reptiles	marsupials	eutherian mammals and birds
0.02	0.3	5	7
0.05	0.7	10	15
0.1	1.2	17	25
0.2	2	29	42
0.5	4	57	83
1	7	96	140
2	11	161	235
5	22	320	468
10	38	540	787
20	63	908	1324
50	126	1805	2632
100	212	3035	4427

Table 23.2: *Estimates of metabolisable energy requirements for maintenance (MER, kcal/day) for animals of a variety of taxonomic groups in relation to body weight (kg).*

The figures are based on the allometric equations listed in Table 23.1.
[1] 1kcal = 4.184kJ.

where (Kirkwood and Bennett, 1992). Perhaps the most important point to emphasise here is that, even when such equations are based on high quality data from a large proportion of the species in a given taxonomic group (which is rarely the case) the upper and lower 95% limits for a prediction often span a wide range. Furthermore, it must be borne in mind that predictions based on interspecies regressions are predictions of species means, and there may be considerable variation among individuals about these means. Allometric equations provide useful first estimates but the actual requirements of an individual may be considerably greater or less.

The steps in estimating the ME requirements for maintenance of an animal are shown in Box 23.1.

Calculating Food Requirements from Metabolisable Energy Requirements

The metabolisable energy densities of foods vary depending on their chemical composition and the digestive efficiencies of the animals eating them. Food requirement (g/day) is equal to the metabolisable energy requirement (kcal/day) divided by the metabolisable energy density of the food (kcal/g fresh weight). Metabolisable energy densities of a wide variety of foods have been measured or calculated and detailed tables are available in the literature. McCance and Widdowson's tables (Paul & Southgate, 1987) are a very useful source of information on the metabolisable energy densities of foods for humans and are probably applicable to many other omnivores. Data for a wide range of laboratory, farm and companion animals are also provided in the series of publications on nutrient requirements published by the National Research Council of the USA (e.g. NRC, 1978). Some data on the metabolisable energy densities of diets fed to birds of prey are given in a review by Kirkwood (1981).

Energy and Food Requirements for Growth

During growth, energy is required both for maintenance functions and for new tissue deposition. The

Food	Carnivore	Omnivore	Herbivore
lean meat	1.5	1.5	-
fat	9	9	9
whole animals	1.5	1.5	-
grass	-	0.5	0.5
hay	-	-	1.8
cereals/grains	-	3.5	3.0
green vegetables	-	0.2	0.3
roots	-	0.4	0.4
fresh fruit	-	0.4	0.4

Table 23.3: *Approximate metabolisable energy densities of some foods (kcal/g fresh weight). (1kcal = 4.184kJ.)*

For example, what is the metabolisable energy requirement of an injured adult red kite *Milvus milvus* likely to be?

1) Weigh the animal and note its weight in kilograms.

   It weighs 0.95kg.

2) Choose a suitable allometric equation for predicting the metabolisable energy requirement for maintenance. Some suitable equations are listed in Table 23.1.

   The red kite is a bird of prey and a member of the family Accipitridae. In this case, the allometric equation for non-passerine birds or for birds of prey or for accipiters could be used (see Table 23.1). In this example, the equation for birds of prey is used (the other two give similar estimates):

   $MER = 109\, W^{0.68}$

   where MER is ME requirement for maintenance in kcal/day and W *is body weight in kg.*

   If there is no suitable equation for predicting MER, first calculate BMR then estimate MER as 1.5 or 2 BMR.

3) Use a calculator with exponent function to solve the equation $MER = 109\, W^{0.68}$.

   First calculate $W^{0.68}$ *which, in this case is* $0.95^{0.68}$

   which equals 0.97.

   Then multiply this value by 109.

   This gives an estimate of MER of 105 kcal/day[1]*.*

4) From this, calculate the daily food requirements.

   To calculate the daily food requirement (g/day), divide the estimate of MER (kcal/day) by the metabolisable energy density of the food (kcal/g fresh weight). See Table 23.3.

   The metabolisable energy density of whole mice is about 1.5 kcal/g fresh weight (see Table 23.3). The food requirement of the kite in this example is calculated as 105/1.5 which is 70g/day of fresh whole mice.

5) Remember this is a first estimate. It is unlikely to reflect the daily requirement exactly but is probably close enough not to cause rapid rates of weight gain or loss.

6) Monitor food consumption, body weight and body condition and adjust this first approximation in the light of the findings.

Box 23.1: *Estimating an animal's daily metabolisable energy and thus food requirement for maintenance.*

* *1kcal = 4.184kJ.*

extent to which the total daily requirement exceeds that for maintenance alone depends heavily on the animal's growth rate and this varies with stage of growth and between taxa (Kirkwood, 1991a). It is therefore impossible to make generalisations about requirements during growth that are, at the same time, both simple and accurate. In all animals, weight gain typically follows a sigmoid pattern with time: the growth rate is initially low, but accelerates to reach a peak when the animal is one third to one half grown, and then declines to zero. In animals which grow very rapidly, such as altricial birds, the total daily energy requirement, at peak growth rates, can exceed the maintenance requirement of a similar-sized adult animal by 2 to 3 times. In contrast, the daily requirements during growth of very slow growing animals, such as many of the anthropoid primates, and especially the great apes (Kirkwood, 1985; Kirkwood and Stathatos, 1992), exceed those needed for maintenance by relatively little.

Estimating the energy requirements of animals during growth is complex (Kirkwood, 1991a; Kirkwood and Mace, 1995) and, for this, it is useful to have data on normal growth curves. However, such data are available for only a minority of species. The following general points may be helpful when it is necessary to estimate energy and food requirements during growth. (a) Except in the very early stages of the growth of altricial birds (before they develop endothermy), total daily requirement during growth is very unlikely to be less than that calculated for maintenance on the basis of body weight as described in Box 23.1. (b) During growth, energy (and food) intake often reaches a peak which is 2 to 3 times greater than the maintenance requirement calculated from body weight. (c) There appears to be a ceiling to ME intake between species of homeotherms at about 400kcal (1680kJ)/d per $kg^{0.75}$ (Kirkwood, 1983) so it is extremely unlikely that requirements will exceed this.

Energy Requirements for Activity and Thermoregulation

The energy requirements for activity and thermoregulation of animals maintained in captivity under comfortable thermal conditions are likely to be small. Estimates of the energy requirements for activity can be derived from allometric equations relating energy cost per kilometre travelled by mammals and birds given by Calder (1994). (I have assumed that ME is used for locomotion with an efficiency of 0.75.)

Birds	ME for activity (kcal/km) = $1.7\, W^{0.77*}$
Mammals	ME for activity (kcal/km) = $3.4\, W^{0.60*}$

These equations indicate that 1kg birds and mammals require 1.7 and 3.4kcal, respectively, for each kilometre covered. In captive animals, activity costs are unlikely therefore to be more than a small proportion of maintenance requirement.

The energy requirements for maintaining body temperature in cold weather (this only applies to endotherms) depend upon the intensity of chilling (which is a function of ambient temperature, radiation, windspeed and wetness) and on the degree to which the animal is adapted to cold conditions. It is not easy to make generalisations or predictions about increments in energy requirements for cold weather. Energy requirements can increase to 2 or 3 times maintenance levels in small birds and mammals in cold conditions but under normal captive conditions, which should include a comfortable thermal environment, demands for thermoregulation are typically much lower than this.

Over- or Underfeeding

Many species of animals (mammals, birds and reptiles) are prone to obesity when fed *ad libitum* in captivity. This may be related to their capacities for deposition of fat stores as an adaption to fluctuating food availability due to seasonal, chance, or other factors. Obesity is therefore not easy to define but it is not usual for wild animals to maintain extensive fat depots throughout the year. There are exceptions to this, for example, marine mammals.

If fed less than required for maintenance, body tissues are metabolised to meet daily energy demands and, if underfeeding persists, the animal will starve to death. Severe loss of condition due to underfeeding rarely occurs in captive animals. There is a danger of its occurrence when inexperienced falconers over-restrict the food intake of their birds whilst regulating intake to keep them 'keen' to return to the fist or lure for food when flown. Underfeeding can also occur when young mammals are bottle-reared using inappropriate milk formulae in which the energy density is too

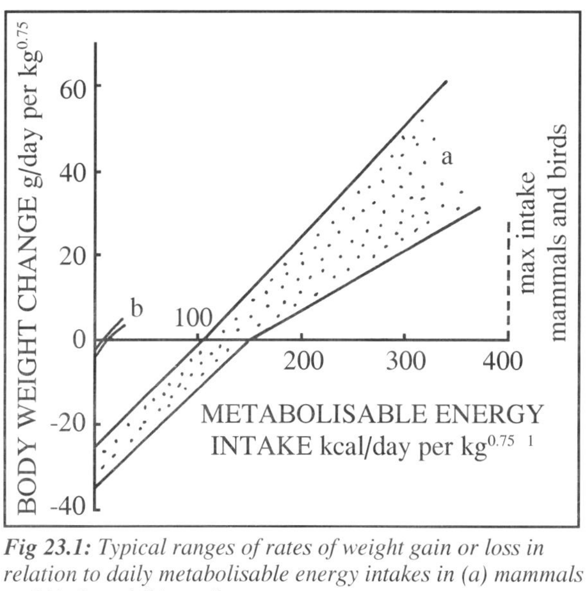

Fig 23.1: *Typical ranges of rates of weight gain or loss in relation to daily metabolisable energy intakes in (a) mammals and birds and (b) reptiles.*

Footnote: Short-term rates of weight loss or gain may be greater than this figure suggests because of fluctuations in gut content. The assumption in this figure is that the latter is constant.

[1] *1kcal = 4.184kJ.*

low, or when the lactose content is too high such that adequate quantities cannot be given without causing nutritional diarrhoea (Kirkwood, 1991b).

The rates of weight gain and loss when adult animals are fed at above or below maintenance level depend on the composition of the tissue being deposited or metabolised. The energy densities of fat and lean tissue (protein and water) are 9 and 1kcal (38 and 4.18kJ)/g, respectively. However, tissue catabolism and anabolism usually involve both fat and lean tissue and measurements of the energy density of weight change have been found to vary widely around 2 to 7 kcal (8.4 to 29kJ)/g and are typically about 2.5kcal (10.5kJ)/g in prolonged fasting (King, 1974; Robbins, 1983; Kirkwood, 1981; Westerterp, 1977). From this, rates of weight gain or loss when fed above or below maintenance level can be estimated (see Fig 23.1). This can be used to provide some guidance as to the relationship between reduced intake and rates of weight loss when attempting to control obesity and also on how rapidly an underfed animal may regain weight.

Specific Nutrient Requirements and Nutrient Composition of Diets

Where available, data on the diets of free-living individuals are a very useful basis from which to devise diets for use in captivity. As a general principle the diet provided in captivity should be as similar to that typically taken in the wild as possible. However, good quantitative data on the composition of the diets of free-living wild animals are scarce. It is important to remember that there may be seasonal changes and also that appetite for particular food items may vary in parallel with changing physiological demands. For example, some birds specifically search for calcium-rich foods (e.g. bone or shell fragments) when laying eggs or to provide to their growing chicks (e.g. Maclean, 1974; Mundy and Leger, 1976). Thus short-term observations of diets of free-living animals may not provide a complete picture of requirements.

When it is possible to provide a diet identical to that normally eaten in the wild, the need to consider individual nutrient intake rates is largely side-stepped because, under these circumstances, nutrient deficiencies or imbalances are unlikely. The risk of specific nutrient deficiencies or imbalances is reduced also when balanced and well tried and tested proprietary feeds are used as part of the daily rations. Specially formulated diets are becoming available for a widening range of species (e.g. Mazuri Zoo Animal Diets, Specialist Diets Services, Witham, Essex).

Care should be taken when supplementing diets with the fat-soluble vitamins (since these can be toxic in high doses). Diseases due to excessive vitamin intakes occur occasionally and can arise when, for example, supplementation rates are miscalculated. Where vitamin preparations are used routinely to supplement diets there is a danger that doses may gradually escalate (because of the naive view that if a little is good, more must be even better). A coagulopathy associated with hypervitaminosis E leading to reduced absorbtion of vitamin K has been observed in pelicans *Pelecanus rufescens* (Nichols *et al.*, 1989). Similarly, hypervitaminosis A was thought to be the cause of deaths associated with a hypovitaminosis K-like coagulopathy in tree shrews *Lyongale tana* (Rivers *et al.*, 1978).

Diet Analyses

Where dietary imbalance or nutritional disease is suspected, detailed analysis of the diet is helpful in assessing the cause and for devising appropriate changes. When the diet is complex and consists of a wide variety of food items, analyses of specific nutrient intakes and determinations of the relative proportions of nutrients in the diet can be a laborious task. For this purpose, the nutrient composition of diets or component foods can be measured directly by laboratory analyses, but it is often sufficient, at least in the first instance, to use data provided in published tables of nutrient compositions (e.g. Paul & Southgate, 1987; NRC, 1978).

Analyses of the nutrient composition are facilitated greatly by the use of software packages such as the Animal Nutritionist (N-Squared Computing, Oregon) (see Products list below). This includes an extensive database of the nutrient composition of foods and permits rapid estimation of the nutrient composition of complex diets. It is important to remember, however, that the nutrient composition of some feeds (e.g. forages) can vary considerably and that specific nutrient densities may differ from the typical values listed in the database.

SOME NUTRITIONAL DISEASES OF CAPTIVE WILD ANIMALS

Nutritional diseases of captive wild animals have been reviewed by various authors (e.g. Scott, 1986; Lowenstine, 1986; Frye, 1981). The subject is too large for systematic review here. In this section, I briefly describe some nutritional diseases which still occur commonly in captive wild animals.

Calcium Deficiency during Growth

Bone disease due to calcium deficiency during growth remains a common problem in captive wild animals. In this, inadequate mineralisation of the growing bones results in predisposition to folding fractures and distortions in the limbs and other parts of the skeleton. The disease can affect any bony animal but is seen perhaps most commonly in carnivores and insectivores fed on diets that do not include bone and also in frugivores and granivores.

The calcium requirements for maintenance are low and it is likely that a dietary calcium concentration of 0.5% in the dry matter is sufficient for all adult animals except laying birds (which may require up to 3%). A concentration of 0.5% is also probably adequate to support normal skeletal development in slow-growing mammals (such as anthropoid primates e.g. macaques or apes). The proportion of calcium required in the diet depends on whether the animal grows relatively rapidly or relatively slowly in relation to its adult size. For animals of a given adult size, those which reach skeletal maturity rapidly need a higher proportion of calcium in the diet because their total food consumption during growth is lower than that of those which grow more slowly. There are few specific data on calcium requirements of wild animals.

A dietary calcium concentration of 0.5 to 1% of dry matter (as recommended for many domestic species) is probably adequate for growth in most mammals and reptiles. Debate continues about the ideal calcium concentrations in the diets of growing birds. Concentrations of 0.7 to 1.3% dry matter are recommended for some domesticated precocial birds (Ullrey *et al.*, 1991), but higher concentrations (at least 1%) may be required for some altricial species with rapid growth rates. It is worthy of note that the calcium density of adult animals is typically about 2.5-3 % of dry matter, so this is the dietary concentration to which carnivores that eat whole animals are normally exposed. Excessive dietary calcium densities should be avoided since these have been shown to lead to disturbances of bone growth in some domestic species (Hazewinkel, 1989). The calcium to phosphorus ratio in diets should be about 1.5:1 to 2:1 and not less than 1:1 (Scott, 1986).

The calcium content of deficient diets can be raised by addition of a suitable supplement. The quantity to be added to the diet should be calculated and weighed out carefully. The calcium content of some calcium supplements are shown in Table 23.4.

Supplement	Calcium content %
Calcium lactate	13
Calcium orthophosphate	38.8
Calcium Phosphorus (PetAg)	19
Vionate	9.4
SA37 (Intervet)	1
Cuttlefish 'bone'	36.2
Bonemeal	30

***Table 23.4:** Calcium content of various calcium supplements.*

Nutritional Diarrhoea in Bottle-Fed Infant Mammals

Infant mammals taken for hand rearing may develop diarrhoea if offered an inappropriate milk replacer. Milk composition varies greatly between mammals (Oftedal, 1984; Jenness and Sloan, 1975) and the most readily available milks (cow's milk and human milk formulae) are poor substitutes for the milks of the majority of other species. Data on milk composition of a range of British wild mammals and also on some milk replacer formulae have been presented elsewhere (Kirkwood, 1991). In general, it is a good principle to use a milk replacer which matches the fat, protein and carbohydrate composition of the milk of the species as closely as possible.

Overnutrition during Growth / Twisting and Bending Deformities of Limb Bones in Precocial Birds

Twisting or bending deformities of the limb bones are common in some species of precocial birds reared in captivity (Kirkwood, 1994). These deformities often affect the leg bones of ratites, waterfowl, and other species (Serafin, 1982; Guittin, 1986) and also affect the wings of waterfowl and others (Kear, 1973). The aetiology is not clear but it appears that animals fed *ad libitum* on high protein or high energy diets are predisposed to these distortions which arise from disturbances to the growth plates. It seems likely that rapid rates of weight gain contribute by causing abnormal loading of relatively immature growth plates. The incidence can be reduced by restricting access to high energy, high protein feeds and by encouraging exercise during growth.

Vitamin D_3 Deficiency in New World Primates

Nutritional bone disease is commonly seen in New World monkeys (e.g. marmosets *Callithrix jacchus*, tamarins *Saguinus* spp. and squirrel monkeys *Saimiri sciureus*). Affected animals typically have a slow, cautious and hunched gait and are thin. The immediate history is often one of sudden deterioration that may be found to be due to pathological fracture of a limb bone or collapse of a lumbar vertebra. These animals have often been fed on diets predominantly of fruit and which are deficient in both calcium and vitamin D_3. New World monkeys need vitamin D_3 and recommended requirements vary from 100 to 400IU/day (NRC, 1978; Escajadillo *et al.*, 1981). The disease can be prevented by providing a diet which contains vitamin D_3 (e.g. Mazuri Primate Diet, Specialist Diets Services, Witham, Essex), or by adding carefully weighed out supplements of the vitamin. Adequate dietary calcium must also be ensured.

PRODUCTS MENTIONED IN TEXT

Animal Nutritionist Software N-Squared Computing, 5318 Forest Ridge Road, Silverton, Oregon 97381, USA.

Calcium Phosphorus PetAg Inc., 30W432 Rt 20, Elgin, IL 60120, USA.

Mazuri Primate Diet Special Diets Services, PO Box 705, Witham, Essex CM8 3AD, UK.

SA37 Intervet UK Limited, Science Park, Milton Road, Cambridge CB4 4FP, UK.

REFERENCES

Bennett AF and Dawson WR (1976). Metabolism. In: *Biology of the Reptilia*. Eds C Gans and FH Pugh. Academic Press, New York **vol 13,** pp 127-223.

Bennett PM and Harvey PH (1987). Active and resting metabolism in birds: allometry, physiology and ecology. *Journal of Zoology* **213,** 327-363.

Blaxter KL (1989). *Energy metabolism in animals and man*. Cambridge University Press, Cambridge.

Calder WA III (1984). *Size, function and life history*. Harvard University Press, Cambridge, MA.

Clarke HE, Coates ME, Eva JK, Ford DJ, Milner CK, O'Donoghue PN, Scott PP and Ward RJ (1977). Dietary standards for laboratory animals: report of the Laboratory Animals Centre Diets Advisory Committee. *Laboratory Animals* **11,** 1-28.

Crandall LS (1964). *The Management of Wild Animals in Captivity*. University of Chicago Press, Chicago.

Dawson TJ, Grant TR and Fanning D (1979). Standard metabolism of monotremes and the evolution of homeothermy. *Australian Journal of Zoology* **27,** 511-515.

Dawson TJ and Hulbert AJ (1970). Standard metabolism, body temperature, and surface areas of Australian marsupials. *American Journal of Physiology* **218,** 1233-1238.

Escajadillo A, Bronson RT, Sehgal PK and Hayes KC (1981). Nutritional evaluation in cotton-top tamarins *(Saguinus oedipus). Laboratory Animal Science* **31,** 161-165.

Evans E and Miller DS (1968). Comparative nutrition, growth and longevity. *Proceedings of the Nutrition Society* **27,** 121-129.

Frye FL (1981). *Biomedical and surgical aspects of captive reptile husbandry*. Veterinary Medicine Publishing Company, Edwardsville, KS.

Garland T (1983). Scaling maximum running speed and body mass in terrestrial mammals. *Journal of Zoology* **199,** 157-170.

Grodzinski W and Wunder BA (1975). Ecological energetics of small mammals. In: *Small Mammals: Their Productivity and Population Dynamics*. Eds FB Golley, K Petrusewicz and L Ryszkowski. Cambridge University Press, Cambridge pp 173-204.

Guittin O (1986). Bow-leg syndrome in ratite birds. *Avicultural Magazine* **92,** 70-79.

Hayssen V and Lacy RC (1985). Basal metabolic rates in mammals: taxonomic differences in the allometry of BMR and body mass. *Comparative Biochemistry and Physiology* **81A,** 741-754.

Hazewinkel HAW (1989). Calcium metabolism and skeletal development in dogs. In: *Nutrition of the Dog and Cat*. Eds IH Burger and JPW Rivers. Cambridge University Press, Cambridge pp 293-302.

Hunt RD, Garcia FG and Hegsted DM (1967). A comparison of vitamin D2 and D3 in New World primates. 1. Production and regression of osteodystropha fibrosa. *Laboratory Animal Care* **17,** 222-234.

Jenness R and Sloan RE (1975). The composition of milks of various species: a review. *Dairy Science Abstracts* **32,** 599-612.

Kear J (1973). Notes on the nutrition of young waterfowl, with special reference to slipped-wing. *International Zoo Yearbook* **13,** 97-100.

Kendeigh SC (1970). Energy requirements for existence in relation to size of bird. *Condor* **72,** 60-65.

King JR (1974). Seasonal allocation of time and energy resources in birds. In: *Avian Energetics.* Ed RA Paynter Jr. Publications of the Nuttall Ornithological Club No 15. Cambridge, Massachusetts pp 4-85.

Kirkwood JK (1981). Maintenance energy requirements and rate of weight loss during starvation in birds of prey. In: *Recent advances in the study of raptor diseases.* Eds JE Cooper and AG Greenwood. Chiron Press, Keighley, England pp 153-157.

Kirkwood JK (1983). A limit to metabolisable energy intake in mammals and birds. *Comparative Biochemistry and Physiology* **75,** 1-3.

Kirkwood JK (1985). Patterns of growth in primates. *Journal of Zoology (London)* **205,** 123-136.

Kirkwood JK (1991a). Energy requirements for maintenance and growth of wild mammals, birds and reptiles in captivity. *Journal of Nutrition* **121,** S29.

Kirkwood JK (1991b) Wild mammals. In: *BSAVA Manual of exotic pets.* Eds PH Beynon and JE Cooper. BSAVA, Cheltenham pp 122-149.

Kirkwood JK (1994). Bone diseases in captive and free-living wild birds. In: *Diseases and Parasites of Birds.* Proceedings of the meeting of the British Ornithologists' Union, September 1993, Madingley Hall, Cambridge.

Kirkwood JK and Bennett PM (1992). Approaches and limitations to the prediction of energy and food re- quirements in wild animal husbandry and veterinary care. *Proceedings of the Nutrition Society* **51,** 117.

Kirkwood JK and Gili C (1994). Food consumption in relation to body weight in captive snakes. *Research in Veterinary Science.*

Kirkwood JK and Mace GM (1995). Patterns of growth in mammals. In: *Wild Mammals in Captivity.* Eds DG Kleiman, ME Allen, KV Thompson and S Lumpkin. University of Chicago Press.

Kirkwood JK and Stathatos K (1992). *Biology, Rearing and Care of Young Primates.* Oxford University Press, Oxford.

Kirkwood JK and Underwood SJ (1984). Energy requirements of captive cotton-top tamarins (*Saguinus oedipus oedipus*). *Folia Primatologia* **42,** 180-187.

Kleiber M (1961). *The Fire of Life.* John Wiley, New York.

Lowenstine LJ (1986). Nutritional disorders of birds. In: *Zoo and wild animal medicine.* Ed ME Fowler. WB Saunders, Philadelphia pp 202-212.

Maclean SF Jr (1974). Lemming bones as a source of calcium for Arctic sandpipers (*Calidris* spp.). *Ibis* **116,** 552-557.

Mundy PJ and Ledger JA (1976). Griffon vultures, carnivores and bones. *South African Journal of Science* **72,** 106-110.

Nagy KA (1982). Energy requirements of free-living iguanid lizards. In: *Iguanas of the World, Their Behaviour, Ecology and Conservation.* Eds GM Burghardt and AS Rand. Noyes Publications, Park Ridge, New Jersey pp 49-59.

Nicholls DK, Wolff MJ, Phillips LJ Jr and Montali RJ (1989). Coagulopathy in pink-backed pelicans (*Pelecanus rufescens*) associated with hypervitaminosis E. *Journal of Zoo and Wildlife Medicine* **20,** 57-61.

NRC (1978). *Nutrient Requirements of Nonhuman Primates.* National Academy of Sciences, Washington D.C

Oftedal OT (1984). Milk composition, milk yield and energy output at peak lactation: a comparative review. *Symposium of the Zoological Society of London* **51,** 33-85.

Paul AA and Southgate DAT (1987). *McCance and Widdowson's the Composition of Foods, 4th edition.* HMSO, Oxford.

Pollock JI (1986). The management of prosimians in captivity for conservation and research. In: *Primates: the Road to Self-sustaining Populations.* Ed K Benirschke. Springer-Verlag, New York pp 269-288.

Rivers JPW, D'Souza F and Hawkey CM (1978). Overnutrition and hypervitaminosis A in the tree shrew (*Lyongale tana*). *Proceedings of the Nutrition Society* **37,** 6A.

Robbins CT (1983). *Wildlife Feeding and Nutrition.* New York, Academic Press.

Ross CA (1989). *Life History Strategies of Primates.* PhD Thesis, University College, London.

Scott ML (1986). *Nutrition of Humans and Selected Animal Species.* John Wiley & Sons, New York.

Serafin JA (1982). The influence of diet composition upon growth and development of sandhill cranes. *Condor* **84,** 427-434.

Ullrey D and Allen ME (1986). Principles of zoo mammal nutrition. In: *Zoo and Wild Animal Medicine.* Ed ME Fowler. WB Saunders, Philadelphia pp 516-532.

Ullrey DE, Allen ME and Baer DJ (1991). Formulated diets versus seed mixtures for psittacines. *Journal of Nutrition* **121,** S193-S205.

Walsberg GE (1983). Avian ecological energetics. In: *Avian Biology*. VII. Eds DS Farner, JR King and KC Parkes. Academic Press, New York pp 161-220.

Westerterp K (1977). How rats economise - energy loss in starvation. *Physiological Zoology* **50,** 331-362.

CHAPTER TWENTY-FOUR

Ornamental Fish Nutrition and Feeding

Alastair Macartney

FEEDING OBJECTIVES AND REQUIREMENTS

Feeding fish is different to feeding terrestrial animals. Food is dispersed into the living environment, and sufficient must be delivered so that it is located and consumed in a volume many times the size of the fish. Feeding too little results in starvation, but excess uneaten food quickly pollutes the environment. Since faeces and excreta are also pollutants, the formulation of the diet must encourage efficient digestion and metabolism.

Fish of more than one species, with different nutritional requirements and feeding habits, are commonly held together in a single tank, and maintained on a single diet. Thus, the diet must be suitable for all tank inhabitants, which may include herbivores, omnivores and carnivores. Not only will these fish have different nutrient requirements, but the digestibility of various components of the diet will differ depending on the natural diet and intestinal morphology. Furthermore the physical characteristics of the diet and the feeding regimen must satisfy the different lifestyles and feeding habits, such as surface, middle and bottom feeders, and diurnal variations in feeding among these groups.

Feeding requirements are dependent on life stage, and also on the requirements of the aquarist. High growth rates are desirable for fry, but in an established tank it may be more suitable to feed closer to the maintenance requirement (the maximum potential adult size is often overlooked when young fish are purchased). These different objectives require diets with both alternative nutrient profiles and physical characteristics, and a change in the feeding regimen.

Whilst the nutrient requirements of food-fish have been the subject of considerable research effort in recent years, ornamental fish have not enjoyed such attention, due of course to their lower sale value. An exception is the koi carp (*Cyprinus carpio*). The nutrient requirements of this fish are relatively well established, but only by virtue of the food value of the common strain of this species. As a result, many of the nutritional data presented here are derived from food-fish. However, it is unlikely that nutrient requirements will vary greatly among species sharing similar habitats and diets in nature. Thus, where the exact requirements of an ornamental fish are unknown, judicious analogy with food-fish can provide valuable information.

ENERGY REQUIREMENTS

Fish are ectotherms and so their maintenance energy requirements change with changing environmental temperature. In general, the maintenance energy requirement of fish is less than 10% of the maintenance energy requirement of birds and mammals (Smith, 1989). Studies at the WALTHAM Aquacentre have shown that the maintenance food requirement of a 5g goldfish (*Carassius auratus*) increased nearly three-fold as water temperature rose from 20° to 24°C. For koi carp in garden ponds, the daily maintenance energy requirement more than doubles when the water temperature increases from 10°C to 20°C. This is an important consideration when planning a feeding strategy for these fish as they virtually stop feeding when water temperatures reach 5°C and lower. Under these conditions their metabolism is reduced to a quiescent level and the fish survive by drawing on their energy reserves until the water temperature rises again in spring. Thus it is vital to prepare pond fish for winter torpor by feeding them a higher level of digestible energy in the late summer and autumn. In contrast, tropical fish are kept at constant temperatures all year round (24°C to 26°C), however they also have an energy requirement far lower than that of endothermic mammalian pets.

Both protein and fat are highly available energy sources for fish. The value of carbohydrate as an energy source is variable between species, depending on the normal diet of the animal (see below). Since fish feed to satisfy their energy requirement, protein and energy in the diet should be balanced. A diet too high in energy will reduce the amount of nutrients ingested, whilst a diet too low in energy will result in protein catabolism for maintenance in preference to growth. Optimum ratios for digestible protein to digestible energy (mg/kcal) for food-fish species are 81–117mg protein/kcal DE (19–28mg

Amino acid	Carp (*Cyprinus carpio*)[1]	Tilapia (*Oreochromis nilotica*)[2]
arginine	1.6	1.2
histidine	0.8	0.5
isoleucine	0.9	0.9
leucine	1.3	1.0
lysine	2.2	1.4
methionine	1.2 [3]	0.8 [4]
phenylalanine	2.5 [5]	1.1 [6]
threonine	1.5	1.1
tryptophan	0.3	0.3
valine	1.4	0.8

Table 24.1: *Indispensable amino acid requirement, as percentage of dry diet, of juvenile common carp and juvenile nile tilapia (Data from Nose, 1979; Santiago and Lovell, 1988).*

[1] 38.5% total dietary protein; [2] 28% total dietary protein; [3] in the absence of dietary cystine;
[4] cystine 0.15% of dry diet; [5] in the absence of dietary tyrosine; [6] tyrosine 0.5% of dry diet

protein/kJ DE) (National Research Council, 1993), and it is likely that ornamental fish species will also fall within this range.

NUTRIENTS

Protein

The protein requirement of fish has two components. First, there is the need to supply the indispensable amino acid (IAA) requirement of the animal, and second, a supply of dispensable amino acids or sufficient amino nitrogen to enable their synthesis.

Fish require ten IAAs, namely arginine, histidine, isoleucine, leucine, lysine, methionine, phenylalanine, threonine, tryptophan and valine. As in mammals, there is a sparing action of cystine on methionine, and tyrosine on phenylalanine. Since the IAA requirement differs between species, in the community environment it would be advisable to supply, for each amino acid, the highest level known for any of the species. However, the known IAA requirements of fish are at present restricted to food-fish species of mainly freshwater origin. As a guide Table 24.1 shows the indispensable amino acid requirement of juvenile carp and tilapia.

The quantitative requirements for IAA are high. As a result, even at high protein intake, marked differences in the nutritional values of different protein sources is observed due to limiting concentrations of certain IAAs (Cowey, 1975). In addition, given that energy is required to synthesise dispensable amino acids, feeding a protein source that closely matches the requirements of the species in question will ultimately lead to the most efficient growth, and reduced protein excretion. Because of its amino acid profile, fish meal, or derivatives, is considered to be the optimal protein source, and alternative protein sources should be selected with care.

The importance of efficient protein utilisation is often overlooked by aquarists, despite the fact that the breakdown products of protein metabolism will directly pollute the living environment of the fish. The majority of excreted nitrogen is in the form of ammonia, with usually insignificant amounts of urea. The toxicity of excreted ammonia is dependent to a large degree on water pH, and to a lesser extent on temperature. This is because ammonia can exist in both the toxic unionised form (NH_3), and the relatively non-toxic ionised form (NH_4^+), and is readily inter-converted between the two. Increasing pH (above pH 7.2) and temperature both favour the conversion of NH_4^+ to NH_3 (Russo, 1985). However, mature biological aquarium filters are colonised by nitrifying bacteria (*Nitrosomonas* spp.) which metabolise ammonia, and the ammonium ion, into nitrite (NO_2^-). The toxicity of nitrite is highly dependent on the chemical composition of the water. For example, nitrite toxicity decreases with increasing chloride ion concentration (Russo, 1985). It is generally accepted by aquarists, however, that in a healthy aquarium both total ammonia and nitrite concentrations should be kept at zero. Fortunately, a further group of nitrifying bacteria (*Nitrobacter* spp.) metabolise nitrite to relatively non-toxic nitrate (NO_3^-). Although nitrates may increase the productivity of an aquatic system, excessive amounts may lead to eutrophication. This is the primary reason for reducing nitrates in aquarium water. However, nitrate may become acutely toxic to the freshwater fish itself at concentrations in excess of 100mg/kg, and at 50mg/kg for marine fish. The bacteria of the biological filter thus play an important role in controlling pollution of the tank with nitrogenous metabolites. Since algae and plants will take up nitrate from the water, they can also be considered part of the biological filter.

The quantity of protein in fish diets is generally high (25–50%), and thus the quality of protein provided in food items should be high to avoid the release of excessive amounts of unmetabolised nitrogen into the tank water. In addition, uneaten food will also add to the nitrogen load in the fishes' environment once it has been metabolised by resident bacteria, and so should be removed from the aquarium after 30 minutes or so. Nitrates are traditionally reduced in the aquarium by performing partial water changes, usually in the region of 10% of the total water volume, when nitrate concentrations, as determined by commercially available test kits, reach unacceptable levels. In static tanks, i.e. those with no filtration equipment, water changes may have to be performed several times per week to reduce ammonia and nitrite. The Aquarian Advisory Service estimates that most queries regarding fish health and disease are related to improper filtration or nitrate build up (D. Sands, personal communication).

Fat

Dietary fat serves as a source of both metabolic energy and essential polyunsaturated fatty acids. Since carbohydrate is a poor energy source in fish, the provision of energy from fat via beta-oxidation in the mitochondria is particularly important. In addition, fat plays an important role as a carrier of fat-soluble vitamins. For these reasons, fish diets should not contain less than approximately 10% fat. However, because of the relatively low energy demand of fish, an upper level of 20% fat is recommended to avoid excessive fat deposition (Cowey and Sargent, 1979). Feeding 'hard' fats high in saturates to fish in a cold environment should be avoided, since solidification in the digestive tract may cause blockage, and subsequent death of the fish.

Essential fatty acids (EFA) requirements of fish depend on the natural environment and feeding habits of the species in question. It is well established that the *n*-3/*n*-6 ratio is higher in marine fish than freshwater fish, and that this reflects the higher dietary input of the more terrestrial in origin *n*-6 series fatty acids in the diets of freshwater fish (Cowey and Sargent, 1979). Freshwater fish are generally able to elongate chains and further desaturate the shorter chain EFA, and thus tend to require either linolenic (*n*-3) or linoleic (*n*-6) acid, or both. In marine fish the situation is more complex. A dietary source of *n*-3 fatty acids is essential for marine fish, and for the marine herbivore and lower carnivores, linolenic acid appears to have full essential fatty acid activity. However, the piscivores require the longer and more unsaturated eicosapentaenoic acid (EPA) (20:5(*n*-3)) or docosahexaenoic acid (DHA) (22:6 (*n*-3)). This pattern of essential fatty acid requirement thus reflects the natural abundance of the longer chain highly unsaturated fatty acids (HUFA) in prey items. Fish eating diets rich in the shorter chain fatty acids are able to desaturate and chain elongate these to HUFA (ultimately DHA), whilst those species consuming large amounts of DHA are generally unable to metabolise DHA from *n*-3 precursors (linolenic acid and perhaps EPA).

In the absence of specific data, essential fatty acid deficiency is best prevented in freshwater ornamental fish by including 1% (w/w) linolenic (*n*-3) and 1% linoleic (*n*-6) acids in the diet. For marine fish the diet should contain 2% linolenic acid for herbivorous and omnivorous species, but this should be replaced by DHA, or a mixture of EPA and DHA, for carnivorous fish. Gross symptoms of essential fatty acid deficiency are manifest as growth retardation, fin rot, myocarditis, increased mortality, and, most profound, a 'shock syndrome' in which the fish lose neuromuscular control (Sinnhuber, 1969).

Carbohydrate

Carbohydrate is only poorly used as an energy source in fish. In general energy metabolism in fish resembles that in a non-insulin-dependent diabetic mammal (Nagai and Ikeda, 1972). Carp react to digestible carbohydrate very much like other teleosts, in that high and prolonged post-prandial glycaemia is observed. Nevertheless, in shallow water aquatic plants and algae do represent a source of carbohydrate for many fish. Most herbivorous fish have developed physiological and morphological adaptations, such as a long intestine:body length ratio, that promotes microbial digestion of carbohydrate. It is thus not surprising that carbohydrate digestion can vary greatly between species, and even between fish of one species, depending on environment.

Vitamins

The characteristic diseases caused by vitamin deficiency in mammals are less well defined in fish species, and are undescribed for practically all ornamental fish, apart from the carp. Values reported for food-fish species are wide ranging, and this reflects the different life stage requirements, as well as nutrient interactions and environmental conditions (National Research Council (NRC), 1993).

The fat-soluble vitamins are only absorbed in the intestine with fat, thus diets high in fat favour absorption. Since fat-soluble vitamins are stored when intake exceeds demand, hypervitaminosis is possible. However, in ornamental fish, only hypervitaminosis A is likely to occur where high levels of fish oil are included in diets. Hypervitaminosis A manifests as slow growth, anaemia and severe necrosis of the caudal fin in brook trout (Poston *et al.*, 1966). Gut microflora have been proposed as an exogenous source of vitamin K in fish, however as yet the specific vitamin K synthesising microflora have not been described.

Vitamin	unit	requirement
A	IU/kg	10000
D	IU/kg	2400
E	mg/kg	100
K	mg/kg	10
B_1 (thiamin)	mg/kg	10
B_2 (riboflavin)	mg/kg	10
niacin	mg/kg	50
B_6 (pyridoxine)	mg/kg	10
B_{12}	mg/kg	0.02
pantothenate	mg/kg	50
folate	mg/kg	10
inositol	mg/kg	440
choline	mg/kg	2000
biotin	mg/kg	1
C	mg/kg	250

Table 24.2: *Estimated minimum vitamin requirements for ornamental fish.*

The water-soluble vitamins are not stored, and thus a constant source is required. Microbial synthesis supplies the requirement of some fish for some water-soluble vitamins, although the effect is more pronounced for herbivores with the longer hind gut; microbial synthesis of vitamins is thought to be insignificant in coldwater carnivores (Hepher, 1988). Thus, during periods of antibiotic treatment, care should be taken to ensure that the full vitamin requirement is met through the diet. Vitamin deficiency symptoms are often not specific to a particular vitamin, and many are species-specific. In general, anorexia, poor growth and poor external appearance may be characteristic of a deficiency.

Table 24.2 gives the range of vitamin concentrations recommended for ornamental fish diets. The data presented are adapted from data for food-fish species (NRC, 1993), and thus is only a guide for ornamental fish. The values in Table 24.2 do not take into account degradation of vitamins during diet processing and storage, nor losses due to leaching of vitamins during feeding.

Minerals

The functions of individual minerals in fish are similar to their functions in terrestrial animals. However, unlike terrestrial animals, fish can absorb some inorganic elements directly from the external environment, either through the gills, fins and oral epithelia, or by drinking in marine fish, thereby reducing or obviating a dietary requirement. Thus, whilst the metabolic mineral requirements of species may not differ markedly, the dietary requirement will vary greatly, depending on whether the fish is marine or freshwater, and on the mineral content of the latter environment, which may vary with geographical location. For this reason, it is recommended that for freshwater fish at least, the total mineral requirement is supplied in the diet.

The quantitative requirements of ornamental fish, especially tropical species, are virtually unknown. Most research to date has concentrated on food-fish species, and these data must be used as a guide for ornamentals until the exact requirements are known. The major mineral requirements are outlined below, however it is generally accepted that the trace elements important in higher animal and human nutrition are also necessary for complete fish nutrition.

Calcium

Minimum requirements have been established for very few species due to the complications of gill and diet interactions, however, calcium deficiency has seldom been detected (NRC, 1993), and it is unlikely in the aquarium environment despite the reduced water turnover. Fish absorb calcium through the gills, the most important site for calcium regulation, and also from dietary input. In marine fish, which drink copiously, the gut is not a major site of calcium absorption due to interactions with other minerals such as magnesium, strontium and zinc. Commercially prepared ornamental fish foods are usually high in calcium because of the high level of fish meal.

Phosphorus

Since the concentration of this mineral in both fresh and salt water is low, dietary sources of phosphorus are essential. Phosphorus availability can be limited. It appears that, from animal meals, such as fish meal, herbivores are less able to extract phosphorus than carnivores, due to the limited gastric secretions of the former (Ogino *et al.,* 1979). In addition, phytin phosphorus is unavailable to fish, thus food items such as soyabean meal are not good phosphorus sources. Dietary requirements ranging from 0.5 to 0.8% of dry diet have been reported for a number of species, including carp (NRC, 1993).

Magnesium

The full requirement can be met either through the gills if present in sufficient concentrations in the external environment, or from dietary supply, including drinking in marine fish. The magnesium requirement for a number of species, including the guppy (Shim and Nag, 1988) has been estimated to range from 400 to 600mg/kg (NRC, 1993). Deficiency signs vary between species, but are generally manifest as anorexia, reduced growth and lethargy.

Sodium, Potassium and Chlorine

The most abundant electrolytes in the body, these minerals are easily absorbed. In addition, because of the high levels in normal diet ingredients, supplementation is unnecessary. The result is that deficiencies of these minerals are rare, and the symptoms largely unknown since it is difficult to induce an experimental deficiency because of the high capacity for absorption from the external environment (NRC, 1993).

Iron

The addition of ferrous sulphate to the water enhanced the growth of swordtails and platys, demonstrating a route for iron absorption through the gills (Roeder and Roeder, 1966). However, most fish environments are low in iron, necessitating a dietary input. A minimum requirement of 200mg/kg diet is advised based on the requirements of food-fish species (NRC, 1993). Deficiency can be determined by morphological and histological examination of the liver, and by reduced haematocrit, haemoglobin and plasma iron concentration. An upper safe level of iron in the diet has been shown to be 1380mg/kg for trout (Desjardins *et al.*, 1987), and in the absence of species-specific data, this should be regarded as a maximum for all ornamental fish.

Copper

A dietary level of 5mg/kg diet is recommended for ornamental fish, again based on the requirements of food-fish (NRC, 1993). Dissolved copper in the water appears to be more toxic than dietary copper, since a concentration of 0.1mg/kg dissolved copper can be acutely toxic to tropical freshwater fish (Stoskopf, 1993).

Iodine

Fish obtain iodine both from the water and diet, however iodine is rapidly depleted in marine aquaria, especially when foam-fractionation filtering systems (protein skimmers) are employed. A dietary requirement of 1–5mg/kg is recommended based on a small number of experiments on food-fish (NRC, 1993).

Zinc

The zinc requirement of fish is in the range 15–30mg/kg diet (NRC, 1993). However, dietary phytate and tricalcium phosphate (present in fish meal) markedly reduce bioavailability, thus up to 200mg/kg may be required to ensure the metabolic requirement is satisfied. Zinc deficiencies have caused growth suppression, cataracts, fin and skin erosion, and ultimately mortality in salmonids (Ogino and Yang, 1979).

Manganese

Based on the requirement for food-fish (NRC, 1993), a minimum of 13mg/kg manganese in the diet is recommended. In salmonids (Yamamoto *et al.*, 1983; Ogino and Yang, 1980) and cyprinids (Ogino and Yang, 1980) manganese deficiency has been associated with reduced growth, skeletal abnormalities, cataracts and dwarfism.

Selenium

Vitamin E has a sparing action on selenium, but cannot replace it entirely, since growth retardation has been observed in rainbow trout fed a selenium-deficient diet with an excess of vitamin E (Hilton *et al.,* 1980). Selenium requirement also varies depending on the lipid content of the diet, and more specifically on the content of polyunsaturated fatty acids, which are prone to oxidation. Selenium is present in fish meal, but the digestibility is low (Bell and Cowey, 1989). Selenium can also be absorbed efficiently across the gills, but whether this can supply in full the requirements of ornamental fish species is unknown. A recommendation based on food-fish requirements (NRC, 1993) is 0.5mg/kg of diet. Toxicity occurs in salmonids at greater than 10mg/kg diet (Hilton and Hodson, 1983), and this should be considered an absolute maximum for ornamental species until the exact toxicity levels are known.

FOOD TYPES

There is an ever increasing range of commercially prepared foods for ornamental fish. These can be classified as those that are nutritionally complete, normally flake, and granular or pelleted diets, and those that are not, such as some pond foods, and frozen insect larvae, bloodworm, cockle etc.

The choice between flake format and granular format complete foods depends on the fish being fed, and the personal choice of the aquarist. Flake formats do offer versatility, in that they can be floated on the water for surface feeders, or submerged to sink slowly for middle and bottom feeders. Since the flakes are easily broken up into smaller pieces, they provide an excellent single food for a range of species and sizes of fish. Granules offer lower nutrient leaching rates (see below), and different granule sizes and densities can be used to target different groups of fish in the aquarium.

Incomplete foods, especially 'live-foods' such as daphnia and bloodworm, either living or pre-frozen, should be fed with care. These foods are good 'treats' for aquarium fish, however feeding too many of these incomplete foods will reduce the intake of complete diet, thus causing a dietary imbalance. They are particularly useful for feeding 'fussy fish' species whilst they are weaned onto flake diets. Species that require exclusively live foods are rare, but those that do are best fed as wide a variety as possible, and it may be necessary to add a vitamin supplement mixture to the live food. Feeding living live food of aquatic origin is best avoided since the animals are often vectors for piscine diseases. Freezing largely neutralises the risk of disease and thus commercially available pre-frozen packs are the safest to feed.

It is seldom necessary to feed a complete food to pond fish stocked in an established pond, since they feed extensively on the pond's natural flora and fauna. Incomplete pond pellets etc. can be used as a supplement, especially in autumn before the winter torpor, and to tempt the fish to the surface for the enjoyment of the pondkeeper. Those fish, for example koi carp, kept in well filtered and relatively bare display ponds, require a complete diet.

Home-prepared diets are frequently incomplete, and care should be taken to satisfy the nutritional requirements outlined above. Usually, vitamin, mineral and amino acid premixes are required to balance the food.

REGIMEN

With the exception of a small number of tropical freshwater carnivorous fish species (Cichlidae), and goldfish and koi carp, ornamental fish are seldom kept in a single-species environment. In a multi-species or 'community' tank, carnivores, herbivores and omnivores share a common environment in which they feed on a single diet. The nutritional requirements of these different groups highlight the need to strike an equilibrium in the dietary formulation; however, equally critical is the ultimate distribution of food between individuals of one species, and between different species, kept in the same aquarium. Intraspecific and interspecific competition are exacerbated during feeding, the latter because of the natural foraging patterns of the individual species. For example, some species will only feed from the water surface, others from midwater, and others from the bottom of the tank. Some fish may be more active at night, with little or no foraging activity during the day.

The **physical characteristics** of the diet also play an important role when species of various weights, from 0.1g (Characidae) to greater than 20g (Cichlidae), are fed on one diet. Food particles need to be small enough for the smaller species to ingest, but large enough to be identified and eaten by the larger species. Many fish do not possess a well defined or large stomach, and are therefore unable to store large quantities of food. These fish are particularly dependent on a regular supply of food throughout the day to achieve proper growth and development. At the WALTHAM Aquacentre the effect of feed frequency on growth of neon tetras (*Paracheiron innesi*) has been examined (Pannevis and Earle, 1994a). These fish have a high metabolic rate, and require a frequent supply of food to sustain growth and maintenance. Fish with an average body weight of 0.2g were fed the same total daily ration of commercial flake food, but with feed frequencies of one to four times per day. In fish fed three small meals per day, 62% higher growth rates were observed compared to those fed one large meal. Interestingly, those fed four times per day had lower growth rates than those fed three times per day. It is thought that this was the result of non-recognition of food given the very small size of the rations.

A further consideration is **nutrient leaching** from food. Experiments conducted at the WALTHAM Aquacentre have shown the potential for water-soluble vitamin leaching from flake format diets (Pannevis and Earle, 1994a). After 30 seconds contact with water, 90% of vitamin B_{12}, 66% of vitamin C, 47% of pantothenic acid, and up to 27% of choline, folic acid and pyridoxine had been lost from the diet. The loss of water-soluble vitamins was dependent on the time of immersion and the surface to volume ratio of the diet. The leached vitamins cannot be absorbed across the gills and so are unavailable to freshwater fish. Although drinking in marine fish represents a method of absorption of the leached vitamins, the volume of tank water into which the vitamins leach, and the lability of the vitamins in solution in tank water, make this route negligible. Vitamin leaching emphasises the importance of feeding small rations regularly as opposed to one large ration where food may remain uneaten for several minutes. However, care should be taken to avoid food rations small enough to promote unacceptable levels of interspecific competition, such that some species do not get the chance to feed.

Leaching is reduced if the surface area to volume ratio of the diet is reduced. This is achieved using a granular or pellet format. However, these formats do

Fish species	Fish size	Maintenance feeding requirement	Maintenance feeding requirement
	g/fish	% BW food/day	mg food/(fish.day)
Goldfish	3.6	0.4	14.4
	4.8	0.2	11.5
	8.1	0.3	25.8
	11.7	0.2	18.3
Neon tetras	0.18	1.9	3.8
Leopard danio	0.31	≤2.4	≤7.2
Kribensis	1.1	≤1.0	≤10.2
Moonlight gourami	1.9	≤1.5	≤28.5

Table 24.3: *Maintenance feeding requirement of five popular species of ornamental fish. (after Pannevis and Earle, 1994b).*

not replace the need for proper feeding, and the same recommendations for flake hold true for granular and pellet diets. Different diet formats may be used together for the most efficient food delivery to the various species in the tank. For example, bottom feeders are particularly vulnerable to both hypovitaminosis and competition from surface and midwater species, which get first access to food. By feeding a combination of flake food for surface and midwater species, and fast sinking pellets for bottom feeders, both groups get rapid access to food with reduced competition. This also gives the opportunity to feed different groups at different times, for example, after the tank lights have been switched off for nocturnal bottom feeders.

As a guide, the maintenance food requirement of selected ornamental fish species has been determined at the WALTHAM Aquacentre (Pannevis and Earle, 1994b). Goldfish maintained at 20°C and tropical species maintained at 26°C were fed Aquarian® fish flakes. Table 24.3 shows the weight of fish and their maintenance food requirement expressed as percent of body weight and weight of food per fish. To put this data into perspective, a single flake weighed approximately 6mg, and had an area of approximately $1cm^2$. Since changes in temperature markedly affect the energy requirement of fish (see above), care should be taken when extrapolating these data to different maintenance temperatures.

If the specific requirements of the fish are unknown, an ideal regimen for feeding fish in a community tank is to feed to satiation, two to three times per day. Although demanding some dedication of time from the aquarist, the method has the advantage that the tank and inhabitants are closely inspected on a regular basis. This allows mortalities or sick fish to be spotted early and removed, or corrective measures or medical treatment to be given. Diseases in fish are no exception to the rule that early diagnosis and treatment improves the prognosis and helps prevent spread to other animals. To feed to satiation, small amounts of food are added continuously to the aquarium until the fish stop feeding eagerly. This usually takes only a few minutes or less, depending on the tank size and stocking density. The procedure is repeated at each feeding.

ASSESSMENT OF SUITABILITY OF FEEDING/NUTRITION OVER TIME

There are many parameters to assess the nutritive values of fish diets, including growth indices, food conversion efficiencies and body composition data. Unfortunately, other than detecting gross changes, measurement of these parameters requires large facilities and analytical equipment not available to the aquarist. In addition, although it is well accepted that nutrition plays an important role in the health and longevity of fish, because the symptoms of malnutrition in the vast majority of ornamental fish are unknown or poorly defined, deficiencies in diets are usually only exposed after significant losses, or during pathological examination.

However, adoption of the correct feeding regimen can result in significant improvements in water quality. Nitrate build-up in aquaria is a very common cause of poor health and reduced longevity in ornamental fish. Unless assimilated into tissue, nitrate is the ultimate fate of all dietary protein added to the aquarium. In association with regular nitrate removal procedures such as partial water changes, the adoption of the feeding practices described above can reduce the rate of nitrate build-up, resulting in reduced stress to fish. Since nitrate is easily measured using inexpensive test kits aimed at aquarists, the fate of protein added to the aquarium can be monitored, and feeding practices or diets modified to reduce nitrate build-up.

SUMMARY

Providing complete nutrition for fish provides many challenges. Not only do fish have different nutrient and energy requirements compared to terrestrial animals, but considerable variation exists between different fish species. Ideally, diet formulations should be tailored to the metabolic requirements of a particular species, and its particular environment (e.g. temperature), however, this is seldom practicable because environmental conditions may vary and because few fish species are kept in mono-species environments. Carnivores, omnivores and herbivores, each with different feeding habits and nutritional requirements, are brought together in community environments and fed a single diet. Formulating these diets is a formidable task, since attractant, palatant, and nutrient properties must satisfy a range of entirely different species. With consideration for each group in the community, a balance can usually be found, however, the value of alternative food formats in allowing species targeting should not be overlooked.

Delivering food into a high volume aquatic environment results in leaching of water-soluble nutrients from the diet. Thus, the feeding regimen is critical to avoid prolonged exposure of food to the environment. Diets may have to be formulated on the basis of predicted loss rates of various nutrients once food is added to the water.

Finally, pollution from nitrogenous waste is a considerable threat to the well-being of fish held in a closed water volume. Filter systems can be employed to reduce the toxicity of nitrogenous waste, however, ultimately even the least toxic forms can reach critical concentrations. Correct diet formulation and feeding regimen can be effectively combined to increase the efficiency of protein utilisation, and thus reduce pollution. In conjunction with good water quality management, this represents a significant tool in improving health and longevity.

REFERENCES

Bell JG and Cowey CB (1989). Digestibility and bioavailability of dietary selenium from fish meal, selenite, selenomethionine and selenocystine in Atlantic salmon (*Salmo salar*). *Aquaculture* **81,** 61-68.

Cowey CB (1975). Aspects of protein utilisation by fish. *Proceedings of the Nutrition Society* **34,** 57-63.

Cowey CB and Sargent JR (1979). Nutrition. In: *Fish Physiology* Vol. VIII. Eds SW Hoar and DJ Randall. Academic Press Inc., San Diego p1-69.

Desjardins LM, Hicks BD and Hilton JW (1987). Iron catalysed oxidation of trout diets and its effects on the growth and physiological response of rainbow trout. *Fish Physiology and Biochem*istry **3,** 173-182.

Hepher B (1988). Vitamins. In: *Nutrition of Pond Fishes.* Cambridge University Press, New York p224-234.

Hilton JW, Hodson PV and Slinger SJ (1980). The requirement and toxicity of selenium in rainbow trout (*Salmo gairdneri*). *Journal of Nutrition* **110,** 2527-2535.

Hilton JW and Hodson PV (1983). Effect of increased dietary carbohydrate on selenium metabolism and toxicity in rainbow trout (*Salmo gairdneri*). *Journal of Nutrition* **113,** 1241-1248.

Nagai M and Ikeda S (1972). Carbohydrate metabolism in Fish. III. Effect of dietary composition on metabolism of glucose and glutamate. *Nippon Suisan Gakkaishi* **38,** 137-143.

National Research Council (1993). *Nutrient Requirements of Fish.* National Academy Press, Washington D.C.

Nose T (1979). Summary report on the requirements of essential amino acids for carp. In: *Finfish Nutrition and Fishfeed Technology.* Eds K Tiews and JE Halver. Heenemann, Berlin, pp 145-156.

Ogino C and Yang GY (1979). Requirement of carp for dietary zinc. *Bulletin of the Japanese Society for Sci. Fish.* **45,** 967-969.

Ogino C and Yang GY (1980). Requirement of carp and rainbow trout for dietary manganese and copper. *Bulletin of the Japanese Society for Sci. Fish.* **46,** 455-458.

Ogino C, Takeuchi L, Takeda H and Watanabe T (1979). Availability of dietary phosphorus in carp and rainbow trout. *Bulletin of the Japanese Society for Sci. Fish.* **45,** 1527-1532.

Pannevis MC and Earle KE (1994a). Nutrition of ornamental fish: Water soluble vitamin leaching and growth of Paracheiron innesi. *Journal of Nutrition* **124,** S2633-2635.

Pannevis MC and Earle KE (1994b). Maintanence energy requirements of five popular species of ornamental fish. *Journal of Nutrition* **124,** S2616-2618.

Poston HA, Livingston DL, Pyle EA and Phillips AM Jr. (1966). The toxicity of high levels of vitamin A in the diet of brook trout, In *Fisheries Research Bulletin* No. 29. State of New York Conservation Dept., Albany, New York pp 20-24.

Roeder M and Roeder RH (1966). Effect of iron on the growth rate of fishes. *Journal of Nutrition* **90,** 86-90.

Russo RC (1985). Ammonia, nitrite and nitrate. In: *Fundamentals of Aquatic Toxicology.* Eds GM Rand and SR Petrocelli. Hemisphere, Washington D.C.

Santiago CB and Lovell RT (1988). Amino acid requirements for growth of Nile tilapia. *Journal of Nutrition* **118,** 1540-1546.

Shim KF and Nag SH (1988). Magnesium requirement of the guppy *Poecilia reticulata* Peters. *Aquaculture* **73,** 131-142.

Sinnhuber RO (1969). The role of fats, In: *Fish in Research.* Eds O Neuhaus and JE Halver. Academic Press, New York, USA pp 245-259.

Smith RR (1989). Nutritional Energetics. In: *Fish Nutrition, 2nd edition.* Ed JE Halver. Academic Press, New York, USA.

Stoskopf MK (1993). *Fish Medicine.* WB Saunders, Philadelphia.

Yamamoto H, Satoh S, Takeuchi T and Watanabe T (1983). Effects on rainbow trout of deletion of manganese or trace elements from fishmeal diet. *Bulletin of the Japanese Society of Science and Fish*eries **49,** 287-293.

PART V

Appendix and Index

APPENDIX I

Summary Tables from relevant chapters

ADULT MAINTENANCE

- Although carnivorous by nature, dogs have adapted to an omnivorous lifestyle and can be maintained on an entirely vegetarian diet if necessary.
- There is a wide range of body weights and body types within the species which complicates the calculation of energy requirements.
- Energy requirements are therefore related to metabolic body size, giving the formula:

$$\text{ME (kcal/day)} = 110W^{0.75} \quad (460W^{0.75}\ \text{kJ/day})$$

- Allowances must be made for different body type and for differences in activity levels.
- Dogs are often fed a single meal per day, although more frequent feeding may be more suitable for some cases.
- Canned, dry and semi-moist foods are suitable for feeding adult dogs.
- Regular assessment of health and body condition will confirm the adequacy of a diet.

Summary Table 3.1: *Feeding adult dogs in maintenance.*

- The cat is an obligatory carnivore which must receive a certain amount of animal tissue in its diet.
- The nutritional peculiarities of the cat include:
  - Higher protein requirement for maintenance and an inability to adapt to a very low protein diet
  - Specific dietary requirement for arginine and taurine
  - Higher dietary requirement for niacin
  - Requirement for pre-formed vitamin A and arachidonic acid, both of which are only found in fat of animal origin.
- The energy requirements of cats can generally be related to body weight as follows:

ME = 70–90kcal/kg body weight/day (293–376kJ) (normal)

or ME = 50–70kcal/kg body weight/day (209–293kJ) (inactive)

- Other essential nutrients must be balanced in relation to the energy content of the diet.
- Canned, dry and semi-moist foods are suitable for feeding adult cats, but not diets intended for use in dogs.
- Cats naturally adopt a pattern of small, frequent meals throughout a 24-hour period, but will readily adapt to an alternative feeding schedule (commonly two meals per day).
- Regular assessment of health and body condition will confirm the adequacy of a diet.

Summary Table 3.2: *Feeding adult cats in maintenance.*

Nutrient	Units	Adult maintenance		Growth		Reproduction	
		Dog	Cat	Dog	Cat	Dog	Cat
Protein	g	16	25	21.7	28	21.7	28
Fat	g	5.5	9	5.5	9	5.5	9
Linoleic acid	g	1.1	1	1.1	1	1.1	1
Arachidonic acid	g	NR	0.02	NR	0.02	NR	0.02
Minerals							
Calcium	g	0.65	0.5	0.65	0.5	1.1	1
Phosphorus	g	0.5	0.5	0.5	0.5	0.89	0.8
Ca:P ratio		0.84	0.5	1.3	0.8	1.3	0.8
Sodium	g	0.07	0.04	0.08	0.2	0.08	0.2
Potassium	g	0.5	0.5	0.5	0.5	0.5	0.5
Magnesium	mg	38.4	30	38.4	500	38.4	50
Iron	mg	4	10	8	13	4.8	10
Copper	mg	0.5	0.5	0.5	0.5	0.7	0.5
Manganese	mg	0.5	1	0.5	1	0.5	1
Zinc	mg	5	4	5	4	5	4
Iodine	mg	0.07	0.1	0.07	0.1	0.15	0.1
Selenium	mg	0.01	0.01	0.01	0.01	0.01	0.01
Vitamins							
Vitamin A	IU	409	267	409	267	499	1,000
Vitamin D	IU	43	20	43	20	50	100
Vitamin E	mg	3	1.4	5	1.4	5	4.8
Vitamin K	mg	[a]	0.01	[a]	0.1	[a]	0.1
Thiamin	mg	0.1	0.4	0.1	0.4	0.1	0.5
Riboflavin	mg	0.25	0.32	0.25	0.32	0.25	0.5
Pantothenic acid	mg	1.1	0.4	1.1	0.4	1.1	1
Niacin	mg	1.2	3.2	1.2	3.2	1.2	4.5
Pyridoxine	mg	0.12	0.32	0.12	0.32	0.12	0.4
Folic acid	ug	21.7	64	21.7	64	21.7	100
Vitamin B_{12}	ug	2.7	1.6	2.7	1.6	2.7	2
Choline	mg	125	200	125	200	125	200
Biotin	mg	[a]	0.01	[a]	0.01	[a]	0.01
Taurine - canned food	mg	NR	250	NR	250	NR	250
Taurine - dry food	mg	NR	100	NR	100	NR	100

Appendix 3.1: *WCPN minimum nutrient requirements for dogs and cats per 400kcal[1] metabolisable energy.*

[1] Multiply figures by 1.67 for results per MJ metabolisable energy
NR No requirement
[a] No requirement when natural ingredients are fed. This is because intestinal bacterial synthesis can generally meet the needs of the animal

REPRODUCTION AND LACTATION

Dietary objectives	To support maintenance in the bitch **plus** fetal growth during gestation and milk production during lactation.
Dietary characteristics	Complete and balanced in energy and nutrient content. In late pregnancy and during lactation diet should be concentrated, highly digestible and highly palatable to ensure an adequate intake.
Energy requirement	
Pregnancy:	Weeks 0–5: Maintenance ration Weeks 5–6: M + 15% Weeks 6–7: M + 30% Weeks 7–8: M + 45% Weeks 8–9: M + 60%
Lactation:	Varies with size and age of the litter, but at peak lactation (3–4 weeks post whelping) may be three or four times the maintenance ration.
Dietary amount of principal nutrients (per 400kcal ME)	Protein (g): 22 Fat (g): 5.5 Linoleic acid (g): 1.1 Calcium (g): 1.1 Phosphorus (g): 0.9 Ca:P ratio: 0.8–1.5 Vitamin A (IU): 500 Vitamin D (IU): 50 Vitamin E (mg): 5.0
Food types	Canned, dry or semi-moist diets are suitable for bitches in reproduction. Concentrated foods (such as puppy food) are of value.

Summary Table 4.1: *Feeding for reproduction and lactation – Dogs.*

Dietary objectives	To support maintenance in the bitch **plus** fetal growth during gestation and milk production during lactation.
Dietary characteristics	Complete and balanced in energy and nutrient content. In late pregnancy and during lactation diet should be concentrated, highly digestible and highly palatable to ensure an adequate intake. The diet must contain some animal-derived tissue.
Energy requirement	
Pregnancy:	100–140kcal/kg BW/day
Lactation:	240+ kcal/kg BW/day
Dietary amount of principal nutrients (per 400 kcal ME)	Protein (g): 28 Fat (g): 9.0 Linoleic acid (g): 1.0 Arachidonic acid (mg): 20.00 Calcium (g): 1.00 Phosphorus (g): 0.80 Ca:P ratio: 0.8–1.5 Vitamin A (IU): 500 Vitamin D (IU): 100 Vitamin E (mg): 8.0 Taurine – canned food (mg): 250 Taurine – dry food (mg): 100
Food types	Canned, dry or semi-moist diets are suitable for adult cats.

Summary Table 4.2: *Feeding for reproduction and lactation – Cats.*

FEEDING PUPPIES AND KITTENS

Dietary objectives	To support maintenance in the puppy **plus** normal development and growth at an optimal rate	
Dietary characteristics	Complete and balanced in energy and nutrient content. Higher levels of energy, protein, minerals and certain vitamins are required, so the diet should be concentrated, highly digestible and highly palatable to ensure an adequate intake	
Energy requirement	At weaning:	2 x maintenance (M)
	40% adult weight:	1.6 x M
	80% adult weight:	1.2 x M
Dietary amount of principal nutrients (per 400kcal ME)	Protein (g):	22
	Fat (g):	5.5
	Linoleic acid (g):	1.1
	Calcium (g):	0.65
	Phosphorus (g):	0.50
	Ca:P ratio:	1.0–1.5
	Vitamin A (IU):	410
	Vitamin D (IU):	44
	Vitamin E (mg):	5.0
Food types	Canned, dry or semi-moist diets are suitable for growing puppies, but dry foods should be moistened with water, milk or gravy for very young animals. Food should be finely divided for small puppies	

Summary Table 5.1: *Feeding for Growth – Puppies.*

Nutrient	per kg diet[1]	per 400 kcal
Protein	240 g	19.7 g
Arginine	10 g	0.82 g
Histidine	3 g	0.25 g
Isoleucine	5 g	0.41 g
Leucine	12 g	0.99 g
Lysine	8 g	0.66 g
Total sulphur-AA	7.5 g	0.62 g
Methionine	4 g	0.33 g
Total aromatic	8.5 g	0.70 g
Phenylalanine	4 g	0.33 g
Threonine	7 g	0.58 g
Tryptophan	1.5 g	0.12 g
Valine	6 g	0.50 g
∑ Essential amino acids	68.5 g	5.65 g
Essential fatty acids		
Linoleic	5 g	0.41 g
Arachidonic	200 mg	16.5 mg
Minerals		
Calcium	5 g	0.41 g
Phosphorus	4 g	0.33 g
Potassium	4 g	0.33 g
Sodium	2 g	0.16 g
Chlorine	3 g	0.25 g
Magnesium	300 mg	25 mg
Iron	80 mg	6.6 mg
Copper	5 mg	0.41 mg
Manganese	5 mg	0.41 mg
Zinc	50 mg	4.1 mg
Iodine	350 µg	28 µg
Selenium	100 µg	8.2 µg
Vitamins		
A	3000 IU	250 IU
D	250 IU	20 IU
E	30 IU	2.5 IU
K	100 µg	8.2 µg
Thiamin	5 mg	0.4 mg
Riboflavin	4 mg	0.33 mg
Pyridoxine	4 mg	0.33 mg
Niacin	40 mg	3.3 mg
Pantothenic acid	5 mg	0.4 mg
Folic acid	800 µg	66 µg
Blotin	70 µg	5.8 µg
B_{12}	20 µg	1.6 µg
Choline	2.4 g	200 mg

Summary Table 5.2: *Nutrient requirements of growing kittens expressed as per kg diet and as per 400kcal of metabolisable energy. No allowance has been made for bioavailability of the nutrients in the diet or for variation of composition of feed ingredients. (Adapted and modified from Morris and Rogers, 1994.)*

[1] *Calculate metabolisable energy value of 4.85kcal/g.*

How to use this table

The following may assist in a comparison of analysed or calculated values of nutrients in a food with those presented in Table 5.2 to determine if a food contains an adequate level of nutrients for a kitten.

1) Check whether the energy intake of the kitten is adequate. Multiply the food intake of the kitten by the energy density of the diet. For example, a 1.5kg kitten eating 77g of an expanded food containing 3.5kcal of metabolisable energy/g has a daily intake of 77 x 3.5 = 270kcal. The energy requirement of a growing kitten of this size is about 180kcal/kg/day or 180 x 1.5kcal/day for this kitten. Therefore the energy intake should be adequate.

2) Calculate the concentration of each essential amino acid in the diet. The amino acid concentrations in Table 5.2 have to be corrected for the bioavailability of the amino acids in the food ingredients used. While overall apparent protein digestibility is not directly equated to bioavailability of each individual amino acid it is a useful first step. Multiply the concentration of each essential amino acid in Table 5.2 by 1/apparent digestibility of the protein in the diet expressed as a decimal fraction. Concentration of each essential amino acid in the diet should exceed this calculated value. Check that the crude protein of the diet is adequate.

3) The variation in bioavailability of minerals in various natural ingredients for cats is unknown. Calcium and phosphorus from bone is readily available to other animals so the requirement values need only be increased by a factor of about 1.1 if the calcium and phosphorus are coming from bone. The calcium content in foods of vegetable origin is generally low and of variable bioavailability. Grains contribute significant amounts of phosphorus in expanded diets but the availability from vegetable sources such as grains is also low, and should be discounted to 0.3 times analytical values. In contrast, magnesium from bone is readily available.

   Sodium and potassium from all sources are readily available, and an analytical value of 1.1 times the requirement appears adequate.

   The availability of zinc from grains and vegetable proteins also is low and the total zinc requirement should come from an available source of zinc, e.g. zinc sulphate.

   The availability of iron depends on the source of iron, but haem iron and ferrous salts of iron are readily available. The bioavailability of copper from animal foods is probably quite good but from some mineral sources, e.g. from copper oxide the copper is totally unavailable. Insufficient information on the bioavailability of the other trace elements is available to make a recommendation.

4) The bioavailability of fat-soluble vitamins is high in normal cats such that analytical values should be adequate. In contrast, the bioavailability of many of the B vitamins from natural sources is low, leading to the recommendation that analytical levels for all the B vitamins be at least 1.5 times the requirements given in Table 5.2.

FEEDING OLDER PETS

1)	Old dogs and cats are a growing sector of the small animal population.
2)	They have requirements which differ from those of younger animals.
3)	These requirements are not well quantified and vary from one to another.
4)	Reduced energy requirement in old age may lead to obesity; reduced appetite may lead to weight loss. Both are treatable.
5)	Maintenance of appetite can be achieved by high quality foods fed two or three times per day.
6)	Age associated disease which reduces appetite e.g. periodontitis should be diagnosed and treated.
7)	Reduced food intake causes reduced vitamin and trace element intake and possibly absorption. Multivitamin supplementation has a place in the old dog or cat diet, particularly after illness.
8)	The quality of raw materials and the availability of nutrients is particularly important to old animals.
9)	Dietary requirements and regimens may change as old age progresses. These require reassessment in order to maintain quality of life.
10)	Dietary enhancement of the quality of life in old age can be effective and rewarding.

Summary Table 7.

THE UNDERWEIGHT PATIENT

Dietary objectives	Diet must meet patient's needs for energy and protein
Dietary characteristics	Food must have adequate energy and nutrient density, palatability, and high digestibility
Energy requirement	Maintenance or specified multiples thereof
Specific nutrient requirements	All essential nutrients must be provided in a diet that is balanced, digestible, and palatable
Food type, nutritional preparation	Commercial pet foods, or, for certain situations, freshly made (home-made) foods
Route and method of feeding	Voluntary or involuntary if warranted
Regimen	Feeding management in general begins at low levels then builds up to maintenance or above maintenance; it should be tailored specifically to each individual

Summary Table 8.

FEEDING THE CARDIAC PATIENT

Cardiovascular Problem	Dietary Recommendation
Advancing age (dogs)	Avoid high salt content diets (over 1% sodium content on a dry matter basis) to help avoid resistance to change to a low salt ration later if it is clinically necessary
Grade I heart failure - murmur present but no clinical signs (common in dogs with endocardiosis)	Feed a complete ration containing less than 0.5% sodium on a dry matter basis to help reduce potential for sodium and fluid retention. (e.g. Science Diet Canine Maintenance (Hill's Pet Nutrition) and Canine Low Sodium Diet (WALTHAM))
Grade II + heart failure (dogs)	Feed a complete ration especially formulated for dogs with clinical heart failure containing: (a) controlled sodium content (less than 0.1% on dry matter basis) (b) high energy density (c) controlled protein content (because of the likelihood of concurrent impairment of renal/hepatic function), and (d) increased water-soluble vitamin content to offset potential losses through concurrent renal insufficieny or diuretic therapy, (e.g. Hill's Prescription Diet Canine h/d and Canine Low Sodium Diet (WALTHAM))
Cardiomyopathy (dogs)	Consider possibility of carnitine deficiency or thiamin deficiency as causes. Feed a complete ration containing adequate amounts of thiamin and carnitine. Supplementation with L-carnitine at a dose of 50-100mg/kg body weight 3 times daily.
Dilated cardiomyopathy (cats)	Consider possibility of taurine deficiency as a cause. Feed a complete ration containing adequate amounts of bioavailable taurine. Taurine supplementation for affected cats at dose 250-500 mg/day. In cats with cardiomyopathy and signs consistent with the diagnosis consider thiamin deficiency as a possible cause.
Concurrent obesity	Feed a ration formulated for weight reduction and reduce body weight to target for breed. (e.g. Canine r/d (Hill's Pet Nutrition) and Canine Low Calorie Diet (WALTHAM)). If necessary maintain target weight by continuous feeding of a reduced calorie ration (e.g. Canine w/d (Hill's Pet Nutrition) and Canine Low Calorie (WALTHAM))
All forms of clinical heart failure	Heart failure is a catabolic state and (unless the animal has severe obesity - see above) a highly digestible, high energy-dense ration should be fed in multiple small meals/day
Concurrent renal insufficiency	Feed a ration formulated primarily for renal failure* with: (a) Controlled protein content (less than 25% on dry matter basis (dogs); less than 35% (cats)) (b) Controlled phosphorus content (less than 0.5% dry matter basis (cats and dogs)) (c) Reduced sodium - indicated if hypertension is present (d) High energy density (e) Increased water-soluble vitamin content to compensate for urinary losses. These dietary characteristics are also appropriate for the management of heart failure (*e.g. Hill's Prescription Diet k/d)
Diuretic use in heart disease	Feed a ration containing adequate concentrations of water-soluble vitamins to avoid depletion due to diuresis and, unless a potassium sparing diuretic is used (e.g. spironolactone), ensure adequate potassium intake - especially in cats - to offset urinary losses due to diuresis

Summary Table 10: *Summary of dietary recommendations in heart disease.*

THE RENAL PATIENT

Parameter assessed	Canine	Feline
Haematological findings		
Non-regenerative anaemia	PCV < 25%	PCV < 27%
Lymphopenia	< 1200 / litre	< 1200 / litre
Biochemical findings		
Creatinine	> 155mol / litre	> 159mol / litre
Serum urea nitrogen	> 10mmol / litre	> 12mmol / litre
Hyperproteinaemia	> 80g / litre	> 80g / litre
Hypercholesterolaemia	> 4.01mmol / litre	> 4.01mmol / litre
Metabolic acidosis	CO_2 < 17mEq/litre	CO_2 < 17mEq/litre
Hyperphosphataemia	> 2.42mmol / litre	> 2.26mmol / litre
Hypokalaemia	< 3.3mEq / litre	< 3.1mEq / litre

Summary Table 11.1: *Abnormal clinicopathological findings associated with chronic renal failure.*

Dietary objectives	To meet nutrient and energy requirements. To alleviate clinical signs of uraemia. To minimise electrolyte, vitamin and mineral disturbances. To try to slow progression of renal failure.
Dietary characteristics	Restricted quantity of high quality protein. Restricted phosphorus, normal to restricted sodium. Supplemented water-soluble vitamins. Supplemented with potassium (cats). High energy. High palatability.
Energy requirement	Unknown. Use normal maintenance values adjusted according to response.
Specific nutrient requirements[1]	Protein – approx. 12–25g/400kcal (dog) – approx. 20–27g/400kcal (cat) Phosphorus – approx. 0.25–0.5g/400kcal[2] Sodium – approx. 0.25–0.8g/400kcal[2] Potassium – >0.65g/400kcal (cat)[3] Water-soluble vitamins – at least double normal minimum recommendations
Food type	Canned, dry or liquid commercial. Home-prepared.
Regimen	Gradual introduction of diet. Regular patient monitoring, with appropriate adjustments made according to clinical response.

Summary Table 11.2: *Dietary management of chronic renal failure.*

1 *Suggested ranges based on references discussed in the text. Adjustments should be made for the individual case. Data are limited for some nutrients, especially for cats.*

2 *100g dry matter contains approximately 400kcal (1674kJ) of metabolisable energy for typical foods, and conversions from literature reports have been made on this basis. However, because of their relatively high fat content, diets designed for CRF patients may contain more than 400kcal/100g (1674kJ/100g) DM.*

3 *Some cats may be hyperkalaemic.*

GASTROINTESTINAL PROBLEMS (DOG AND CAT)

Condition	Oropharyngeal disease	Oesophagitis	Oesophageal stricture
Dietary objectives	Enteral nutrition by-passing localised disease process	Reduce trauma to mucosa and reduce gastric reflux	Enteral nutrition by-passing localised disease process
Dietary characteristics	Suitable for tube feeding	Soft, moist blended food	Suitable for tube feeding
Energy requirement	Maintenance	Maintenance	Maintenance
Specific nutrient requirements	None	None	None
Food type / nutritional preparation	Liquid	Food blended to slurry or gruel	Liquid
Route and method of feeding	Naso-oesophageal or gastrostomy tube	Oral (Gastrostomy if severe)	Gastrostomy (or naso-oesophageal) tube
Regimen	See chapter 17	Small meals 3–4 times per day	See chapter 17

Summary Table 13.1: *Gastrointestinal problems (dog and cat).*

Condition	Megaoesophagus	Gastric dilatation / volvulus	Acute (gastro)enteritis
Dietary objectives	Deliver food to stomach without aspiration	Reduce aerophagia, gastric distension and bacterial fermentation	Initial bowel rest then gradual regrading
Dietary characteristics	Slurry or particulate depending on individual capabilities	Highly digestible	Highly digestible, bland diet
Energy requirement	Maintenance	Maintenance	≤ Maintenance
Specific nutrient requirements	None	None	None
Food type / nutritional preparation	Any food, but usually blended	Good quality, highly digestible food	Commercial or home-cooked 'intestinal diet'
Route and method of feeding	Oral, from raised bowl	Oral	Oral
Regimen	Normal	Small, frequent meals with no peri-prandial exercise	Small frequent meals, gradually returning to staple diet

Summary Table 13.2: *Gastrointestinal problems (dog and cat).*

Condition	Chronic gastritis	Halitosis, borborygmi and flatulence	Small intestinal bacterial overgrowth
Dietary objectives	Reduce gastric distension and food retention	Reduce substrates available for bacterial fermentation	Reduce substrates, especially fat, available for bacterial fermentation
Dietary characteristics	Bland, low fat, and finely ground	High digestibility, low fat, reduced protein, and lactose-free	High digestibility, low fat, reduced protein, and lactose-free
Energy requirement	Maintenance	Maintenance	≥ Maintenance
Specific nutrient requirements	None	None	Multivitamins ± parenteral B_{12}
Food type / nutritional preparation	Home-cooked or commercial 'intestinal diet'	Commercial reduced protein diet	Commercial low fat diet (not obesity diet)
Route and method of feeding	Oral	Oral	Oral
Regimen	Frequent small meals	Normal	3 divided meals per day

Summary Table 13.3: *Gastrointestinal problems (dog and cat).*

Condition	Dietary sensitivity	Inflammatory bowel disease	Lymphangiectasia
Dietary objectives	Exclude dietary component to which animal is sensitive	Reduce antigenic load and fat malabsorption, and aid digestion	Reduce fat malabsorption and replace protein loss
Dietary characteristics	Single protein and carbohydrate source	High digestibility, 'hypoallergenic' low fat and lactose-free	High digestibility, low fat
Energy requirement	Maintenance	Up to twice maintenance if PLE exists	Up to twice maintenance
Specific nutrient requirements	None	Multivitamins	MCT oil Multivitamins ± parenteral fat-soluble vitamins
Food type / nutritional preparation	Commercial or home-cooked exclusion diet	Home-cooked or commercial 'hypoallergenic intestinal diet'	Home-cooked or commercial low fat diet (not obesity diet)
Route and method of feeding	Oral	Oral	Oral
Regimen	Normal	Frequent, small meals	Frequent small meals

Summary Table 13.4: *Gastrointestinal problems (dog and cat).*

Condition	Idiopathic colitis	Irritable bowel syndrome	Constipation
Dietary objectives	Reduce substrates for fermentation and antigenic load ± increase fibre content	Regulate intestinal motility	Improve colonic motility
Dietary characteristics	Highly digestible, reduced fat, single protein source, ± high fibre	Low fat, high insoluble fibre	High fibre
Energy requirement	Maintenance	Maintenance	Maintenance
Specific nutrient requirements	± added fibre (isphagula, bran)	None	± bulk laxative (sterculia, isphagula, bran, methylcellulose)
Food type / nutritional preparation	Home-cooked or commercial hypoallergenic ± high fibre	Commercial high fibre diet	Commercial high fibre diet, or add fibre supplement
Route and method of feeding	Oral	Oral	Oral
Regimen	Normal	Normal	Normal

Summary Table 13.5: *Gastrointestinal problems (dog and cat).*

THE EXOCRINE PANCREAS

Dietary objectives	Re-establish normal nutrient absorption (particularly protein/calories)
Dietary characteristics	Low fibre content Avoid excessive fat content
Energy requirement	Approximately 10–15% above anticipated maintenance requirements for normal animals
Specific nutrient requirements	Parenteral cobalamin, parenteral vitamin K_1, and oral supplements of tocopherol and perhaps other vitamins may be required
Food type / nutritional preparation	Highly digestible, moderate or reduced fat content diet supplemented with powdered pancreatic extract immediately prior to feeding. Consider medium chain triglyceride supplementation if weight gain is suboptimal.
Route and method of feeding	Oral
Regimen	Two or three meals daily until normal body weight is attained. One or two meals daily to supply maintenance requirements.

Summary Table 15.1: *Dietary strategy in exocrine pancreatic insufficiency.*

Dietary objectives	Rectify or prevent hyperlipoproteinaemia and obesity. Avoid excessive stimulation of pancreatic secretion.
Dietary characteristics	Low fat content, moderate protein content, carbohydrate rich diet
Energy requirement	Meet maintenance requirements if patient is not obese. Feed at below maintenance requirements to correct obesity.
Specific nutrient requirements	Parenteral nutrition may be required (particularly in cats) if patients cannot tolerate oral feeding for an extended period of time.
Food type / nutritional preparation	During recovery from acute pancreatitis feed a commercial low fat content diet or rice-, pasta- or potato-based home-made diet. Patients with chronic pancreatitis may benefit from addition of pancreatic enzyme extract to a low fat content diet.
Route and method of feeding	Oral if tolerated. Parenteral nutrition if oral intake is not tolerated for a prolonged period.
Regimen	Multiple small feedings during recovery from acute pancreatitis to minimise pancreatic stimulation.

Summary Table 15.2: *Dietary strategy in pancreatitis.*

CANINE AND FELINE DIABETES MELLITUS

Dietary objectives	Coordinate effects of meal with effects of insulin
Dietary characteristics	Consistent caloric density and nutrient composition, high nutrient composition, high palatability, appropriate texture
Energy requirement	As for maintenance but individual variation dictates increased or decreased demand
Specific nutrient requirements	Preferably high in complex carbohydrates (consider dietary fibre up to 40g/1000kcal) (40g/4184kJ) and low in fat (<30g/1000kcal) (<30g/4184kJ)
Food type	Unprocessed traditional composition with added fibre or various commercial products of suitable palatability. Once weekly raw bone
Administration	Standard feeding process
Regimen	Feed half daily caloric requirements one to two hours after porcine or human lente insulin given 12 hourly

Summary Table 16.1: *Dietary strategy in diabetes mellitus.*

FEEDING THE SICK ANIMAL

Dietary objectives	Assess nutritional status using: Subjective criteria - body condition score, history, physical exam; Objective criteria - body weight, serum protein, haematology Address requirements for protein, carbohydrate and fat.
Dietary characteristics	Highly digestible meat or milk-protein based diets. Nutrient requirements; Protein 20–22% of IER (dogs), 24–30% of IER (dog with increased protein requirements), 28–40% (cats); Fat 40–70% IER; Carbohydrate 10–40% IER.
Energy requirement	MER (kcal)[1] = 125 x ($W_{kg}^{0.75}$) or MER (kcal)[1] = 2 x ([30 x W_{kg}] + 70). Multiply MER by an illness factor (0.65–1 for dogs, 1.0 for cats) to determine energy requirements.
Food type/nutritional preparation	Home-produced diets: Protein sources - chicken, white fish, liver, egg, cottage cheese; Carbohydrate sources - rice, potato. Fat sources - beef, corn/sunflower oil, tuna in oil, cheese Commercial diets: Tinned foods (meat-based) or liquid diets containing adequate amounts of protein, fat and carbohydrate.
Route and method of feeding/administration	Voluntary intake if possible. If inappetant or anorectic consider syringe feeding or tube feeding. If GI tract non-functional use parenteral feeding.
Regimen	Initiate nutritional support at earliest opportunity. If anorectic: 1. Return to own environment if possible. 2. Hand feed. 3. Ensure food is fresh and at room/body temperature. 4. Use strong smelling food. 5. Diazepam (dogs and cats) or oxazepam (cats) to increase appetite. 6. Syringe or tube feeding if anorexia persists for greater than 3 days. Continue until patient eats 75% of daily requirement voluntarily. Feed 3-4 times a day.

***Summary Table 18.1:** Feeding the sick animal.*

[1] *1kcal = 4.184kJ.*

UROLITHIASIS - A NUTRITIONAL PERSPECTIVE

Dietary objectives	Urine pH < 6; Specific gravity < 1.015; Low urinary urea, magnesium and phosphorus; BUN 0.8–1.6mmol/litre.
Dietary characteristics	Low protein, magnesium and phosphorus; high sodium.
Energy requirements	As normal
Specific nutrient	A commercial diet contains:1.47g protein/100kcal (418kJ) Requirements ME; 3.3mg magnesium/100kcal ME; 24mg phosphorus/100kcal ME; 23.3mg sodium/100kcal ME.
Food type/nutritional preparation	Commercial diet formulated for struvite dissolution.
Route and method of feeding/administration	Standard.
Regimen	No specific requirement.

***Summary Table 19.1:** Struvite dissolution – Dogs.*

Dietary objectives	Urine pH < 6.5.
Dietary characteristics	Low magnesium; low phosphorus; acidic ash.
Energy requirements	As normal
Specific nutrient requirements	A typical commercial ration formulated for this purpose contains: 14.8mg magnesium/100kcal (418kJ) ME; 89mg phosphorus/100 kcal ME.
Food type/nutritional preparation	Commercial diet formulated for struvite prevention.
Route and method of feeding/administration	Standard feeding regimen. Fast for 8 hours prior to checking urine pH.
Regimen	No specific requirement.

Summary Table 19.2: *Struvite prevention – Dogs.*

Dietary objectives	Urine pH < 6; Low urinary magnesium and phosphorus.
Dietary characteristics	Low magnesium; low phosphorus; acidic ash; added acidifier
Energy requirements	As normal
Specific nutrient requirements	A commercial diet contains: 11.2mg magnesium/100kcal (418kJ) ME and 100–110mg phosphorus/100kcal ME.
Food type/nutritional preparation	Commercial diet formulated for struvite dissolution.
Route and method of feeding/administration	Standard.
Regimen	No specific requirement.

Summary Table 19.3: *Struvite dissolution – Cats.*

Dietary objectives	Urine pH < 6; low urinary magnesium and phosphorus.
Dietary characteristics	Low magnesium; low phosphorus; acidic ash.
Energy requirements	As normal
Specific nutrient requirements	< 20 mg magnesium/100kcal ME; < 140mg phosphorus/100 kcal (418kJ) ME; acid ash.
Food type/nutritional preparation	Commercial diet formulated for struvite prevention.
Route and method of feeding/administration	Standard.
Regimen	No specific requirement.

Summary Table 19.4: *Struvite prevention – Cats.*

Dietary objectives	Reduce ammonium and urate excretion; urine pH 7.0–7.5.
Dietary characteristics	Low protein; low sodium; potassium citrate added.
Energy requirements	As normal
Specific nutrient requirements	1.9–2.1g protein/100kcal (418kJ) ME; potassium citrate until urine pH 7.0–7.5. Suggested dose 100–200mg (0.25–0.5mEq)/kg PO bid.
Food type/nutritional preparation	A commercial diet formulated for ammonium urate urolith dissolution.
Route and method of feeding/administration	Standard.
Regimen	No specific requirement.

Summary Table 19.5: *Ammonium urate urolith dissolution and prevention – Dogs.*

Dietary objectives	Reduced cystinuria; urine pH >7.5.
Dietary characteristics	Low protein; low sodium; potassium citrate added.
Energy requirements	As normal
Specific nutrient requirements	1.9–2.1g protein/100kcal (418kJ) ME; 45–55mg sodium/100kcal ME.
Food type/nutritional preparation	A commercial diet formulated for cystine urolith dissolution.
Route and method of feeding/administration	Standard.
Regimen	No specific requirement.

Summary Table 19.6: *Cystine urolith dissolution and prevention – Dogs.*

Dietary objectives	Reduce urine calcium excretion; urine pH 7.0 - 7.5.
Dietary characteristics	Low protein; low sodium; potassium citrate added.
Energy requirements	As normal
Specific nutrient requirements	1.9–2.1g protein/100kcal (418kJ) ME; 45–55 mg sodium/100 kcal 70–80mg calcium/100kcal ME; 25–30 mg phosphorus/100kcal ME.
Food type/nutritional preparation	A commercial diet formulated to prevent calcium oxalate urolith formation.
Route and method of feeding/administration	Standard.
Regimen	No special requirement.

Summary Table 19.7: *Calcium oxalate urolith prevention – Dogs.*

Dietary objectives	Reduce urine calcium excretion; urine pH 7.0–7.5.
Dietary characteristics	Low protein; low sodium.
Energy requirements	As normal
Specific nutrient requirements	5.0–5.5g protein/100kcal (418kJ) ME; 65–70mg sodium/100kcal ME. 100–110mg calcium/100kcal ME; 80–85mg phosphorus/100 kcal ME.
Food type/nutritional preparation	A commercial diet formulated to prevent calcium oxalate urolith formation. Add potassium citrate 100–200mg (0.25–0.5mEq)/kg PO bid.
Route and method of feeding/administration	Standard.
Regimen	No specific requirement.

Summary Table 19.8: *Calcium oxalate urolith prevention – Cats.*

NUTRITION RELATED ORTHOPAEDIC DISEASES

Prevalence:	Common in most large breeds, occasionally in middle and smaller breeds.
Age:	Clinical symptoms seen already at 6 weeks in severely affected individuals; more commonly at 6 months to 1 year and also often in older animals because of degenerative arthroses. Diagnosed with accuracy from 12 months.
Symptoms:	Lameness, pain on manipulation of hip joint.
Dietary history:	Inconclusive
Clinical biochemistry:	Inconclusive
Diagnosis:	By radiology. (Conformation and secondary arthroses)
Therapy:	Various surgical and medical techniques to relieve pain
Prognosis:	Depends on severity of changes, type of work, care and training.
Prevention:	Selection of breeding stock. Avoidance of overfeeding.
DIET	
During growth:	Complete and balanced diet in restricted amounts.
When diagnosed:	Complete and balanced diet in restricted amounts to prevent overweight.

Summary Table 20.1: *Hip dysplasia.*

Prevalence:	Extremely rare nowadays. Large sized breeds more prone than smaller.
Age:	Weaning to 6 months of age.
Symptoms:	Broadened metaphyses. Bulging costrochondral junctions. Bowing of long bones.
Dietary history:	A diet deficient in vitamin D, often low in calcium and high in phosphorus; i.e. an all-meat diet.
Clinical biochemistry:	Inconclusive although both serum calcium and serum phosphorus might be low, whereas urinary phosphorus might be strongly elevated.
Diagnosis:	By dietary history and by radiology.
Therapy:	Institute a complete and balanced diet as soon as possible. Corrective surgery if needed later.
Prognosis:	Depends on severity of changes. Bowing of bones.
Prevention:	By feeding a complete and balanced diet.
DIET	
During growth:	Complete and balanced diet.
When diagnosed:	Complete and balanced diet in restricted amounts to ensure proper mineralisation.

Summary Table 20.2: *Rickets.*

Prevalence:	Common in most large breeds, occasionally in middle sized breeds, rarely in smaller sized breeds.
Age:	Clinical symptoms seen as early as 4 months but also at much older age; more commonly at 6 months and at older ages due to secondary arthrosis.
Symptoms:	Lameness, pain on manipulation of joint involved.
Dietary history:	Inconclusive.
Clinical biochemistry:	Inconclusive.
Diagnosis:	By radiology.
Therapy:	Surgery.
Prognosis:	Depends on severity of changes and age at surgery.
Prevention:	Selection of breeding stock. Avoidance of overfeeding and oversupplementation.
DIET	
During growth:	Complete and balanced diet in restricted amounts.
When diagnosed:	Complete and balanced in restricted amounts to avoid overweight.

Summary Table 20.3: *Osteochondrosis.*

Prevalence:	Occasionally in large sized breeds. Some breed predisposition - Boxers, Great Danes.
Age:	Clinical signs may be seen as early as 2 months of age and as long as longitudinal growth is allowed for.
Symptoms:	Metaphyseal enlargement. Pain on palpation of metaphyseal regions of long bones. Reluctance to move. Fever.
Dietary history:	Inconclusive.
Clinical biochemistry:	Inconclusive.
Diagnosis:	By radiology.
Therapy:	Supportive only, as long as aetiology is unknown. Cage rest. Restricted feeding of a complete and balanced diet to minimize defective bone formation. Antibiotics and pain relief to be considered depending on course of disease.
Prognosis:	Most commonly favourable, but guarded, with extensive changes and repeated relapses.
Prevention:	Unknown.
DIET	
During growth:	Complete and balanced diet in restricted amounts.
When diagnosed:	Complete and balanced diet in restricted amounts.

Summary Table 20.4: *Metaphyseal osteopathy.*

Prevalence:	Occasionally in large sized breeds. Some breed predisposition - German Shepherd Dogs. Affects males more frequently than females.
Age:	Most commonly first seen at about 6 months of age but may be seen earlier and sometimes also in adult dogs.
Symptoms:	Shifting lameness. Pain on palpation of diaphyses.
Dietary history:	Inconclusive.
Clinical biochemistry:	Inconclusive.
Diagnosis:	By radiology (or scintigraphy).
Therapy:	Only supportive as long as unknown aetiology. Pain relief may be considered. Restricted feeding of a balanced diet to minimise defective bone formation.
Prognosis:	Most commonly favourable but occasional cases are seen with long-lasting symptoms.
Prevention:	Unknown
DIET	
During growth:	Complete and balanced diet in restricted amounts.
When diagnosed:	Complete and balanced in restricted amounts.

Summary Table 20.5: *Enostosis.*

Prevalence:	Occasionally in large sized breeds.
Age:	During periods of most rapid growth.
Symptoms:	Deviation of bone axis. Broadening of metaphyseal regions of long bones.
Dietary history:	Inconclusive, but commonly affecting individuals allowed to meet rapid growth potentials by excessive food intake.
Clinical biochemistry:	Inconclusive.
Diagnosis:	By radiology.
Therapy:	Complete and balanced diet in restricted amounts. Corrective surgery if needed later on.
Prognosis:	Favourable if changes not too pronounced.
Prevention:	By feeding a complete and balanced diet in restricted amounts.
DIET	
During growth:	Complete and balanced diet.
When diagnosed:	Complete and balanced diet in restricted amounts.

Summary Table 20.6: *Retained cartilage.*

SMALL PETS - FOOD TYPES, NUTRIENT REQUIREMENTS AND NUTRIONAL DISORDERS

		Rats and Mice		Gerbils	Rabbits		Guinea Pigs	Hamsters
Nutrient	Unit	Breeding	Maintenance		Breeding	Maintenance		
Digestible energy	kcal/g[1]	2.6-3.2	2.4-3.2	2.6-3.9	2.5	2.1	1.8-3.0	2.7-4.2
Metabolisable energy	kcal/g[1]	2.5-3.0	2.2-3.0	2.5-3.7	2.4	2	1.7-2.9	2.5-3.9
Crude protein	%	17-20	13-14	17-18	15-18	12-13	18-20	18-22
Fat	%	2-5	1-3	10-12	2-4	2-3	2-4	4-5
Crude fibre	%	4	4	4	10-14	14-16	7-11	4-8
Minerals								
Calcium	%	0.8	0.6	0.8	0.8	0.6	0.6	0.8
Phosphorus	%	0.6	0.4	0.6	0.5	0.4	0.5	0.6
Magnesium	%	0.2	0.25	0.2	0.3	0.3	0.2	0.2
Potassium	%	0.5	0.5	0.5	0.6	0.6	0.5	1.0
Sodium	%	0.25	0.25	0.25	0.5	0.2	0.5	0.3
Chloride	%	0.25	0.25	0.25	0.5	0.3	0.5	0.3
Cobalt	mg/kg	0.4	0.4	0.4	0.4	0.4	0.4	0.5
Copper	mg/kg	5.0	5.0	5.0	10	10.0	6	17.0
Zinc	mg/kg	30	30	30	50	50	20	50
Iron	mg/kg	100	100	100	50	50	50	140
Manganese	mg/kg	75	75	75	30	30	40	70
Iodine	mg/kg	0.2	0.2	0.2	0.2	0.2	1	1.6
Selenium	mg/kg	0.1	0.1	0.1	0.1	0.1	0.1	0.1
Vitamins								
Vitamin A	iu/g	7	5	7	10	10	23	14
Carotene	mg/kg	nr	nr	nr	0.83	1	nr	nr
Vitamin D	iu/g	1	0.80	1	1	1	1	2
Vitamin E	mg/kg	60	60	60	50	50	50	60
Vitamin K	mg/kg	2	2	2	2	2	5	4
Vitamin C	mg/kg	nr	nr	nr	nr	nr	200	nr
Thiamin (B_1)	mg/kg	4	4	4	10	10	2	20
Riboflavin (B_2)	mg/kg	5	4	5	10	10	3	5
Pyridoxine (B_6)	mg/kg	6	6	6	15	15	3	6
Vitamin B_{12}	mg/kg	0.05	0.05	0.05	0.01	0.01	0.01	0.01
Folic acid	mg/kg	1	1	1	1	1	4	2
Pantothenic acid	mg/kg	10	10	10	20	20	20	20
Niacin	mg/kg	10	10	10	50	50	10	50
Biotin	mg/kg	0.20	0.20	0.20	0.2	0.2	0.3	0.20
Choline	mg/kg	1000	1000	1000	1500	1500	1000	1500

Summary Table 21.1: *Summary of recommended nutrient requirements of small pets.*

nr not required.

[1] *1kcal = 4.184kJ.*

SMALL PETS AND EXOTICS - FEEDING METHODS & TECHNIQUES

	Rodents and Lagomorphs	Reptiles	Birds
Dietary objectives	To allow growth, breeding or maintain weight without causing obesity.	To allow growth, breeding or maintain weight without causing obesity. All species should be maintained at their correct temperature to allow adequate digestion.	To allow growth, breeding or maintain weight without causing obesity. Should not be used to alleviate boredom and should be as varied as possible. Raptors may have their diets further restricted during hunting seasons to maintain a 'flying weight'.
Dietary characteristics	Herbivores, granivores, frugivores and insectivores.	Snakes arc mainly carnivores. Chelonia are herbivores or omnivores. Terrapins are often carnivores. Lizards may be herbivores, frugivores, carnivores, insectivores or omnivores.	Passerines - mainly frugivores or insectivorous. Psittacines - granivores, frugivores and insectivores. Raptors - carnivores and insectivores.
Food types (brief description)	Seeds, vegetables, fruit.	Carnivores - rodents, chicks, fish, amphibians, snakes or lizards. Herbivores - vegetables and fruit. Insectivores - Meal worms, crickets, locusts, wax mouth larvae. Avoid abnormal food types (i.e. milk, cheese, cake etc.).	Passerines and psittacines - Seeds, fruit and vegetables. Raptors - Chicks, birds, rodents, earthworms and insects.
Special nutrient requirements	Vitamin B requirements provided by intestinal bacteria. Guinea pigs require added Vitamin C.	With the exception of carnivores, all food types need to be supplemented with Vitamin D_3 and calcium to prevent osteodystrophy. Fish-eating reptiles need additional Vitamin B_1 to prevent thiamin deficiency. Excessive protein intake in non-carnivorous species can lead to gout. Some species will not drink from bowls, but require their vivaria to be 'misted'.	Grit availability is a debatable requirement. Should be provided for passerines. Psittacines have a high requirement for vitamin A. All seed diets may lead to calcium deficiencies and thus require supplementation. Raptors reared on pieces of meat will require calcium supplementation.
Route and method of feeding	*Ad libitum* of commercially produced low energy density food or twice daily of high energy seed diets. Most practice coprophagy.	Live feeding (other than insects) should be avoided. Feeding frequency may vary with age, size, temperature and individual species but may be twice daily to twice monthly. Records should be kept of feeding frequencies, as this varies with seasons, shedding or reproductive cycles.	*Ad libitum* if fruit and vegetables but restricted access to seeds to prevent obesity. Raptors - usually once a day.

Summary Table 22.1: *Feeding the healthy animal – Feeding techniques.*

ORNAMENTAL FISH NUTRITION AND FEEDING

	Goldfish (5g body weight, 20°C maintenance temperature)
Dietary objectives	To support maintenance in the fish with minimal pollution to the water.
Dietary characteristics	Complete and balanced in energy and nutrients. Easily digestible for omnivorous-herbivore.
Energy requirement	9.5kcal/kg (40kJ/kg) body weight
Dietary amount of principal nutrients	30–40% protein (balanced amino acid profile) 10–15% fat 1% linoleic acid, 1% linolenic acid
Food types	Flake, granular or pelleted commercially prepared diets
Daily amount of typical food type per unit body weight	11.5mg flake per fish per day, in three daily rations (approximately 0.5% body weight)

Summary Table 24.1: *Typical summary table for fish feeding – Goldfish. Figures are for maintenance. It is recommended to feed slightly above maintenance level. Growth rates can be increased by feeding up to 4% body weight with most commercially prepared flake mixtures.*

Index